Ontario, M3C 0H5

w.oupcanada.com

Complimentary Copy /
Exemplaire gratuit

Invoice No / No de facture		Page No / No de page	
90964507	03.10.2011	1 of / de	1

Shipped Via / Mode d'expédition	Canpar LTL
Delivery / Livraison	80827563

Brian McGuinness
Tel: 519-709-0652 ext   email: brian.mcguinness@oup.com

	Author / Auteur - Auteure
	NEENA CHAPPELL

a@oup.com, visit us on the Web at www.oupcanada.com/contact.html, or contact your
w.oupcanada.com.

urriel à customer.service.ca@oup.com, nous visiter sur le Web à l'adresse
ventes local. Vous pouvez trouver un catalogue complet des titres de OUP à la page

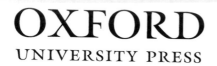

OXFORD
UNIVERSITY PRESS

8 Sampson Mews, Suite 204, Don Mills
Tel: (416)441-2941, Fax: (416)444-0427
SAN # 1150731, G.S.T./T.P.S. # R122319775, w

Ship-To / Destinataire

DEBORAH FITZSIMMONS
98 NORMAN ST
STRATFORD ON   N5A 5R7
CANADA

Account / No de compte

187760

The following examination copies are sent to you compliments of your
Oxford University Press representative:

Votre représentant d'Oxford University Press a le plaisir de vous faire
parvenir les exemplaires gratuits suivants :

Qty / Qté	ISBN ISBN-10	Title / Titre
1	9780195424768 019542476X	UNDERSTANDING HEALTH, HEALTH CARE P

We welcome your comments on our titles. Please e-mail us at customer.service.
local sales representative. A complete catalogue of OUP titles is available at wv

Vos commentaires sur nos titres sont les bienvenus. Veuillez nous envoyer un c
www.oupcanada.com/contact.html,, ou communiquer avec votre représentant des
www.oupcanada.com.

UNDERSTANDING HEALTH,
HEALTH CARE,
AND
HEALTH POLICY IN CANADA
Sociological Perspectives

NEENA L. CHAPPELL AND MARGARET J. PENNING

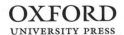

OXFORD
UNIVERSITY PRESS

OXFORD
UNIVERSITY PRESS

70 Wynford Drive, Don Mills, Ontario M3C 1J9
www.oupcanada.com

Oxford University Press is a department of the University of Oxford.
It furthers the University's objective of excellence in research, scholarship,
and education by publishing worldwide in

Oxford   New York

Auckland   Cape Town   Dar es Salaam   Hong Kong   Karachi
Kuala Lumpur   Madrid   Melbourne   Mexico City   Nairobi
New Delhi   Shanghai   Taipei   Toronto

With offices in

Argentina   Austria   Brazil   Chile   Czech Republic   France   Greece
Guatemala   Hungary   Italy   Japan   Poland   Portugal   Singapore
South Korea   Switzerland   Thailand   Turkey   Ukraine   Vietnam

Oxford is a trade mark of Oxford University Press
in the UK and in certain other countries

Published in Canada
by Oxford University Press

Copyright © Oxford University Press Canada 2009

The moral rights of the author have been asserted

Database right Oxford University Press (maker)

First published 2009

Library and Archives Canada Cataloguing in Publication

Understanding health, health care, and health policy in Canada:
sociological perspectives / Neena L. Chappell, Margaret J. Penning.

Includes index.

ISBN 978-0-19-542476-8

1. Social medicine—Canada—Textbooks.   2. Medical care—Canada—Textbooks.
3. Medical policy—Canada—Textbooks.   I. Penning, M.   II. Title.
RA449.C43 2008   306.4'610971   C2008-902099-5

Cover Photo: Getty Images/Ira Brock

1 2 3 4 - 12 11 10 09

This book is printed on permanent (acid-free) paper ∞.
Printed in Canada

Contents

Preface and Acknowledgements

Health, health care, and health policy are of major importance to us as individuals and to the society within which we live. Collectively, these topics also represent an area of major sociological interest and activity in Canada and internationally. The sociology of health, health care, and health policy, also frequently known as medical sociology, represents one of the largest sections within Canadian, American, and international sociological associations; courses in the area are popular among undergraduate and graduate students alike. Canada is both similar to and yet distinct from other countries such as the United States and Britain when it comes to issues of health, health care, and health policy. Yet, too often, we rely on books written about and research conducted elsewhere to inform our understanding of the Canadian situation. To date, there are few contemporary Canadian texts available, particularly at an introductory level. However, the depth of Canadian academic scholarship in this area is notable.

This book is part of a series of concise texts designed to highlight recent research and trends in sociology and written by Canadian scholars. It attempts to reflect the range and diversity of sociological approaches to health, health care, and health policy in Canada and to examine major issues and debates within the contemporary context. We agreed to write this text because we felt there were topics and issues within the sociology of health and health care that other Canadian authors do not cover. In addition, we perceived a need to draw attention to some of the central theoretical issues of concern to sociologists in our approach to these topics and issues. Therefore, this book draws attention to one of the major challenges facing the discipline (namely, the integration of structure and agency) then proceeds to present a broad, balanced understanding of sociological debates and issues within health and health care. Both experiential and structural perspectives are consistently presented around concrete issues in a Canadian context. The text also emphasizes issues of social inequality, focusing on multiple inequalities (including social class, gender, racial/ethnic, age, and others).

This book is intentionally written at a level that ensures complex concepts are easily understandable. It does so in a condensed text to allow instructors the opportunity to supplement with in-depth readings. Thus, it is not intended to be comprehensive nor to provide a detailed examination of the issues but is meant to serve as a foundation for such examination. Our intent is to provide a brief introduction to the area, one that reflects the range and diversity of sociological approaches and provides evidence of their application to an understanding of health, health care, and health policy in the Canadian context. By highlighting some of the key issues, debates, and areas of research in the Canadian setting and demonstrating the value of both macro structural and micro social psychological approaches to the area, we provide a foundation for more in-depth studies of the sociology of health and health care. The purpose of the book is to help students better understand issues in health, health care, and health policy from a sociological perspective and to point out how and why a sociological perspective is critical to an understanding of health, health care, and health policy.

We would like to express our thanks to the series editors—Drs Lorne Tepperman, Susan McDaniel, and the late James Curtis—for their invitation to contribute a book on the sociology of health, health care, and health policy to the series. We would also like to thank those at the University of Victoria who contributed their thoughts and expertise to the work (Dr Moyra Brackley, Nancy Davis, and Carren Dujela) as well as those at Oxford University Press (Rachael Cayley, Jennifer Charlton, Janna Green, and Lisa Meschino) who worked with us at various stages to see this project through to completion.

This book was written while the senior author was a Canada Research Chair in Social Gerontology. Both authors have received support for their research activities over the years from agencies such as the Social Sciences and Humanities Research Council of Canada (SSHRC), the Canadian Institutes of Health Research (CIHR), Health Canada, the Michael Smith Foundation for Health Research (MSFHR), and the Alzheimer's Society of Canada. We are greatly indebted to each for their ongoing support of our academic endeavours.

Finally, we would also like to thank our colleagues, mentors, friends, and family members (especially Kristen and Michael B. and Sean, Ryan, and David C.) for their continuing encouragement and support of our work and of our health while we were working on this project.

Neena L. Chappell, PhD
Margaret J. Penning, PhD
University of Victoria

Chapter 1

Health and Health Care: Sociological History and Perspectives

Learning Objectives

In this chapter, you will learn that:

- In the past, sociologists typically approached the study of health and health care from a medical perspective, adopting a view of health as the absence of disease. More recently, however, they have become critical of this view and have shifted toward a broader focus on the topic.
- Several theoretical perspectives have guided sociological understanding of health and health-care issues, including social structural and social psychological.
- While structural functionalists focus attention on societal norms and roles as affecting health-related behaviour, political economy perspectives emphasize larger socio-political and economic influences. Gender-based approaches draw attention to gender as a basic organizing principle of society; race and ethnic studies do so for race/ethnicity.
- Social psychological perspectives have been drawn upon ever since sociologists began to consider health and health care; this interest continues with an added focus on understanding the construction of meaning in everyday interaction.
- While most theoretical perspectives in sociology emphasize either the structural or the individual interaction level, a major challenge for the discipline lies in integrating both into one perspective. This challenge also characterizes the sociology of health and health care.
- Attention to social inequality is foundational to sociology; the sociological study of health and health care is no exception. This area examines relationships between inequality and the differences in the health of individuals and populations, as well as differential access to health-care services.

A SOCIOLOGICAL PERSPECTIVE

A **sociological perspective** addresses interactions or relationships between individuals; between individuals and groups, communities, or larger social structures; and between different social structures (such as families and the health-care system). By focusing on connections between the individual and the social, as well as among elements within the social, this perspective increases our understanding of both individuals and societies and in so doing reveals the importance of social construction. As C. Wright Mills (1959) expressed it, sociology conceptualizes private troubles 'of milieu' in relation to public issues of social structure. A sociological perspective, therefore, is interested in such things as the relationships between health beliefs and culture, health behaviours and education, health needs and health care, and economic structures and health-care services. Because it probes beneath the surface to examine the how and why of these relationships, it tends to question assumptions about how the world operates and allows us to envision alternative relations within and among societies. The new knowledge thereby created can be considered a vehicle for social change.

This book addresses these relationships within the field of health and health care in Canada. It is premised on the view that sociology is uniquely situated to enhance our understanding of health and the provision of care as shaped by while simultaneously shaping the social structures within which both are embedded. We embrace the multiplicity of theoretical perspectives within the discipline as not only valid but also preferred for a more comprehensive understanding of the area. In this chapter, we begin with a brief review of sociological thinking about theoretical approaches to health and health care and conclude with a discussion of social inequalities, an underlying theme in this area. The chapters that follow address the role of social structural factors in influencing Canadians' health and health care, while also considering the social construction of meaning and the exercise of human agency and choice. Chapter 2 examines these factors in relation to the actual levels of health and illness, while Chapters 3 and 4 focus on the provision of care, beginning with that provided by individuals themselves (self-care) and by the family members and friends located within people's informal social networks (informal and formal care) and then proceeding to an examination of the care provided by the various health-care providers and settings located within the formal health-care system. Building on this discussion, Chapter 5 then analyzes health-care policy and its implications for health and the various types of care that are available to us. We conclude with a discussion of future directions in health and health care as well as for sociological thought in this field. Our intent is to provide a brief introduction to the discipline, one that reflects the range and diversity of sociological approaches and provides evidence of their application to an understanding of health, health care, and health policy in the

Canadian context. By highlighting some of the key issues, debates, and areas of research in the Canadian setting and demonstrating the value of both structural and social psychological approaches to the area, we provide a foundation for more in-depth studies of the sociology of health and health care. (See Suggested Websites for a selection of websites on health and health care, some specific to sociology.)

A BRIEF HISTORY OF SOCIOLOGICAL THINKING ABOUT HEALTH AND HEALTH CARE

Medicine's central importance within modern industrialized societies such as Canada arose during the late nineteenth and early twentieth centuries. With the emergence of the germ theory of disease, it became accepted that each disease had its origins in a particular microorganism. In the process, health became synonymous with the absence of disease. At the same time, modern inventions such as the stethoscope, clinical thermometer, and hypodermic syringe; techniques for sterilizing operating procedures; and vaccines for smallpox and other infectious diseases were introduced. Medical licensing laws were passed, medical schools were standardized, restrictions were placed on entry into the medical field, and the income and status of the profession increased (Brown, 1979; Bryden, 1974). During this period, the occurrence of infectious disease decreased, which was attributed to the success of modern medical science.

As the incidence of infectious diseases declined and the risks of illness became increasingly predictable (i.e., relatively constant rather than fluctuating cyclically or changing suddenly), the Canadian government, along with many others in developed nations, believed that the risks of sickness within the population should be underwritten by the community as a whole and that universal health insurance should be made available to every citizen. In the 1950s, the federal government established a program to assist in funding hospital construction, thereby making hospitals the primary location for accessing medical care. National hospital insurance followed in 1957 to cover the medical and other types of care (e.g., pharmacy, nursing, and physiotherapy) provided within these settings. The hospital became the only place where health services like pharmacy or physiotherapy were insured, as long as they were performed under the supervision of a physician. Physician care was publicly insured in 1968, providing Canadians with universal access to medical care outside of hospital settings and adding the second and final piece to Canada's Medicare system (Coburn et al., 1983). As a result, physicians evolved as the gatekeepers to our health-care system, becoming the only health-care practitioners whose services were included in universal public insurance and who could certify our illnesses, order prescription medications and medical tests, or admit someone to hospital.

It was after health was equated with the absence of disease and health care with medical care that sociologists began to study it. The initial focus, known as **medical sociology,** was on the social and social psychological factors that influenced medical care utilization. In the late 1950s, Straus (1957), a sociologist, drew a distinction between sociology *in* medicine and sociology *of* medicine. **Sociology *in* medicine** refers to sociological research in which the researcher studies questions of interest to and often defined by the medical profession. The intent is to try to solve problems of importance from a medical perspective. Examples include research on patient compliance (who follows doctor's orders, who does not, and why or why not) and program effectiveness (whether immunization programs in schools are successful in ensuring that most children become immunized or how diabetes can be treated cost-effectively). Research from this perspective takes the relevance of the research questions for granted; it does not critically evaluate the questions posed or medicine itself.

Sociology *of* medicine takes a more distant and critical approach to studying medicine, its workers, and its methods of delivery. The primary objective is to enhance sociological knowledge and understanding. Thus, the research questions pursued are more likely to be posed by sociologists than by health-care professionals. Examples include research on power relationships involving doctors, nurses, and patients; research on the quality of health care delivered by for-profit companies versus care delivered by not-for-profit companies; and research on the results of medical trials funded by pharmaceutical companies versus those funded by public monies.

To date, medical sociology has produced a considerable amount of important research. Segall and Chappell (2000) summarize much of this research as focusing on four areas:

- the distribution of illness and disease among different populations (e.g., social classes, ethnic groups, age cohorts, gender);
- the social patterning of illness behaviour and variations in how people think about, experience, and respond to similar symptoms and diseases (e.g., cultural differences in the meanings of various symptoms or experiences with pain);
- the social institutions established for dealing with disease (e.g., traditional folk healers and modern hospitals); and
- the broader social organization and delivery of health services (e.g., the regulating of alternative medicines, determining which services should be included in provincial health care, and setting the levels at which pharmacare premiums should be set).

However, as research in the area grew, so too did a reflective sociological critique. In the 1970s, sociologists began to reflect critically on the power of the medical profession to define the research that was being conducted, both through the articulation of the questions to be studied and through permitting or denying access to the locations and participants needed for study (see Pflanz, 1974, 1975). In the process, they also became critical of the tendency for research to focus largely on illness rather than on its prevention of illness or on a broader conception of health. Both academics and the grassroots populace began to question the narrowness of a health-care system that operated almost exclusively from an individualized medical perspective (Chappell et al., 2003). Wilkinson (1996) used the analogy of the physician in war—while they are very necessary to treat battlefield wounds, they play no role in preventing the war in the first place. This period of self-criticism was followed by the emergence of sociology of health and health care as a distinct area from medical sociology.

In contrast with its predecessor's primary interest in individual illness (who gets sick, how it is treated, and how that treatment is delivered), the sociology of health and health care emerged in the 1980s with an emphasis on health in addition to illness; on alternative forms of care (including self-care and informal care) and practitioners such as midwives, homeopaths, and naturopaths in addition to traditional medical care and medical care providers; on community-based as well as hospital and institutional settings for care; and on analyses from structural and societal perspectives (e.g., population health) in addition to individual and personal perspectives. There was a shift from a narrow preoccupation with patient illness behaviour to a broader focus that included population health behaviour.

The sociology of health and health care arose within a societal context in which medicine was becoming increasingly criticized, not as useless, but as not being the *only* important perspective or approach when it comes to the health of individuals and nations. Our medically oriented health-care system also came under attack as treating illness only after it occurred, as not facilitating health promotion and illness prevention, and as providing the most expensive form of care available (Evans, 1994; Rachlis and Kushner, 1989). Not only academics but also the grassroots populace began to question the narrowness of a health-care system that operated almost exclusively from an individualized medical perspective (Chappell et al., 2003). The 1990s witnessed a firm acceptance and an expansion of interest in the sociology of health and health care. By 2000, the Medical Research Council of Canada, the country's major funder of medical research, was transformed into the Canadian Institutes of Health Research, funding the four pillars of health research: biological research, clinical research, health-services research, and population and public health research. The transformation of Canada's leading public funder of research signified a shift in the nation's (and indeed the world's) thinking about health.

At the present time, the sociology of health and health care could be viewed as 'healthy', co-existing alongside the traditional interests of medical sociology and bringing a broader focus to the discipline that acknowledges the importance of both social structures and social interactions for individual and population health. As such, it ensures attention beyond the individual to communities and larger societal structures when examining questions related to illness, a focus inclusive of health and illness as well as traditional medicine and other types of care. The sociology of health and health care allows for both agency on the part of the individual and the influences of social structure.

THEORETICAL APPROACHES TO HEALTH AND HEALTH CARE

Not surprisingly, definitions of health and the questions chosen for study are influenced by researchers' theoretical orientations and reflect the theoretical approaches in vogue at a given time. There is no one sociological perspective. Instead, sociology is a diverse discipline with many theoretical perspectives, which primarily focus either on the individual and interactions among individuals or on the social structure. The former asks research questions such as the following: What is the experience of illness for those with cancer? Are health beliefs related to health-maintenance behaviours? Does our peer group influence our health behaviours? Do spouses share similar health beliefs? Do teenagers reflect health habits more similar to their parents or to their friends? The latter asks: How does the economy affect the organization and delivery of health-care services? Is health-care service delivery organized differently in rural than in urban areas? How do health behaviours differ between ethno-cultural groups, social classes, genders, and ages? Sociologists often refer to a focus on the individual or on interactions among individuals as a micro level of analysis and that on social structure as a macro level. An intermediate focus, as on groups or communities, is referred to as being at the meso level.

Currently, a major challenge for sociologists of health and health care is the integration of the individual and the social structural levels of analysis into a coherent whole, since both are widely acknowledged as necessary for a comprehensive understanding of social life. Here we briefly discuss several theoretical perspectives and the emphasis each places on the individual social psychological level or on more macro social structures. We begin with a focus on social structural perspectives, including structural functionalism and conflict approaches, followed by a discussion of social psychological perspectives that emphasize individual interaction in the social creation of meaning and experience. We then discuss more contemporary views that attempt to integrate both perspectives and conclude with a discussion of social inequalities in health and health care.

Social Structural Perspectives

The concept of **social structure** has been referred to as 'one of the great blocks on which the architecture of the social sciences has been built' (Williams, 2003: 132). Thus, unlike disciplines such as economics that tend to focus on the individual as a rational actor free of social constraints, sociologists tend to be more concerned with constraints upon individual action (van Krieken, 1997, cited in Deacon and Mann, 1999: 414).

This insight has also had important implications for our understanding of health and health care. In epidemiological circles (epidemiology deals with the incidence, distribution, and control of disease in a population), attempts to understand health and health care have focused on various attributes or characteristics of individuals. Similarly, in medical, public-health, and health-policy circles, attempts to improve health and to reduce inequalities have often targeted individuals to alter their behaviour (i.e., eat better, smoke less, etc.). Those who emphasize individual responsibility tend to view health inequalities as the outcome of differences in how people make choices (e.g., the decision to start smoking). Yet, as Lynch and colleagues (1997) have noted, understanding why people behave poorly when it comes to their health requires a shift toward the realization that behaviours often thought of as within the realm of the individual and therefore under individual control occur within a social context that also has an impact. This effect occurs in various ways: by shaping norms, enforcing patterns of social control (which may be health-promoting or health-damaging), by providing or not providing opportunities to engage in certain behaviours, and by reducing or producing stress for which certain behaviours may be an effective coping strategy.

Structural Functionalism

When sociologists began studying medicine in the 1950s and 1960s, the dominant paradigm in North American sociology was **structural functionalism** (Parsons, 1951). From this perspective, society is viewed as consisting of a number of social institutions (social structures) that are interdependent and when functioning properly, ensure social order and stability. These include familial, educational, economic, political, and health-care institutions. Within these institutions, people are socialized to play out roles that meet the needs of society. Thus, the behaviours prescribed within these roles help ensure societal functioning. This applies to health and illness no less than to other social roles. From this point of view, the individual is considered relatively passive, more a product of social influences assisting the overall functioning of society than being an active architect in its creation.

Early studies from this perspective viewed health, and especially illness, as social roles with highly structured behavioural expectations attached. In the early 1950s, Parsons (1951) described the institutionalized behavioural expectations associated with being sick—**the sick role**—as encompassing both rights and duties:

- a right to exemption from responsibility for illness (it is assumed that, except in rare instances such as sexually transmitted diseases due to unprotected sex, one is not personally at fault for being sick);
- a right to exemption from normal role responsibilities such as having to work or go to school when one is sick;
- a duty to try and get well (one is expected to view illness as undesirable and to resume normal roles as soon as possible); and

- a duty to seek technically competent help (such as a physician) and to comply with instructions in order to recover as quickly as possible.

Within structural functionalism, the sick role represents a temporary and medically authorized deviation from roles that facilitate the smooth functioning of society. From this point of view, those in the medical profession serve as agents of social control; only physicians can certify the fact that we are sick. Yet their motives are altruistic; it is their job to help us get well so that we can return to the roles that enable a stable society.

With the evolution of the sociology of health and health care and the broadening of interest beyond medicine, Parsons's sick role concept was criticized on several grounds, including its normative assumptions and failure to address issues of power and conflict; its narrow focus on only temporary acute illness episodes to the exclusion of chronic illness and the psychosocial aspects of health and illness; its underestimation of the roles of self- and informal care within the overall provision of health care; and its overestimation of the roles played by formal and professional services, particularly physicians. To overcome some of these limitations, Segall (1997) proposed a modification of Parsons's concept to a non-medicalized sick role that takes everyday health and illness behaviour into account. This modified sick role concept also includes rights and duties, some of which overlap with those identified by Parsons:

- one has the right to make decisions about health-related matters;
- one is exempt from performing well roles when sick;
- one should make use of social support and depend on lay others when sick;
- one has an obligation to maintain one's health and manage one's illness;
- one has a duty to engage in routine self-health management; and
- one has a duty to make use of available health-care resources.

This health concept is broader than the original sick role concept. It acknowledges lay health beliefs and health behaviours as well as the informal network of social interaction in which we all participate. It recognizes each of us as an active agent in our everyday lives, choosing some behaviours and avoiding others. It includes health promotion as well as illness care. It reflects the thinking within a sociology of health perspective that differs from medical sociology while staying within a structural functionalist approach.

Conflict and Power
Conflict and power approaches (including Marxist theorizing and political economy perspectives, as well as gender-conflict and race-based approaches),

have also been applied to the area of health and illness. Similar to structural functionalism, conflict theories also focus on the societal level, but with a concentration on competing interest groups, viewing society as characterized by groups with different levels of access to power and associated resources. The emphasis on power relations within societal political and economic structures (Navarro, 1976) is a common theme, as are the implications of power differentials for generating inequality, exploitation, and alienation as well as social change. The dominance of the medical profession in the health area is a major topic of interest: how it attained its power, how it maintains its power, and how its power affects our views and behaviours with regard to health and illness. In the 1970s, Freidson (1970a, 1970b) wrote extensively about how medicine negotiated its position of dominance with regard to health-related matters (through licensure, imposing restrictions on entry to medical school, obtaining exclusive rights to diagnose and treat disease, etc.). Medicine's ability to expand its domain has also received considerable attention (Conrad, 1975; Illich, 1975). Over the years, mental illness, alcoholism, gambling, and childbirth have all come to be defined as diseases to be diagnosed and medically treated. The expanding boundaries of medical care led some sociologists, such as Zola (1972), to argue that everyday life was becoming medicalized.

Marxist theory is an example of a conflict perspective, emphasizing the primary importance of class structures and economic inequalities in the production, distribution, and treatment of illness (Navarro, 1985). Here, the capitalist pursuit of profit is seen as responsible for exploiting those in the working class and consequently for the negative health effects that result. The practice of medicine not only reflects class inequalities (with those who practise medicine coming from the bourgeoisie) but also reinforces them. Physicians are private entrepreneurs who seek profit at the expense of workers and also act as agents of social control (certifying who and how long people are considered sick, restricting their access to health services, and so on).

More recent thinking along these lines is evident in the **political economy perspective** on health and health care. This perspective assumes that our experiences of health and of illness are shaped by and inextricable from the larger socio-political and economic contexts within which they are embedded. For example, Conrad and Kern focus on the importance of understanding relationships between social structure and health outcomes: 'We must investigate how social factors such as the political economy, the corporate structure, the distribution of resources, and the use of political, economic, and social power influence health and illness and society's response to health and illness' (1986: 2). The structural contexts of the economy, the state, the labour market, and class, gender, race, and age divisions within society are of paramount importance for the health and illness of its citizens (Estes, 1991; Myles, 1984). Proponents note that the economic mode of production shapes social conditions and relations within it (Armstrong, 2001) and these evolve over time. Canada, like other Western nations, is an advanced industrial and capitalist country; it has slowly transitioned from competitive to monopoly to global capitalism. This transition, as will become evident in later chapters, has had important implications for individual and population health and health care.

Gender-conflict approaches also emphasize structural inequalities and issues of power and conflict but take gender rather than social class inequalities as their point of departure. For example, **feminist theorizing** in the areas of health and heath care often reflects this approach. Here, gender (see Box 1.1) is considered a fundamental organizing principle of society that operates over the life course. Gender relations are embedded within social organization and are socially constructed power relations immersed within social processes and institutionalized into everyday life, thereby affecting men's and women's life chances (Calasanti, 2004; Fine, 1996). Gendered relations are entwined within social stratification and inequality, patterning advantage and disadvantage, typically with women being disadvantaged. As a whole, women have lacked social, economic, and political power, often translating into a lack of agency at the individual level. This lack is reflected in the tendency for women to concentrate on the helping professions (nursing, social work, home care attendants, etc.) rather than the more powerful physician occupation. When they do become physicians they tend to practise general medicine and a few lower status specialties such as pediatrics or family medicine rather than higher status specialties such as surgery and not to occupy more powerful positions such as heads of teaching hospitals (Riska and Wegar, 1993).

These tendencies do not mean, however, that all women lack agency in all circumstances. A feminist approach assumes women's everyday knowledge is legitimate and valuable, an assumption that fuelled women's lobbies to take account of women's perspectives in the treatment of breast cancer and in childbirth, both of which had been medicalized. Similarly, attention to empowerment is inherent within a feminist approach. Feminist researchers view legitimizing women's voices and helping them to use new knowledge for advocacy as inherent within their role. Sharing experiences can facilitate women's awareness while simultaneously empowering new knowledge as researchers learn about their experiences in health and in illness.

More recently, **lesbian, gay, bisexual, and transsexual (LGBT) studies** has emerged to advance the interests of these groups and to contribute culturally and intellectually to their movements. Both gender-based approaches, feminism and LGBT studies seek to expose the injustices and harm that result from heteronormativity (the practices and structures that legitimize and support heterosexuality as natural within society; see Cohen et al., 2005). However, both have been criticized for their lack of emphasis on the social forces that create and maintain gender inequality (Kirsch, 2000; Williams, 2006), even though their focus is often on the structural force of gender as a societal organizing principle.

Box 1.1
Sex and Gender Defined

Sex-/gender-sensitive research examines the interaction of sex and gender and its subsequent health effects, essential components to understanding the complexity and diversity of human health. Such research requires an understanding of the differences between the terms:

Sex refers to the biological characteristics such as anatomy (e.g., body size and shape) and physiology (e.g., hormonal activity or functioning or organs) that distinguish males and females.

Gender refers to the array of socially constructed roles and relationships, personality, traits, attitudes, behaviours, values, and relative power and influence that society ascribes to two sexes based on a differential basis. Gender is relational—gender roles and characteristics do not exist in isolation, but are defined in relation to one another.

Source: Canadian Institutes of Health Research. 2007. *Gender and Sex-Based Analysis in Health Research: A Guide for CIHR Researchers and Reviewers*. Available at: http://www.cihr-irsc.gc.ca/e/32019.html#toc2.

Just as gender-based perspectives expose and question master narratives about gender and sexuality, a race/ethnic focus does so for race and ethnic relations. Those who apply a race/ethnic lens consider race/ethnicity a fundamental organizing principle of society, one that is socially constructed, pervasive, and that operates throughout the life course. Indeed, Blau et al. (1979) have argued that race/ethnicity is the most fundamental division within American society, a more pervasive and more powerful organizing principle than social class or socio-economic status (SES). Embedded within social organization, this division is inherently about power relations that are reflected in social processes and institutionalized into our everyday lives. The advantage/disadvantage pattern and lack of social, economic, and political power that we saw with the gender approach also applies here and affects all areas of social life, including health and health care. Members of ethnic minorities are more likely to live in poverty, which is related to poor health (Chappell, 2007b), and they are more likely to work in jobs where they exercise little control and are exposed to rigid work schedules, poor air quality, or crowded quarters, all of which can result in stress and impact health. Similar to feminist approaches, race/ethnic approaches are about empowerment and social justice. Sociologists conducting this type of research often try to use it to help those involved understand the consequences of their circumstances and to gain greater control within their lives.

A unique problem encountered by health researchers interested in race/ethnic issues is the **race relations problematic**, initially identified by Miles (1982). This refers to the reification of race or race relations through its use—the use of the term tends to imply that race is biologically based, when in fact science has rejected this notion. On the other hand, the social construction of race reflects reality, and dropping the use of the term may make the real consequences of race relations more invisible (Barot, 2006). As expressed by Nayak: '[H]ow do we discuss race in a way that does not reify the very categories we are seeking to abolish?' (2006: 415)

Indeed, Bonilla-Silva (2000) argues that the new racial ideology, or **new racism**, is making race even more invisible throughout Western societies. This new racism has resulted from the **interiorization of race** (significant increases in the size and diversity of racial minorities in Western countries in recent years) and the extension of national capitalist economies into a world system whereby Africa, South America, and Asia have been racialized as underdeveloped and inferior when compared with the white supremacy of the West. This new world order, created through globalization, emerged in the mid-1960s and resulted in sizeable migrations to Western countries, where these minorities often lived as second-class citizens. Also known as **laissez-faire racism**, this new ideology of equality for all within unequal class-based systems allows people to believe they are not racist, yet the countries they live in enact **institutional racism** (policies and practices that are embedded within societal institutions and serve to disadvantage those in particular racial or ethnic groups). The challenge in the health area is to expose and study the relevance of race/ethnicity for health and health care, without either suggesting its roots are biological or making the concept more invisible.

Gender and race/ethnicity are but some of the structural characteristics that have profound effects on the lives and health of our citizens. Social class and age are two more. Although sociologists have tended to study each separately, there is increasing recognition that they co-exist and interact with one another in influencing our lives. Consequently, while some argue for the need to theorize one overarching structure of domination (e.g., Collins, 1990), others call for the discipline to study the **intersectionality** of these statuses to better understand their relevance to our health.

Social Psychological Perspectives

Thus far, all of the approaches we have discussed have emphasized the macro or structural level. They differ from one another in the assumptions they make about societies and how societies operate, but they share a lack of major focus on the social psychological level. As a result, they are criticized as overly deterministic and as according insufficient attention to human agency or potential for individuals to influence their situations. From a purely structural perspective, social factors such as unemployment cause ill health: 'Deprivation causes disease. Society . . . is held to be at fault. . . . The individual is relegated to being nothing more than a system outcome, not a thinking and acting human being' (Kelly and Charlton, 1995: 83).

However, recent years have seen a resurgence of interest in the importance of **human agency**—the 'actions, activities, decisions, and behaviours that represent some measure of meaningful choice' (Deacon and Mann, 1999: 413). Proponents point out that this does not mean that such choices are uninfluenced by any structural constraints, but rather that options exist, albeit also restrained. According to Popay and colleagues (1998), those who focus on inequalities in health tend to ignore the complexity of social processes, failing to consider social context and creative human agency. In their view, one of the main limitations of the literature on health inequalities is a lack of attention to understanding why individuals and groups behave the way they do within broader social structures. That is, what is the link between agency and social structure and how does it operate (Williams, 2003)? In particular, the subjective dimensions of health inequalities have often been neglected by structuralists.

Social psychological approaches have long been central to sociology, so their application to health and illness is not new. Perspectives and related methodological approaches include symbolic interaction, phenomenology, ethnography, and interpretive inquiry, to name but a few. They share an interest in social interaction and a belief that we construct meaning and interpret the world through our social interactions. While largely ignoring more macro social structures, these perspectives add a valuable dimension to health research through their pursuit of knowledge on such issues as how we define when we are healthy and when we are not, whether the factors we believe influence our health (for example, beliefs regarding the importance of what we eat) are actually related to our health, whether we act on the basis of our beliefs, and what our experience of different types of illnesses includes.

Symbolic Interaction
One of the first theoretical perspectives to draw attention to such matters was **symbolic interaction**, still popular today. Its founder, George Herbert Mead (1934), argued that the self is formed not at birth but only through our interactions with others, that we are actors as well as reactors, helping to create the world that in turn influences us. Thus, it is through our interactions with others that reality is created and re-created. Socialization is a key term for symbolic interactionists; it is through symbolically mediated interaction that we learn to take the attitudes, values, and affectivity of specific social situations. While interpreting and responding to others, we also reflect on and form our own assessments of situations (Blumer, 1969). Societal roles have received much attention within this perspective because they provide expectations that influence behaviour, telling us what we should and should not do and acting as internalized guides to behaviour. Role changes tend to mark life transitions such as graduating from school and

beginning a job, getting married, having children, or becoming sick with a serious illness. Each of us at the same time can reflect and act against society's prescriptions. In addition, society is comprised of many reference groups, not all of which promote consistent norms and expectations—our family may teach us that smoking is unhealthy, but our friends may smoke.

Following in this tradition, Goffman (1959, 1963) used **dramaturgical analysis** to enlighten our understanding of how we adopt certain behaviours in everyday face-to-face interactions, including those involving health and health care. He described life as a stage, with ordinary people enacting their social roles as scripted performances that change depending on the context; his metaphor included recognition of the actions we take when we are backstage and the actions that depend on the audience. He also included non-verbal communication as part of our behaviour. Part of the difficulty for those with mental illnesses, as opposed to more definitively diagnosed physical ailments, is convincing others that they 'really' are sick because they do not enact the role of a sick person as conventionally scripted. Even those with many physical ailments are sometimes not believed by others to be sick (consider, for example, when we refer to someone as a hypochondriac). When we become ill we are expected to act in certain ways if others are to accept and respond to our self-identity as ill.

According to Goffman, failure to succeed at impression management can lead to stigma (negative labelling) or a discredited identity, with important consequences for how others treat us and, in some instances, for how we perceive ourselves (for example, if we adopt the discredited identity as our self-identity). We all label others with language, and certain words become shorthand imbued with fuller meaning. **Labelling theory** has also been used in sociology, primarily to discuss the consequences of stigma, especially in relation to criminology and mental illness. To be called a criminal or mentally ill defines you as a deviant, simultaneously defining others as 'normal'. Others treat you based on this identity, and your own self-identity and behaviour can be created and/or influenced through this interaction. Some early sociologists, such as Scheff (1966), argued that mental illness is entirely created by society; an individual so labelled and treated eventually comes to believe the label and act accordingly— there is no other cause (e.g., a biological basis of the disorder). However, the consequences (e.g., being shunned and/or isolated from others, being refused rental accommodation, being refused jobs) of labelling can follow even if these illnesses have physiological causes. That is, a belief in the biological causes of mental illness does not preclude the importance of labelling.

Social Constructionism

Consistent with this approach is modern-day **social constructionist sociology**, in which interest focuses on how people interpretively produce and organize their lives as they make everyday experiences meaningful. As such, the social constructionist digs under our everyday lives to understand how that world is constructed,

Box 1.2
A Social Constructionist Example

Mrs F. was married to a 35-year-old taxi driver. For some time, Mrs F. normalized her husband's sometimes strange behaviour in terms of his past experiences or the type of person he was. He started to work only sporadically then hardly at all. She initially interpreted this as his desire to spend more time with his new wife, typical of newlyweds. As the behaviour continued, she saw it as typical of other taxi drivers who also did not like to work hard. As time passed, she noticed behaviours that were uncharacteristic of him: he complained the TV set was 'after him'; he talked about a worm growing out of his grandfather's mustache. This was confusion from his watching little worms in their fish tank. He claimed his genitals had been blown up and covered him in little seeds; he said he killed his grandfather and begged his wife to forgive him and wondered if his wife were his mother or God. This was understandable given his wartime experiences. To Mrs F., her husband was normal, with occasional troubles.

However, when Mr F. stopped taking baths and changing clothes and one night woke his wife to tell her that the book he was writing had nothing to do with science but was about him solving the problems that had been bothering him for 10 years, she reinterpreted his behaviour. Mrs F. decided his behaviour was 'rather strange', providing an entirely different framework for understanding his behaviour. She reinterpreted much of his past behaviour in terms of a person who was 'crazy' and had been from the start. He was subsequently admitted to a mental institution.

Source: J.F. Gubrium and J.A. Holstein, eds. 2000. *Aging and Everyday Life*. Oxford: Blackwell Publishing.

sustained, and changed. Interpretive practice is the constellation of procedures, conditions, and resources through which we apprehend, understand, and convey reality in everyday life (Gubrium and Holstein, 1997). For example, instead of taking for granted that you will go from university to the work force, constructionists ask how you have come to adopt that interpretation. Thus, the focus is on the 'public construction of private lives' (Gubrium and Holstein, 2000: 205).

The social constructionist does not deny the existence or importance of social structure but focuses on the individual level and the 'local enactment' of the broader culture. It is a matter of emphasis—the social constructionist is interested in how individuals interact with, interpret, and re-construct meanings within the context of culture as it presents itself locally. Interest is directed to the individual as an active participant in his or her own life, choosing from among the contradictory complexities of his or her own experiences and those of the culture. Box 1.2 provides an example of how a wife's interpretation of her husband's behaviour is transformed over time.

The focus here is on what we normally take for granted and an understanding that meanings are socially constructed and not objective truths. Especially in the area of mental illness, judgment and interpretation define whether one is mentally healthy or not. The reverse also occurs; we interpret the actions and motivations of a convicted criminal in one light but reinterpret the person when DNA evidence finds she or he was innocent all along. Persons who behave strangely (e.g., suddenly become anxious and obsessive) are seen in a different light when it is learned that their medications made them act this way, but once they are off the medications they are back to their own or 'real' selves. One more example: 30 years ago, Illich (1976) discussed how the depersonalization of diagnosis and therapy has resulted in medical malpractice no longer being viewed as an ethical problem. Rather, it is now considered a technical problem where, within complex technological medical environments, negligence is translated as 'random human error' or 'system breakdown', callousness becomes 'scientific detachment', and incompetence becomes 'a lack of specialized equipment'.

Social psychological approaches are popular when studying gender and race/ethnic relations and health issues because they provide an understanding of the language, norms, and experiences of members of these groups as well as the social circumstances that impact the production of localized facts and debunk myths about group members as irrational, inferior, and disorganized (Esposito and Murphy, 2000). They allow study of the ongoing and unfolding definition of the 'colour line', constantly mediated and constantly specified, giving voice to minority members so they are no longer 'others' within a cultural standard of white normalcy. In their efforts to empower as well as study, social psychological researchers have contributed to the development of **participatory action research (PAR)**. While there are many varieties of PAR, they tend to share an interest in involving study participants (not only the researchers) in the research enterprise and aim to assist in restructuring local power arrangements. Participants gain new knowledge that they can use to improve their own living conditions. The Aboriginal community in Canada has embraced these principles for research in which they are involved. Box. 1.3 includes some of the Canadian Institutes of Health Research (CIHR)'s guidelines for health research involving Aboriginal people.

Research focusing on the intersectionality of more than one status is also beginning to appear, using social psychological approaches as well as structural approaches. Few (2007), for example, studied black women using an intersectionality matrix (a specific location of multiple systems of oppressions, simultaneously operating to oppress and marginalize to define them as 'others') to understand the lived and dynamic subjectivities of these lives. **Black feminists** politicize their situatedness in relation to oppressive hierarchies of social relationality and in so doing balance both gender and race consciousness. They recognize the multiple locations and identities that intersect within the lives of black women.

Box 1.3
CIHR Guidelines for Health Research Involving Aboriginal People

Aboriginal people refer to Inuit, Métis, and members of First Nations. The Canadian Institutes for Health Research articulates several ethical principles of Aboriginal health research. These include the following:

- A researcher should understand and respect Aboriginal world views, including responsibilities to the people and culture that flow from being granted access to traditional or sacred knowledge. These should be incorporated into research agreements, to the extent possible.
- A community's jurisdiction over the conduct of research should be understood and respected.
- Communities should be given the option of a participatory-research approach.
- A researcher who proposes to carry out research that touches on traditional or sacred knowledge of an Aboriginal community, or on community members as Aboriginal people, should consult the community leaders to obtain their consent before approaching community members individually. Once community consent has been obtained, the researcher will still need the free, prior, and informed consent of the individual participants.
- Concerns of individual participants and their community regarding anonymity, privacy, and confidentiality should be respected and should be addressed in a research agreement.
- The research agreement should, with the guidance of community knowledge holders, address the use of the community's cultural knowledge and sacred knowledge.
- Aboriginal people and their communities retain their inherent rights to any cultural knowledge, sacred knowledge, and cultural practices and traditions, which are shared with the researcher. The researcher should also support mechanisms for the protection of such knowledge, practices, and traditions.
- Community and individual concerns over, and claims to, intellectual property should be explicitly acknowledged and addressed in the negotiation with the community prior to starting the research project. Expectations regarding intellectual property rights of all parties involved in the research should be stated in the research agreement.
- Research should be of benefit to the community as well as to the researcher.
- A researcher should support education and training of Aboriginal people in the community including training in research methods and ethics.
- A researcher has an obligation to learn about, and apply, Aboriginal cultural protocols relevant to the Aboriginal community involved in the research.

- A researcher should, to the extent reasonably possible, translate all publications, reports, and other relevant documents into the language of the
  community.
- A researcher should ensure that there is ongoing, accessible, and understandable communication with the community.

Source: Canadian Institutes of Health Research. 2007. *CIHR Guidelines for Health Research Involving Aboriginal People.* Article 1 to Article 11.3. Excerpts from Section IV—Articles. Ottawa: Canadian Institutes of Health Research. Available at: http://www.cihr-irsc.gc.ca/e/29134.html. Reproduced with the permission of the Minister of Public Works and Government Services Canada, 2008.

Contemporary Theorizing

Sociologists have recognized the two solitudes that have characterized the discipline. Increasingly, they have been directing attention to developing theories to
bridge the social structural and social psychological divide. In later chapters we
shall see that much more attention has been given to integrating the two general
approaches at the theoretical level than at the empirical level. In this chapter we
look briefly at some of the theoretical attempts to integrate structure and agency.

Life Course Perspective as Applied to Health and Health Care

When we talk about health and health care (and other social structures), we tend
to restrict ourselves to the here and now; the focus tends to be static rather than
dynamic. For example, when we think about the importance of income inequalities, we act as if current inequalities are at issue, forgetting that their impact is
tied not only to current circumstances but also to the past. Similarly, when we
talk about social construction, we tend to refer to current reality, seldom taking
the influence of the past into account or taking a life course perspective. Yet
some argue that life course effects are fundamental to understanding health-
related issues, for example the origins of health inequality: 'Life course effects
refer to how health status at any given age, for a given birth cohort, reflects not
only contemporary conditions but embodiment of prior life circumstances . . .'
(Kawachi, Subramanian, and Almeida-Filho, 2002: 650).

The **life course perspective** emerged in the 1970s (Elder, 1975), becoming a
dominant perspective by the 1990s. This perspective includes a focus on both
biography and history as well as the intersections of these two within social
structure; it thereby attempts to link both the micro and the macro levels (Elder,
1985). Elder defines the **life course** as

> trajectories that extend across the life span, such as family or work; and by
> short-term changes or transitions, such as entering or leaving school, acquiring
> a full-time job, and the first marriage. Each life course transition is embedded
> in a trajectory that gives it special form and meaning. (2000: 1615)

Proponents of a life course perspective argue that, to understand individuals' current circumstances, we must consider the major social and psychological forces that have operated throughout their lives. Researchers who use this perspective focus on the following: (1) life as dynamic, contextual, and processual; (2) age-related transitions and life trajectories; (3) the relationship between the life course and social contexts, cultural meanings, and social structural location; and (4) the influence of time, period, and cohort on life course transitions for individuals and groups (Bengtson, Elder, and Putney, 2005).

Understanding the differing effects of age, period, and cohort is an essential part of this perspective. An **age effect** refers to changes that occur because one is getting older—an example is the graying of one's hair or the gradual decline in one's eyesight. One of the important questions concerning age effects is which ones are inevitable and which ones are amenable to lifestyle or other influences (such as drug use). A **cohort effect** refers to a historical event that differentially affects people of different ages, i.e., a cohort. For example, the Vietnam War fuelled the counterculture among 1960s youth, but had a different effect on middle-aged and older adults of the time. However, a historical event that affects persons of all ages in a similar manner is called a **period effect**. The events of 11 September 2001 might prove to have a period effect (Chappell, McDonald, and Stones, 2007).

According to Elder (2000), the life course perspective contains four organizing principles. First, the life course of individuals is embedded in and shared by their historical and geographical placement. That is, the life courses of different cohorts vary because of economic, cultural, and geographic differences. For example, the children of the baby boom generation entered the job market during an economic recession where jobs were difficult to come by. In contrast, those entering the job market five years from now will find a plentitude of jobs left by a retiring baby boom generation. Today's older adults grew up during the Great Depression, while the youth of today are immersed in a consumption culture. (See Box 1.4 for Duxbury's four generations in the workplace.) Geographic variations are also important; youth in the Atlantic provinces often must migrate to other provinces to find work. At the present time, youth in Alberta often choose not to complete high school, seduced by the availability of well-paying jobs created by that province's economic boom.

Second, the impact of a transition or event depends on when it occurs in a person's life (referred to as the **life-stage principle**). Having cancer as a child could seriously affect the rest of your life by delaying or preventing educational opportunities and leaving you with frail health. Having cancer as an older adult, while not preferable, will not affect your life chances in terms of education, work, or marriage. A woman who has a baby at age 15 will lessen her likelihood of furthering her education and of having a well-paying job. A woman who has her first child at age 30 is unlikely to experience the same effects. At an individual level, a life course perspective therefore sees health at any point in time as

Box 1.4
Duxbury's Four Generations in the Workplace

The Veteran Generation, born before 1946, had parents who lived through the Great Depression. These children lived through the Second World War and post-war reconstruction, typically in a traditional family with a single male worker, wife at home, four children, economic prosperity, and a job for life. They believed that if you work hard, are loyal and dependable, all will be well. These are the parents of the baby boom generation.

The Baby Boomers, born between 1946 and 1964, experienced a shift from a seller's market to a buyers' market for labour and grew up in economically prosperous times, resulting in optimism and an attitude of entitlement. Many boomers will soon be retiring from the labour force.

Generation X, born between 1961 and 1974, entered the labour market during a period of economic recession followed by a brief recovery, and followed by yet another recession. Competition for employment was fierce and permanent work was elusive, leading to underachievement and apathy. Their situation was not of their own doing.

Generation Y, also known as Millennials or Nexus Generation, were born in 1975 or later and are currently the youngest generation in the labour market. This generation is influenced by their parents' hard times but also see that things are getting better for themselves. They have been taught to think independently. They are about to experience a sellers' labour market in which there will be more jobs available than people to fill them.

Source: K. Foster. 2006. 'Mind The Gap', *Carleton University Magazine* Spring: 14–17. Kris Foster is the editor of *Carleton University Magazine*.

reflecting accumulated advantages and disadvantages associated with social position and the social processes structured by such position.

Third, lives are interdependent (also referred to as **linked lives**). Our lives are enmeshed with multiple others—what we do affects others and vice versa. If a working parent decides to take a job in another city, the family moves as well. A new job in the same city can affect all members of the family, in terms of income and time availability. When sons and daughters grow up, leave home, and begin a family all have repercussions for the parents. Parents who are active campers take their children with them when they are young. What our university peers do influences what we do.

Fourth, individuals construct their own life courses through their choices and actions, contingent upon the constraints and opportunities provided by history and social circumstance. That is, we are agents of our own lives. While recognizing that there are constraints on our actions, individuals are not viewed as passive recipients of societal scripts. Rather, we all participate in the construction of our lives. Different individuals in the same circumstances may choose to act differently: one may refuse a job promotion, another may take it; one may choose to visit a physician for certain ailments, another may choose to do nothing, and still another may choose a naturopathic route.

When applied to health and health care, the life course perspective draws our attention to how individuals' early experiences, their particular circumstances at present, and the timing of various events in their lives can all affect their current health. In addition, the life course perspective also embraces the idea that, within their unique biographical history, individuals have agency and can choose to act in different ways that can impact their health. It is, in other words, a comprehensive theoretical orientation that seeks to combine social structure and agency over time.

In recent years, much important research emanates from a life course perspective (Hertzman et al., 2001; Mhccn et al., 1999; Wadsworth and Kuh, 1997). However, as is the case with other theoretical perspectives, the life course approach is not without its critics. One of these criticisms is that a clear notion of social structure has not been articulated and that, instead, much of the research from this perspective has been micro or individually focused (Hagestad and Dannefer, 2001). Even within the individual focus of most research in this area, Settersten and Hagestad (2001) are critical of the assumption that agency is necessarily good (for example, what about agency that puts the individual at risk or creates stresses?) and the lack of interest in how individuals affect social structures. After all, it is individuals who construct the health-care system and other governmental structures.

It is also interesting to note that a particular life course or developmental framework is often adopted by various health professions as a basis for helping those who come to them. For example, self-help programs such as Alcoholics Anonymous adopt a notion of a linear life course—one is an alcoholic for life, always 'recovering'. The manifestations can be interpreted as 'one day at a time'. Other examples include our conceptualizations of domestic abuse as a 'cycle' of violence, transmitted from one generation to another. As Gubrium and Holstein say, 'a model of how lives are structured in some continuous fashion underpins both the diagnosis of, and solution to, the problem' (2000: 212).

Foucault's Post-Structural Analyses of Power, Knowledge, and the Body

Michel Foucault (1926–1984), a French social and historical philosopher, had a major theoretical influence over the sociology of health and health care, including our thinking about issues of structure and agency. He is perhaps best known for his theory and analyses of power, wherein he not only challenged Marxist conceptualizations of power as a macrostructure (e.g., the state) that served to support industrial capitalism but also existential notions of a free and fully empowered individual (Turner, 1997). Unlike Marxist, political economist, and feminist scholars who tended to see power as concentrated in the hands of capitalists (bourgeoisie or patriarchs) and as coercive and suppressing those over whom it is wielded (e.g., the working class, women), Foucault saw power as something that was diffused and embedded within social relationships, operating at a micro level in everyday routines and practices. Thus, it was not a possession of only certain individuals or groups but 'like a colour dye diffused through the entire social structure and . . . embedded in daily practices' (Turner, 1997: xii). According to Foucault, people internalize state-sanctioned professional models and are 'active subjects' who willingly participate in these power relations:

> He who is subjected . . . assumes responsibility for the constraints of power; he makes them play spontaneously upon himself, he inscribes in himself the power relation in which he simultaneously plays both roles; he becomes the principle of his own subjection. (Foucault, 1979: 202–3)

Foucault's ideas regarding power influenced his work on such topics as the medical profession and discourses of health and disease, the body, and the self. For example, he was interested in the (everyday) power of medical knowledge and discourse/practise to determine how individuals understand, experience, and deal with their own health and illness. According to Foucault, what we think of as objective and factual knowledge about ourselves and about society changes over time, including our knowledge about medicine. For example, eighteenth-century medicine was conducted at patients' bedsides and required their involvement in diagnosis and treatment through reports of their symptoms. As Western societies modernized, new and distinct forms of medical knowledge developed that gradually saw care relocated to hospital settings. At the same time, the need to rely on patients' reports of symptoms increasingly gave way to identifying underlying pathology as the dominant focus of diagnosis and treatment. As a result, patients' experiences became increasingly irrelevant to an understanding of health and illness because, unlike symptoms, underlying disease pathologies were not visible to patients. Consequently, a shift to hospital medicine meant that patients became somewhat removed from their own illness experiences.

On the one hand, Foucault saw modern institutions like medicine (also law, religion, etc.) as coercive and as exercising social control on behalf of the state through the '**power/knowledge**' of medical experts in contemporary Western societies (Foucault, 1972, 1982). He saw power as embedded within the routine practices of the medical profession. Thus, the '**medical gaze**' had the power to create a discourse on its subject matter (the human body) and to provide guidelines about how patients should understand, regulate, and experience their bodies (Lupton, 1997: 99). Yet, at the same time, he argued that doctors were not simply figures of domination with patients as their passive subjects. Instead, both parties were linked in a set of power relations (Foucault, 1984b: 247). Foucault also directed considerable attention to the body, paving the way for subsequent writers to propose a 'sociology of the body' as a specific sub-field within the sociology of health and health care and within sociology more generally (Featherstone et al., 1991; Turner, 1997). To Foucault (1973, 1977), the body was a social and cultural construct, created and reproduced through medical discourse, rather than a biological phenomenon. In modern medical discourse (as well as other power/knowledge processes) people are classified and objectified. Thus, he considered the body a target of power, the intent and outcome of which was to render it obedient and docile (Fox, 1997; White, 2002). Yet Foucault rejected the idea that individuals were wholly constrained and compelled to act on the basis of externally-imposed dictates. Instead he argued that we also experience ourselves, including our bodies, as subjects.

Foucault's work is often described as controversial and has been widely criticized. For example, some criticize him for his lack of attention to factors such as gender (Bunton and Petersen, 1997). More often, the criticisms focus on his arguments with regard to the structure–agency divide. According to some theorists, his perspective tends to reduce social agents to docile bodies. In their view, patients are likely to be more active than Foucault suggests. However, others assert that Foucault's **post-structural approach** effectively addresses the limitations inherent in previous structuralist approaches (that de-emphasize agency), by rejecting notions of 'sovereign power' and thereby overcoming the determinism evident within these approaches (Fox, 1997: 39). Yet this may be truer of his later rather than earlier works (Fox, 1997; Frank, 1998). While Foucault is widely known for focusing on the body as a site for the exercise of power, his later work is said to shift focus away from the body and toward 'the self' and 'reflective subjectivity'. Here individuals are conceptualized as 'reflective, living, speaking beings' (Foucault, 1985: 7) with the capacity to resist prevailing discourses of power. Box 1.5 provides an overview of Queer Theory, one example of a post-structural approach.

The Social Model of Disability and Disability Theory

The critiques levelled by Foucault and others on the power of the medical profession to define and treat illness, to thereby medicalize much of social life and social problems, and to serve as a mechanism for social control had a major impact on sociological theorizing in all areas of health and illness. For example, in the 1980s, a **social model of disability** was proposed based on a critique of the medical and individualistic approach that saw social restrictions for disabled people as resulting from their bodily physical impairments. In other words, individuals' physical impairments led to restrictions on activities, making it difficult for them to participate fully within mainstream social life (the essence of disability). In contrast to the medical approach, proponents of a social model

Box 1.5
Queer Theory

Queer theory, an outgrowth of both feminist and LGBT research, focuses on a search for knowable meanings by uncovering an essentiality masked by the dominant narratives of identity. As a post-structural perspective, it opposes the normalizing forces of master narratives by arguing for and exposing the multiple and fluid subjectivities experienced at the local level. Specificity of context and the dynamic nature of selves are emphasized through the deconstruction of master narratives (Lovaas et al., 2006). Plummer (2003) notes that queer theory applies poststructuralism to sexualities and genders.

According to Lovaas and colleagues (2006), queer theory differs from feminist and LGBT studies in that the former focus on destabilizing and deconstructing sexual and gender identifies rather than embracing a notion that they are fixed. All three gender-based approaches, however, expose the injustices and harm from heteronormativity. Queer theory has been criticized for a lack of emphasis on structural influences on inequality (Kirsch, 2000; Williams, 2006).

argued that disability was socially constructed and a product of social organization rather than a problem rooted in individual impairment (Oliver, 1983; Barnes et al., 1999). They drew a distinction between **impairment** and **disability**—where impairment refers to biological dysfunction and disability is socially produced through processes of social exclusion. It was argued that people with impairments were disabled, not by their own individual physical impairments but by a social system that creates barriers, marginalizing and excluding them from full participation in society (Hughes and Paterson, 1997). For example, someone in a wheelchair becomes disabled only when she or he is required to enter inaccessible buildings. Similarly, those who are blind become disabled only when the required information is not provided in a form (e.g., Braille, auditory) required for their participation in social affairs.

In recent years, the social model has come under considerable criticism for its primary emphasis on structural constraints and separation of impairments from disability and therefore of bodily experiences from social life (e.g., Corker and Shakespeare, 2002; Shakespeare and Watson, 2001). For example, some critics charge that the social model has too completely severed disability from physical limitations and also has erroneously accepted the view that the body is purely biological: 'The social model—in spite of its critique of the medical model—actually concedes the body to medicine and understands impairment in terms of medical discourse' (Hughes and Paterson, 1997: 326). These and other authors point to the need to recognize the impaired body as part of the domains of history, culture, and meaning and not only as a purely natural object as medicine would see it (Hughes and Paterson, 1997). Instead, various disability theorists have argued for a more holistic model that acknowledges the intersections and interactions between impairment (as a socially situated or 'embodied' experience) and disability (as social oppression) (Thomas, 2001). In other words, the body is both a physical or biological (corporeal) phenomenon and a social construction—shaped by our own individual sensory experiences (e.g., the effects of living with pain, mobility limitations, exhaustion) as well as by social relations.

The relationship between bodily and social experiences is a reflexive one (Butler and Bowlby, 1997). Socially shared understandings and expectations about disability influence individuals' bodily experiences. As well, individuals make sense of their bodily experiences (impairments) and this in turn affects their views of themselves, their identities, and their actions. Finally, as one author puts it, recent disability theorists attempt to combine a focus on structure, agency, and meaning. They focus on individuals' understandings of experience (such as how impairment and disability are experienced) to restore a focus on agency and identity (Mulvany, 2000).

Structuration Theory

Structuration theory, developed by British sociologist Anthony Giddens (1979, 1984), represents another attempt to link structure and agency, this time using the concept of **duality**. Duality refers to the fact that structure and agency are two ways of considering the same phenomenon, namely social action. From this perspective, agency consists of social action and interaction of situated actors whereas structures consist of the rules, resources, and social relationships created, recreated, and transformed through social interaction. While structure provides the context for action (because agents utilize structural rules and resources), it is also itself the outcome of action and can always transform. People create social systems through repeated interactions with one another, interactions that are guided by rules and resources (power relationships) that constitute social structure. Systems and structure are in a reciprocal relationship referred to as **structuration**, defined by Giddens as 'the structuring of social relations across time and space, in virtue of the duality of structure' (1984: 376). Social structure organizes interaction and, as interaction continues over time, the structure is either reproduced or transformed. Agency therefore can change institutions, but it is never totally free of its influence.

The focal point of structuration theory is neither the experience of individuals nor the larger social structure but social practices as they are ordered across time and space. Structure in this perspective is not objective and external to individuals (i.e., outside of social action or practice) but exists only because of and through this action. Social structures are both the result of these actions and are also the medium of it. Actors in each social situation behave in habitual, reflexive, reflective, and conscious ways. Thus, structure and agency represent a mutually dependent duality. In relation to health and health care, this perspective suggests that we behave in certain ways, often but not necessarily in a taken-for-granted manner, within the rules and resources in which we have been social-ized—our eating habits, our activity levels, and our use of health-care services tend to be consistent with those of our social position and of our family and friends in a relatively structured way. However, within parameters, we can choose the extent to which we deviate from the lifestyles and actions we were socialized to and enacted by our associates.

Structuration theory instructs us to view the rules and resources (the structure) of social relations and the agency of individuals as part of the same phenomenon rather than as distinct entities or dualisms. In order to accom-plish this, it directs our attention to examining individuals' health actions (practices or behaviours) to understand the essential intertwining of the two. We may choose to eat more nutritionally and to seek the services of alternative practitioners rather than of medical doctors even though everyone we know eats poorly and uses the services only of the medical profession when they are ill. Over time, if enough of us choose to eat organically grown food (as an example) and to visit alternative practitioners, the expected rules of behaviour (social practice) change. Indeed, many alternative practitioners enjoy flourish-ing businesses today compared with 25 years ago precisely because the actions of sufficient numbers of people have changed the structure of health care in Canada.

Despite its recognition of structure, this theory has been criticized as neglecting hierarchy both in terms of individuals' differential impact on the reproduction and transformation of social systems and their differential impact on individuals' lives. The stratified nature of social reality and the constraints on people's lives are neglected. It has also been criticized because it sees structure as existing only in the minds of individuals and their enactment of its rules and resources. Critics argue that structure exists independently; that is, rule gov-erned actions exist and persist over time even while no one is enacting them (Vaughn, 2001). Another criticism refers to the lack of human motivation or emotions within Giddens's actors. Callahan (2004) argues that structuration theory views emotions as issues or problems but not substantive elements of the process. He proposes a form of structuration theory that incorporates human emotion as both structuring and being structured by social systems.

Another example of the use of structuration theory to bridge the struc-ture–agency divide is evident in the writings of French sociologist Pierre Bourdieu (1977, 1984). Bourdieu envisioned agency as the embodiment of social structures and symbolic orders. He argued that each of us is situated in a multi-dimensional social space defined by the amounts of different kinds of capital (including social, cultural, and symbolic capital) we possess. Our social position, though, is situated within social hierarchies, of which some dominate. He focused on how social classes are maintained and reproduced, how ruling classes preserve their social privileges through **symbolic violence**—mistakenly interpreting the social construction of hierarchies as the 'natural' order of things. This term refers to the imposition of ways of thinking and perceiving onto others, who then interpret these ways of thinking as just and right rather than taken-for-granted, pre-reflexive norms and attitudes. Bourdieu revealed how social domination is maintained and reproduced through cultural capital and its subtleties of language (including, for example, grammar and accent) and bodily know-how (how one dresses, walks, carries one's body). This view of symbolic violence is similar to that of Antonio Gramsci's (1977) concept of cultural hegemony, in which one class dominates within an otherwise diverse culture. Gramsci argued that daily actions and beliefs were the building blocks for complex systems of domination and that the masses had a false consciousness in adopting the culture norms of the elite. In present-day society, the adoption of compulsory schooling, mass media, and popular culture can all be seen as representing the ruling class, adopted by the masses because of the infiltration of the ruling culture. Gramsci claimed that the masses have false consciousness in adopting the cultural norms of the elite.

Contrary to both an economic model of rational man and a Marxist emphasis on economic conflicts between social classes, Bourdieu argued that we act according to practical logic. His notion of practical logic is captured in his concept of **habitus**—a lasting, acquired system of dispositions (habitual schemes of perception, thought, and action). We draw on habitus in our everyday lives and act unconsciously on the level of bodily logic; habitus is essential to social reproduction and the generation and regulation of social life. The arena in which we perform our social actions is referred to as a **field**, consisting of a system of social positions not synonymous with social classes but often autonomous spaces of social activities (i.e., social conditions). Habitus tends to reproduce the structures of the fields. Habitus represents objective structures within the subjective thoughts and actions of the agents whereas a field consists of the agents participating in it—this is Bourdieu's reconciliation of objective and subjective or of the structure–agency divide.

Bourdieu's attempts to integrate structure and agency reorient sociology away from treating the body as an object of scrutiny to a thinking and acting subject, albeit one lodged within and shaped by the social. Bourdieu's fields are embodied spaces of practice (Entwistle and Rocamora, 2006). As Howson and Inglis (2001) point out, the sociological actor had been disembodied when cognitive abilities were placed in the mind as an entity separate from the physical body. A new **embodied sociology** argues that the body is a source of personal knowledge and understanding relevant and essential to our disciplinary knowledge. That is, sociology of the body seeks to transcend the structure–agency dualism by positioning the body as a site of knowledge and intention, experience and action influenced by social structure but not determined by it. Subjectivity and the body (corporeality) are the same and cannot be separated one from the other. To quote Howson and Inglis: 'Thus the embodied agent is both a producer of society and yet society creates the embodied agent' (2001: 305). The term **lived body** (Crossley, 2001) conveys a similar notion, that structure and the experiencing body are intertwined.

Structuration theory and embodied sociology have important implications for the sociology of health and health care because they make explicit an assumption that body, mind, and spirit are inseparable from one another. Even though, in everyday language, we may speak of our minds and our bodies as if they are different entities, adopting a structurationist perspective means acknowledging that this is a false dichotomy. Rather, when we study health, we should focus on each as related to the other and do so by focusing on social action (practices) with an eye to understanding how individual agency works within that action, how our actions recreate or modify social structure, and how social structure is embedded within our actions. The health beliefs and health behaviours we adopt can be analyzed in this fashion.

Bourdieu, though, also has his critics. Notably, he has been criticized for privileging social structure over agency (Howson and Inglis, 2001) and for his lack of attention to how fields are reproduced through agency in daily practice (Entwistle and Rocamora, 2006). Even Crossley (2001), who argues against this criticism, concedes that Bourdieu might occasionally lapse into determinism. Chodos and Curtis (2002), for example, point out that despite Bourdieu's insistence on agency and the dynamic nature of habitus, his writings on masculine domination seem to lead to the conclusion that gendered structures are fixed. Other criticisms include a failure to distinguish between economic and political power (Hesmondhalgh, 2006).

Summary

A major theme emanating from these theoretical approaches that is central to sociological thinking and research in the areas of health and health care is the importance of both social structure and individual human agency. We tend to think of structure and agency in terms of dichotomies, as either/or dualisms. In the past, different theoretical traditions within sociology have tended to emphasize one or the other, while at the same time often acknowledging the relevance of the other. In addition, most research is conducted in the present, at one point in time. Yet our lives evolve over time; that which occurred in the past has consequences for the present and the future.

More recently, sociologists have begun to acknowledge the equal value of both structure and agency, recognizing that opportunities for agency are variously structured (e.g., depending upon one's position within the social structure and how much access one has to resources) and that we need to understand the complex interplay between social structure and individual agency. Thus, we need to see how they play out differently over time and in the lives of men and women, different social classes, and diverse racial/ethnic groups. According to Kelly and Charlton (1995: 83), for example, we need to understand interaction between individual experiences, actions through which people create the world around them, and the power structures within which people are embedded. Simultaneously, the contexts that make the structures are constantly being recreated, constantly evolving (Frolich, Corin, and Potvin, 2001). There are also times and circumstances when structural forces can be overwhelming (Williams, 2003). More recent theorizing has led to assertions of the inseparability of structure and agency within theories such as life course and structuration. Research that takes both perspectives into account may be increasing in importance as life course arrangements are less standardized and more self-directed than in the past (Heinz and Kruger, 2001).

SOCIAL INEQUALITIES IN HEALTH AND HEALTH CARE

Another theme that is central to the sociology of health and health care, as it is for sociology generally, is inequality. Although implicit thus far in our discussion, inequality has been described as the 'stock and trade' of sociology since the discipline's earliest days (Allen and Chung, 2000). One of the central tenets of the discipline has been the view that social stratification results in the unequal distribution of desirable resources and rewards in society (Williams, 1990). Sociologists have therefore sought to address inequality's origins, its persistence over time, the movement of individuals and groups within structures characterized by inequality, and its implications for individuals and the societies in which they live.

Given the importance of inequality within the discipline as a whole, it is not surprising that it has also emerged as a core concern within sociological studies of health and health care, although not continually. On the one hand, the direct association between economic and occupational factors and health status has been recognized for centuries. According to Lynch and Kaplan (2000), for example, Paracelsus noted unusually high rates of disease in miners in medieval Europe. By the nineteenth century, systematic investigations were studying associations between rent levels and mortality in Paris while, in England, Engels (1848) decried the impact of the new working conditions of the Industrial Revolution on the health of the poor. At the same time, Virchow (1848) noted that the factors leading to infectious epidemics of typhus and other illnesses were closely tied to socio-economic position and therefore that social and economic policies were major instruments for combating disease and promoting health. He concluded that medicine is a social science (cited in House, 2001).

Over time, however, the emphasis on the importance of social factors was overshadowed by an emphasis on biological determinants and the germ theory of disease. Some attribute this to political influences, arguing that attention to the role of social influences was attacked and undermined by proponents of the germ theory of disease. In addition, during the 1950s, there was a tendency to view poverty and class divisions as declining in increasingly affluent post-World War II North American and European societies. Thus, as noted by House

(2001), attention to social inequalities generally and to health in particular was often muted if not absent in sociology during the 1950s and the early 1960s. It was believed that social inequalities in health were tackled through national medical insurance programs.

Whatever the reasons for the lack of attention directed to inequalities in health during the middle years of the twentieth century, the 1960s saw a resurgence of interest in the subject. Most continued to believe that these differences could be largely explained and resolved by equalizing access to medical care (House, 2001). However, more recent evidence (e.g., the Black report) revealed that national health insurance programs did not appear to be effective in reducing inequalities in health and, in fact, these inequalities seemed to be increasing (during the period from 1960 to 1986) despite increasing equalization of access to care.

In 1950–51, Canada's first national survey on the distribution of health and illness revealed that those in high-income groups consistently reported fewer days of disability than those in medium- or low-income groups (Canadian Sickness Survey, 1960). In the early 1960s, Harding and colleagues (1963) conducted a large study in rural Nova Scotia and concluded that the risk of psychiatric disorder increased as occupational disadvantage increased. This was true for both hospitalized patients and individuals living in the community.

While several such studies were taking place throughout the Western world, the Black Report from Great Britain was the first to receive international acclaim. It indicated that men and women with the lowest occupational status were approximately 2.5 times more likely to die before retirement age than those in the highest occupational grouping. Similar findings were evident for morbidity (illness) levels, with stronger relationships for chronic illness than for acute or short-term illness (Townsend and Davidson, 1982). In 1986, Whitehead (1988) reviewed the growing number of studies on the question of inequality and health for the British government. She concluded that lower occupational groups are generally disadvantaged in terms of mortality, subjective and objective measures of illness, and both chronic and acute conditions compared with higher occupational groups. As well, those who are unemployed have poorer physical and mental health than those who are employed.

Since that time, numerous findings of a similar nature have been reported. These findings hold despite different conceptualizations and measures of social class and socio-economic status (e.g., income, education, occupation, or combinations of these) and different conceptualizations and measures of health (e.g., specific diseases, functional disability, days sick in bed, days in hospital, perceptions of one's health, or death rate). And, even though as age increases the number of both chronic and acute illnesses also increases, social status differences in heath are evident at all age levels (Hay, 1994).

These studies show that the structure of opportunities within society and the availability of positions are relevant to our health. The importance of the relationship between social structure and health lies in the fact that social structure is modifiable, thus at least some of illness is potentially preventable. Much of illness is humanly made. Wilkinson (1996: 54) has dramatically described the relationship between social structure and health as the power of social structure over life and death.

Social class and social relations have a long-standing history of attention within sociology generally, and the sociology of health and health care specifically, which continues today. More recently, sociologists have been interested in other inequalities, including those discussed earlier in this chapter. Although social-class inequality still receives much more attention, there is growing awareness of the importance of these other inequalities, which also brings a greater focus onto the experiences of those who are disadvantaged and, with some of the new approaches, an explicit attempt to empower these groups through the research process. With the recognition of many inequalities, a new question has arisen: What is the relationship between social class and other inequalities? There is increasing awareness that any analysis of socio-economic, class, and income inequalities is incomplete without consideration of characteristics such as gender and race/ethnicity (Kawachi, Subramanian, and Almeida-Filho, 2002) and, more recently, of age, sexual orientation, religion, and disability (Estes, 2005; Whittle and Inhorn, 2002).

This increased awareness of various sources of inequality has led researchers to ask whether these are separate forms of inequality that each exert an independent and therefore additive effect on health outcomes or whether they overlap so that some inequalities (e.g., race, ethnicity) can be explained, in part or in whole, by others (e.g., social class). More recently, it has also led scholars to highlight the importance of addressing more complex relationships, based on notions of **intersectionality**, noted earlier, among different types of inequality. For example, the feminization of poverty may not be totally separate and distinct from other oppressions such as race, ethnicity, class, and sexuality. As Patricia Hill Collins states, these are 'interrelated axes of social structure' and not 'just separate features of existence' (Estes, 2005: 552) that may shape the health and well-being of all women (Whittle and Inhorn, 2002). Instead, race is gendered and gender is racialized. Race and gender may be so inextricably tied that understanding their relationship to health and health care necessitates an understanding of their complex confounding with one another (Browne and Misra, 2003:1). Similarly, social class expresses itself in a gendered form (Hilary Graham, 2000).

CONCLUSIONS

This introductory chapter has emphasized the importance of both social structure and agency for an adequate understanding of health and health care from a sociological perspective. The importance of inequality has also been noted. It is not, however, only sociologists who believe all of these components are necessary.

Box 1.6
Canadian Health Network

The Public Health Agency of Canada's Canadian Health Network website contains health information on several groups, including children and aboriginal peoples.

Groups

Children
Youth
Seniors
Aboriginal Peoples
Women
Men

Disease Prevention

Cancer
Cardiovascular Disease and Stroke
Diabetes
HIV/AIDS
Respiratory Diseases

Topics

Active Living
Complementary and Alternative Health
Environment and Health
Health Promotion
Health System
Healthy Eating
Injury Prevention
Living with Disabilities
Mental Health
Sexuality/Reproductive Health
Substance Abuse/Addictions
Tobacco
Violence Prevention
Workplace Health

Source: Public Health Agency of Canada. 2008. Available at: www.canadian-health-network.ca/servlet/ContentServer?cid=1044475860190&pagename=CHN-RCS%2FPage%2FGTPage Template&c=Page&lang=En.

Rather, they reflect much of the thinking about health and health care within society. For example, the importance of both in regards to our health was recognized by the World Health Organization (WHO) as early as 1948, when it defined health as more than the absence of disease. WHO's definition of health as 'a state of complete physical, mental, and social well-being and not merely the absence of disease or infirmity' includes social well-being of both the individual and the collectivity (1948: 100). The organization also views health as a resource for living, not simply an end unto itself. Health promotion is a mediating strategy between people and their environments, integrating personal choice and social responsibility and including physical and social environments that promote health (WHO, 1984).

In the 1980s, the WHO set the year 2000 as the target for *Achieving Health for All* for a number of European countries. The goal was to provide people with a positive sense of health, emphasizing health promotion and the prevention of disease (Asvali, 1986: 113). Achieving this goal requires tackling social inequalities. In many ways, the Canadian government also appears to recognize the importance of both social structure and agency, as seen by the Public Health

Agency of Canada's listing of governmental, academic, and other websites in Canada and elsewhere (see Box 1.6).

In the following sections of this book, we turn our attention to the role of structural factors in influencing health and health care while also addressing the construction of meaning and the exercise of human agency and choice. In other words, we are also interested in social psychological perspectives within sociology that draw attention to the social construction of meaning, of experience. It is through this social construction that individuals exercise agency. As will become evident, empirical research tends to integrate the two perspectives less than we saw in recent attempts at theorizing.

Questions for Critical Thought ──────────────────────────

1. It has been noted that the sociology of health and health care arose within a societal context in which medicine was becoming increasingly criticized. Discuss the nature, origins, and implications of the criticisms involved.
2. Compare and contrast structural and social psychological approaches toward an understanding of health and health care. Describe a theory that exemplifies each approach and then critique it from the other perspective.
3. It has been suggested that behaviours that are often thought of as being under individual control occur within a social context that also has an impact. Discuss the relative importance of individual control and social context with reference to adolescent smoking or drinking behaviour.
4. A life course perspective draws our attention to the importance of changing social contexts for people's health and health care. Describe some of the ways (or pathways) that the social context experienced in one's early childhood might affect one's health in later life.
5. Inequality has been described as foundational to sociology. Illustrate your understanding of the concept from a social psychological perspective and a social structural perspective using an example within the sociology of health and health care.

Suggestions for Further Reading ──────────────────────────

Armstrong, P.A., H. Armstrong, and D. Coburn. 2001. *Unhealthy Times: Political Economy Perspectives on Health and Care in Canada*. Don Mills, ON: Oxford University Press.

Coburn, D. 2004. 'Beyond the Income Inequality Hypothesis: Class, Neo-liberalism, and Health Inequalities', *Social Science & Medicine* 58, 1: 41–56.

Gubrium, J.F., and J.A. Holstein, eds. 2000. *Aging and Everyday Life*. Oxford: Blackwell Publishing.

Lovaas, K.E., J.P. Elia, and G.A. Yep. 2006. 'Shifting Ground(s): Surveying the Contested Terrain of LGBT Studies and Queer Theory', in *LGBT Studies and Queer Theory: New Conflicts, Collaborations, and Contested Terrain*. Binghamton, NY: Harrington Park Press, 1–18.

Petersen, A., and R. Bunton. 1997. *Foucault, Health and Medicine*. London: Routledge.

Williams, G.H. 2003. 'The Determinants of Health: Structure, Context and Agency', *The Sociology of Health & Illness* 25: 131–54.

Health and Illness

Learning Objectives

In this chapter, you will learn that:

- While life expectancy doubled globally over the course of the twentieth century, there were major differences in life expectancy and mortality across and within countries.
- Significant inequalities in health are associated with social structural location, as indicated by such factors as area of residence; social class and socio-economic position; race, ethnicity, and immigration status; gender; and age.
- Social class and socio-economic status differences in health are found in every country. These differences cannot be explained by poverty alone. Possible explanations focus on materialist, neo-materialist, and psychosocial factors.
- Although recent immigrants appear to be healthier than non-immigrants, their health advantage declines over time.
- In Canada, women's life expectancy is greater than that of men, but their physical and mental health is widely considered to be poorer.
- People's experiences with health and illness are subjectively as well as objectively defined. People are actively involved in giving meaning to their experiences and in shaping their personal identities and sense of self.
- Being ill can result in biographical disruption leading to a search for meaning in our experiences. It can also result in positive change in personal identity and a liberating experience.
- We know much more about the experience of illness than the experience of being healthy, although people distinguish between 'health' and 'being healthy'.

DEFINITIONS OF HEALTH AND ILLNESS

How healthy are Canadians today? The answer to this question depends on how health is defined and the standards against which and the contexts (e.g., historical, national) within which it is assessed. As noted in the previous chapter, Canadians tend to define health based on a biomedical model, equating it with the absence of disease and especially with avoidance of and survival from acute life-threatening disease. Mishler (1981) characterizes **the biomedical model** in terms of four key assumptions: (1) that disease can be explained by deviations from normal biological functioning and consequently that health represents the absence of disease; (2) that each disease is caused by a single and identifiable biological agent (e.g., germ), also called the 'doctrine of specific etiology'; (3) that diseases are generic and do not vary over time, across cultures, or societies; and (4) that medicine is scientifically neutral and objective. Thus, the model holds that disease is an objectively observable, biological phenomenon, is situated within the individual human body, is universal in its expression, and can be effectively diagnosed and treated by medicine using objective scientific techniques.

Consistent with our reliance on a biomedical definition of health, we frequently assess the health of the population by focusing on such things as morbidity, mortality, and life expectancy. **Morbidity** refers to the level of disease within a given population at a particular point in time and tends to be assessed in terms of incidence and prevalence. **Incidence** refers to the number of new cases of a specific disease or health problem within a particular population during a specified period of time and tends to be used when we are concerned about the spread of a disease or other health problem. It is calculated by dividing the number of new cases of a disease reported within the population of interest during a given period of time by the total number of people considered to be at risk. In contrast, **prevalence** refers to the total number of cases of a disease or health problem within the population during a specified time period. It includes new cases (incident cases) as well as those previously present and is therefore used as an indicator of how common or widespread a particular disease or health problem is within the population. Prevalence rates tend to be calculated by dividing the total number of cases of a disease reported within the population of interest during a given period of time by the total number of people considered to be at risk of the disease during that period. Figure 2.1 shows recent prevalence rates for some of the major chronic diseases reported by the Canadian population. **Chronic conditions** are those that are expected to persist or recur over time (usually a year or more). Over one-half of all Canadians currently report having a chronic health problem, most commonly back and other musculoskeletal problems (e.g., arthritis), allergies, high blood pressure and other cardiovascular conditions, and asthma.

Mortality rates capture the number of deaths within a particular population. While crude death rates often refer to the total number of deaths evident in the population, one of the most used indicators of the physical health of the

Figure 2.1   Prevalence of Chronic Conditions within the Canadian Population, 2001

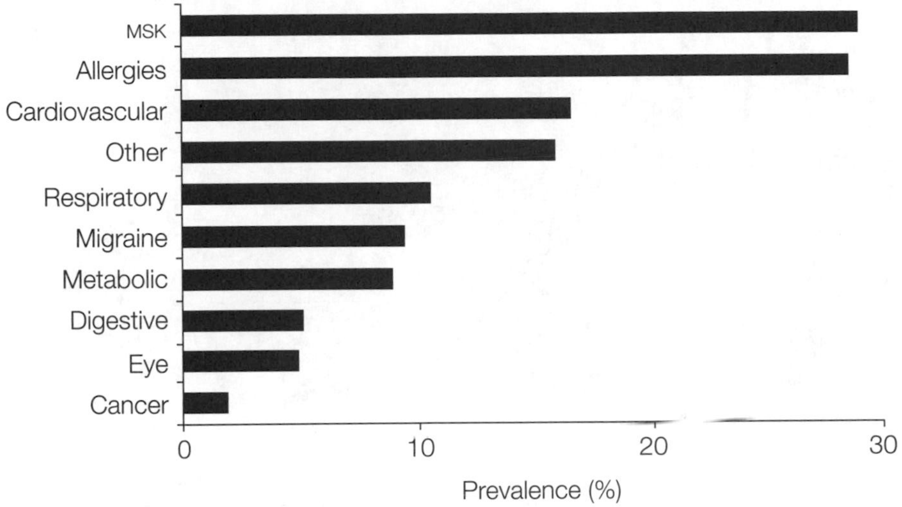

Source: CIHR's Institute of Musculoskeletal Health and Arthritis. 2007. 'Prevalence of Chronic Conditions within the Canadian Population, 2001'. Ottawa: Canadian Institute of Health Research. Available at: http://www.cihr-irsc.gc.ca/e/18976.html. Reproduced with the permission of the Minister of Public Works and Government Services Canada, 2008.

population is the **infant mortality rate** (i.e., the number of deaths of children under the age of one reported for every 1,000 live births) evident in a given year. As shown in Figure 2.2, Canadian infant mortality rates have dropped dramatically over the past century, particularly during the first half of the twentieth century. In 1895, there were about 145 deaths for every 1,000 live births in Canada. By 1960, this figure had declined to 27.3 (Statistics Canada, 1995); it now stands at about 5.3 (Statistics Canada, 2006a). This decline is often interpreted as evidence of the improving health of the Canadian population.

As mortality rates declined, life expectancy increased. **Life expectancy** refers to the average number of years that individuals at a given age can expect to live before death and is usually, but not necessarily, measured from birth. In 1831, the average life expectancy of Canadians was approximately 39 years of age (Statistics Canada, 1992). Those born a century later could expect to live to over 60 years of age (62.1 years for women and 60.0 years for men). Since then, life expectancy has increased by a further 20 years for women and 17 years for men (Statistics Canada, 2002e). Thus, in 2004, the average life expectancy of women in Canada was 82.6 years while for men it was 77.8 years (Statistics Canada, 2006a; see Figure 2.3).

Changes in life expectancy in Canada and other Western industrialized nations have been accompanied by changes in the major causes of death. During

Figure 2.2   Infant Mortality Rates, Canada, 1890–2004

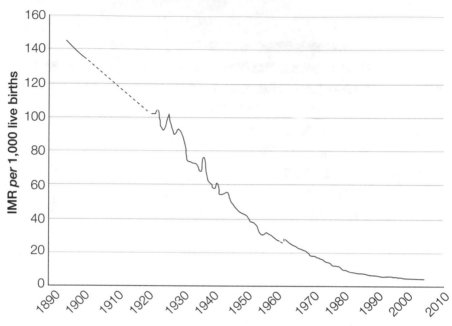

Source: Statistics Canada data. Data for 1900–1920 and 1960 not available.

the early twentieth century, major causes of death among Canadians included a number of infectious diseases (influenza, bronchitis, pneumonia, tuberculosis, measles, whooping cough; see Table 2.1). Although cardiovascular diseases (heart disease, stroke) and cancer also caused death during this time, they did not account for the majority of deaths, as they do today. Over the years, deaths due to infectious as well as many other diseases have decreased considerably. Today, most of the major causes of death tend to be chronic conditions, including various types of cancer, heart disease, stroke, and chronic respiratory diseases (Statistics Canada, 2002e). Currently, over 40 per cent of Canadians will develop cancer at some point in their lives (usually in later life) and one in four will die of some form of the disease (see Table 2.2).

Demographers and epidemiologists often refer to this shift in causes of death as reflecting an **epidemiological transition,** or gradual change in patterns of disease and mortality in a country associated with development. According to Omran (1971), who originally developed the concept, societies tend to experience three stages as they undergo development and industrialization: (1) an 'age of pestilence and famine' characteristic of ancient societies and dominated by frequent famines, plagues, and other lethal infectious diseases; (2) an 'age of receding pandemics' during which major disease pandemics gradually disappeared; and (3) an 'age of man-made (*sic*) and degenerative diseases'. By the middle of the

Figure 2.3   Life Expectancy in Canada

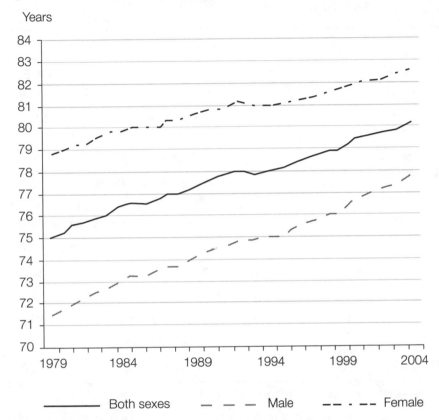

Years

Source: Statistics Canada. 2006a. Adapted from Statistics Canada Publication *The Daily*, catalogue 11-001, 20 December 2006. Available at: http://www.statcan.ca/Daily/English/061220/d061220b.htm. Accessed 14 December 2007.

nineteenth century, Canada and other Western industrialized countries entered the third stage, during which people tend not to die from acute infectious diseases and consequently live longer (see Figure 2.4 for resulting changes in the Canadian age structure that occurred during this period). The hope was that this was the final stage—once reached, societies could cease worrying about the misfortunes created by famines and disease epidemics and begin directing their energies toward the chronic and degenerative diseases that tend to characterize more affluent societies (e.g., cancer, heart disease, diabetes).

Currently, however, there is recognition that chronic illnesses are not limited to affluent societies, but also affect low- and middle-income countries. In addition, there is debate over the implications of new and re-emerging infectious diseases (such as Mad Cow Disease, West Nile Virus, Legionnaire's Disease, HIV, Ebola, and Bird Flu) as well as increasing resistance to immunizations in an increasingly globalized, industrialized, and environmentally fragile world.

Table 2.1   Changes in Leading Causes of Death in Canada, 1921–25 and 2004

1921–25		2004	
CAUSE OF DEATH	MORTALITY RATE	CAUSE OF DEATH	MORTALITY RATE
All causes	**1030.0**	**All causes**	**571.9**
Cardiovascular, renal diseases	221.9	Malignant neoplasms (cancer)	173.7
Influenza, bronchitis, pneumonia	141.1	Diseases of the heart	126.8
Diseases of early infancy	111.0	Cerebrovascular disease (stroke)	34.9
Tuberculosis	85.1	Chronic lower respiratory disease	24.8
Malignant neoplasms (cancer)	75.9	Accidents (unintentional injuries)	24.7
Gastritis, enteritis, colitis	72.2	Diabetes meilitus	19.6
Accidents (unintentional injuries)	51.5	Influenza and pneumonia	13.4
Communicable diseases (e.g., diptheria, measles, whooping cough, scarlet fever)	47.1	Alzheimer's disease	12.7
		Suicide and homocide	12.5
		Renal failure	8.3

Note: Age-standardized rates (per 100,000 population)

Sources: Statistics Canada, CANSIM, Table 102-0552 and Catalogue no. 84F0209X for 2004 data; S. Crompton (2000). '100 Years of Health', *Canadian Social Trends*, Statistics Canada, Catalogue 11-008, No.

Whether this represents a need for the model to recognize that the old health problems never went away or reflects the possibility of yet another epidemiological transition is at present unclear (see Barrett et al., 1998).

SOCIOLOGY AND THE SOCIAL CONSTRUCTION OF HEALTH AND ILLNESS

Biomedical indicators (of morbidity, mortality, and life expectancy) point to major and continuing improvements in the health of the Canadian population over the course of the past century or more. However, sociologists have long been critical of biomedical definitions of health, largely because, as Mishler points out, the 'biomedical model strips away social contexts of meaning' and thereby individualizes what are often broader social problems (1981: 153). He and others assert that health is more than the absence of disease and that the biomedical model neglects broader domains of health, including social, psychological, and spiritual well-being. Early work within the sociology of health and

Table 2.2   Lifetime Probability of Developing and Dying from Cancer

	LIFETIME PROBABILITY OF:	
	DEVELOPING	DYING
Male	%	%
All cancers	**44.5**	**28.5**
Prostate	13.5	3.7
Lung	8.6	8.0
Colorectal	7.4	3.7
Bladder	3.5	1.1
Non-Hodgkin Lymphoma	2.2	1.1
Leukemia	1.7	1.1
Kidney	1.5	0.7
Stomach	1.4	0.9
Oral	1.4	0.5
Melanoma	1.3	0.4
Pancreas	1.3	1.3
Multiple Myleoma	0.8	0.5
Brain	0.8	0.6
Esophagus	0.7	0.8
Larynx	0.6	0.3
Liver	0.6	0.3
Female		
All cancers	**39.3**	**24.1**
Breast	11.0	3.6
Colorectal	6.4	3.3
Lung	6.2	5.4
Body of uterus	2.4	0.6
Non-Hodgkin Lymphoma	1.9	1.0
Ovary	1.4	1.1
Pancreas	1.3	1.5
Thyroid	1.2	0.1
Leukemia	1.2	0.7
Bladder	1.2	0.4
Melanoma	1.1	0.2
Kidney	1.0	0.4
Stomach	0.8	0.6
Cervix	0.7	0.2
Oral	0.7	0.3
Multiple Myleoma	0.6	0.4
Brain	0.6	0.5

Source: Canadian Cancer Society/National Cancer Institute of Canada. *Canadian Cancer Statistics,* Toronto, 2008.

Figure 2.4   Canadian Population Structure 1851–2001

Population in thousands by age group

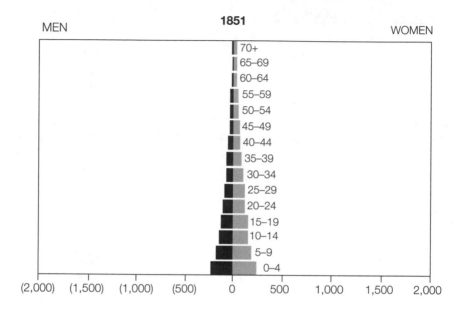

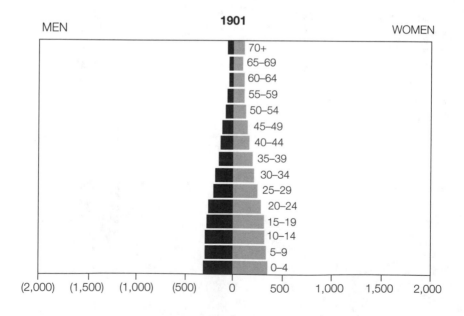

Figure 2.4   (continued)

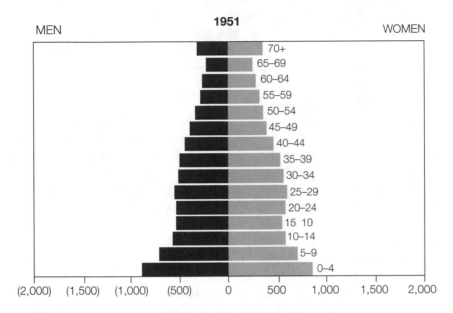

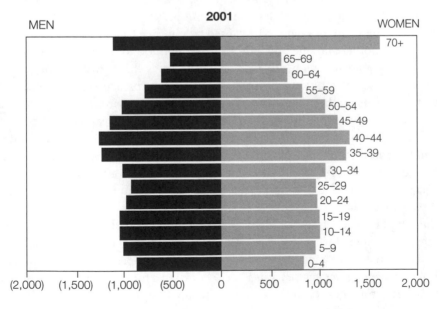

Sources : Statistics Canada, Series A78-93, 'Population (thousands), by age and sex, census dates, 1851 to 1976'. Available at: http://www.statcan.ca/english/freepub/11-516-XIE/sectiona/A78_93.csv; BC Stats, 'Population Estimates for Canada by Age and Gender: 1956–2003'. Available at: http://www.bcstats.gov. bc.ca/data/pop/pop/CanPop5y.htm.

illness often failed to question the separations established between body and mind or between individual and society. Instead, they generally argued for the need to recognize both. More recent work (e.g., sociology of the body) rejects assumptions of mind–body dualism or complete separation of mind and body, arguing that there is a need to see such relationships as dialectical: 'there is a feedback in operation in which social environments construct bodies, which impact back on social behaviour, which then further modify the body' (Annandale, 1998: 57).

Another criticism often levelled against a biomedical definition is that not only does it exclude broader domains of health but it also assumes a standard of 'normality' in biological functioning that is unclear and difficult to define. In other words, what is normal? Is it the average or does it represent some ideal level of biological functioning? How do we know it when we see it?

Other assumptions of the biomedical model have also been challenged. The doctrine of specific etiology (Dubos, 1959) is said to follow from the germ theory of disease and the early work of people like Louis Pasteur and others, showing that specific micro-organisms were responsible for specific infectious diseases. However, researchers have noted that there is no necessary or direct connection between exposure to disease-causing agents and disease (i.e., not everyone who is exposed to a disease-causing agent actually experiences the disease). As well, the search for disease-causing biological micro-organisms is considered overly simplistic and often inappropriate when applied to chronic diseases. These illnesses tend to be caused by multiple factors that often interact with one another and often include socio-economic and environmental factors (e.g., inadequate nutrition, asbestos, smoke). Critics charge that the model also results in a search for biomedical 'magic bullets' (i.e., pharmaceutical solutions) to treat disease rather than for socio-economic and environmental solutions. This is no less true for chronic than for acute infectious diseases.

The notion that diseases will have the same symptoms regardless of social and historical settings has also been refuted by research evidence suggesting that, far from being universal, illnesses may be experienced very differently in one society or time period than another. For example, the nature and implications of diseases like measles, chicken pox, or HIV will differ greatly depending on whether they affect individuals in Canada or in some of the world's poorest nations; what may be considered harmless or at least treatable in one context can be viewed as a death sentence in another. Another example is menopause. Within a biomedical framework, menopause tends to be considered a hormone-deficiency disease treatable through estrogen replacement therapy (Kaufert and Gilbert, 1986). Yet cross-cultural studies point to variations in how women respond to menopause; the experience and severity of various symptoms typically said to be associated with menopause in our society (e.g., hot flashes, insomnia, depression) may not be evident in societies where menopause is associated with freedom from the restrictions within women's lives (Kaufert and Gilbert, 1986; Lock, 1986).

Our social constructions of disease and the factors associated with it also shift over time. For example, some diseases of the past are no longer considered diseases at all. Childhood masturbation (known as onanism), a frequently diagnosed disease in the eighteenth and nineteenth centuries in Britain and believed to cause insanity and epilepsy, is no longer identified as a disease (Engelhardt, 1974; Hunt, 1998). Another more recent example is homosexuality, which was removed from the International Classification of Diseases (WHO, 2007) in the 1990s following political pressure by gay rights groups. Conversely, transsexualism and other so-called gender identity disorders (e.g., dual-role transvestitism) currently remain included. As well, newly discovered diseases are constantly being added to the list. A fairly recent example is Chronic Fatigue Syndrome (see Box 2.1).

Finally, it has also been argued that medicine, far from being independent of the larger societal context, is in fact deeply embedded within it. From a sociological perspective, medical ideas about health and illness are seen as socially constructed and situated within specific socio-historical and political contexts. For example, some argue that the need to redefine health stems from the changes in the field. When we take care of one type of health problem, new ones come into prominence, thereby limiting the usefulness of prevailing definitions. As one author notes, with the improvements that have taken place over the past 150 years, we have gradually moved away from viewing health in terms of mere survival to a period when we defined it in terms of freedom from disease, to an emphasis on one's ability to perform everyday social roles and activities, and, more recently, to an emphasis on individual quality of life, happiness, and overall well-being (McDowell, 2006). It is only where problems of premature mortality are no longer a pressing social concern does it become relevant to think of health in the World Health Organization's (WHO) terms of 'physical, mental, and social well-being, and not simply the absence of disease and infirmity' (McDowell, 2006: 11).

From a sociological perspective, our ideas regarding health and illness are developed and transmitted as part of a political process (Freund and McGuire, 1999: 206). Sociologists often refer to this process as one of **medicalization**—a social and political process wherein more and more areas of life come under the purview of medical science and consequently under medical authority and control (Zola, 1983). Often this includes the medicalization of everyday events and experiences (such as sexuality, childbirth, menopause, aging) as well as those defined as deviant (including addictions, pathological disorders, general conduct disorders, attention deficit disorders, sleep disorders, eating disorders, gender-identity disorders, and sexual dysfunctions). Box 2.2 provides an example of conduct disorders as currently defined within the International Classification of Diseases.

The medicalization of particular diseases may or may not involve or be intentional on the part of the medical profession (Conrad, 1992). On the one

Box 2.1
Chronic Fatigue Syndrome Recognized

Sharon Baillie once loved to read. Not any more. By the time she gets to page three of a book, she has generally forgotten what she read on page one. She used to enjoy 25-kilometre hikes on weekends. Now, she can barely manage a 20-minute walk with her golden retrievers, Buddy and Dusty. Baillie, 54, . . . suffers from Chronic Fatigue Syndrome (CFS), a debilitating condition with symptoms that include exhaustion, memory loss, and aching muscles. Diagnosed in May 1991, Baillie won a precedent-setting legal decision when Alberta Court of Queen's Bench Judge Philip Clarke ruled that she is entitled to disability benefits from her former employer, Regina-based Crown Life Insurance Co. 'At times, I wondered if I could stick it out', she said after the 2 March decision was made public last week. 'But I paid into their plan, and I'm entitled to benefits.'

Victims of CFS—more than 70 per cent of them women—applauded the ruling, the first in Canada to recognize the disease as a physical rather than a psychological condition. Although as many as 30,000 Canadians are believed to suffer from the disease, insurance industry executives say they have no way of estimating the number of claims that could be filed as a result of the decision. Meanwhile, a Crown Life spokesperson said the company is considering an appeal, and other industry representatives said they will still deal cautiously with chronic fatigue claims because the condition is difficult to diagnose and symptoms can vary widely. In fact, doctors who treat the syndrome concede the causes are unknown, and they can only treat it, not cure it. 'This is an emerging illness', says Calgary physician Beverly Tompkins, 43, who developed it herself 10 years ago and now devotes her practice to the syndrome. 'Many physicians can't recognize it in a patient.' . . .

But it took more than four years of legal wrangling to get the case to court last February. Baillie's lawyer, Mark Feehan, called several doctors to testify about the severity of her disability and the physical nature of the disease. Crown Life called one medical witness, Cochrane, AB, psychiatrist Keith Pearce, who told the court that Baillie suffers from a mental condition called conversion disorder, in which an overloaded central nervous system turns stress into physical symptoms.

The judge's decision was unambiguous. 'CFS is not a psychoneurotic injury', Clarke ruled. 'It is organic.' And he said Baillie is entitled to disability benefits, yet to be specified. . . .

Source: D'Arcy Jenish, 'Chronic Fatigue Syndrome Recognized', *Maclean's* 4 May 1998. Reprinted by permission of the publisher.

hand, the increasing prominence of the biomedical model for understanding and treating disease historically occurred in conjunction with a political process that gave the medical profession legitimacy and then dominance relative to other health-care providers (Freund and McGuire, 1999: 206). (See Chapters 1 and 4.) On the other hand, medicalization does not necessarily nor only serve the medical profession's interests. Instead, it is a process that has not always been

Box 2.2
International Classification of Diseases and Related Health Problems, 10th Revision

Conduct Disorders

Disorders characterized by a repetitive and persistent pattern of dissocial, aggressive, or defiant conduct. Such behaviour should amount to major violations of age-appropriate social expectations; it should therefore be more severe than ordinary childish mischief or adolescent rebelliousness and should imply an enduring pattern of behaviour (six months or longer). Features of conduct disorder can also be symptomatic of other psychiatric conditions, in which case the underlying diagnosis should be preferred.

Examples of the behaviours on which the diagnosis is based include excessive levels of fighting or bullying, cruelty to other people or animals, severe destructiveness to property, fire-setting, stealing, repeated lying, truancy from school and running away from home, unusually frequent and severe temper tantrums, and disobedience. Any one of these behaviours, if marked, is sufficient for the diagnosis, but isolated dissocial acts are not.

Source: WHO. 2007. *International Classification of Diseases and Related Health Problems*, 10th Revision.

initiated or even embraced by the medical profession (e.g., the debate surrounding active euthanasia) and one that, at various times, has come to serve the interests of other professional groups (e.g., psychologists), societal institutions (e.g., legal institutions, schools), private interests (e.g., health insurers, pharmaceutical companies), as well as patients and organized grassroots organizations (e.g., those interested in legitimating various forms of deviance, such as alcoholism, by having them redefined as illnesses [Conrad, 1992]). A recent Canadian study by Malacrida (2004) examines how Attention Deficit (Hyperactivity) Disorder (ADD/ADHD) often comes to be medicalized through the activities of educators (including teachers and psychologists) working within school settings. The fact that Medicare in Canada covers only medically defined conditions also increases the likelihood that patients will seek or at least support the medicalization of various conditions (as exemplified in Box 2.1).

Together, criticisms such as these and increasing dissatisfaction with the limitations of the biomedical model have generated ongoing debate regarding the definition of health as well as attempts to develop alternative definitions. Yet a clear and concise definition of health and a means of assessment remain elusive. It is now widely accepted that health is a multi-dimensional concept that includes biological, psychological, and social components. This is most clearly articulated in the WHO's definition discussed above. As such, health is both objective and subjective. Moreover, there is recognition of the reciprocal interactions between a healthy body, a healthy mind, and a healthy social situation at the individual level as well as between a healthy individual and a healthy social and physical environment. For example, in more recent years, the WHO has modified its definition of health to include people's abilities to lead 'socially and economically productive lives' (WHO, 1977; Yach, 1998).

SOCIAL STRUCTURAL FACTORS IN HEALTH AND ILLNESS

Examining health and illness from a social structural perspective involves posing questions like the following: What are the factors that are related to and influence our health? To what extent is it influenced by social and economic conditions such as income levels, home environments, personal relationships, and treatment as a result of gender, race/ethnicity, sexual preference, or age? What about social policy decisions that are reflected in the health services we receive?

A biomedical approach draws our attention to the importance of genetic and physiological factors as well as improvements in medical and surgical care for improvements in the physical health of the population over the past 100+ years. Certainly, the genetic characteristics of the population will not have changed much over such a short period of time, making it extremely unlikely that they can account for such improvements. Also, with the exception of mass immunizations against diseases such as smallpox, diphtheria, and tuberculosis, it is difficult to imagine how improvements in medical and surgical care could solely account for much of the overall improvements in life expectancy during the last century. For example, although surgeries undoubtedly save lives among those requiring such care, relatively few people in the overall population require surgery in any given year.

Evidence accumulated over the course of the twentieth century suggests that the improvements in longevity in countries such as Great Britain, the United States, and Canada were due to declines in acute infectious diseases (McKeown, 1975, 1976; McKinlay and McKinlay, 1977). Although these results were widely believed to be caused by improved immunization and medical therapies, these treatments accounted for approximately 10 per cent of the increase in life expectancy. Despite the importance of immunizations, most were discovered after the declines in mortality were already well under way. The major factors thought to be responsible for these improvements were not tied to medical discoveries or care but to changing social and economic conditions of life reflected in improvements in the population's nutrition and hygiene. Overall, about one-half of the increase in life expectancy over this period was attributed to improvements in nutrition and one-sixth to improvements in hygiene (e.g., safe water supplies). Subsequent studies have supported McKeown's findings, indicating the greater importance of socio-economic than medical resources for the health of the population (Kim and Moody, 1992; McKinlay and McKinlay, 1987).

Since the early 1970s, the importance of social determinants of health has been increasingly acknowledged. As well, the list of social factors considered important to health has been expanded. For example, in 1974, Canada's Minister of Health (Marc Lalonde) issued a health policy document that for the first time formally acknowledged that non-biological factors also contributed to the health of the population. He identified three such factors as important: lifestyle, environment, and health care. Just over a decade later, in 1986, a subsequent Minister of Health (Jake Epp) acknowledged the importance of social, economic, and physical environments as well as lifestyle and health services. Since then, Canadian governments and the population as a whole have focused much of their attention on individual behavioural or lifestyle factors such as smoking, drinking, dietary practices, and physical activity levels, together with health services as predictors of health outcomes.

The attention paid to social, economic, and other environmental factors has been recent. Yet it has become increasingly well-established that social factors such as the percentage of the population that is Aboriginal or a member of a visible minority, unemployment rates, population size, percentage of the population aged 65 and older, average income, and average education are also related to our population's health (Shields and Tremblay, 2002). A shift of attention away from individual lifestyle factors toward broader social and economic factors associated with people's location in the social structure is evident. A **social determinants of health** approach therefore informs much of recent research in this area. From this perspective, the major factors that influence health are social and economic in nature. According to Raphael:

> [S]ocial determinants of health are the economic and social conditions that influence the health of individuals, communities, and jurisdictions as a whole. Social determinants of health determine whether individuals stay healthy or become ill (a narrow definition of health). Social determinants of health also determine the extent to which a person possesses the physical, social, and personal resources to identify and achieve personal aspirations, satisfy needs, and cope with the environment (a broader definition of health). Social determinants of health are about the quantity and quality of a variety of resources that a society makes available to its members. (2004: 1)

There are several different approaches to understanding the social determinants of health. All are concerned with the organization and distribution of social and economic resources. However, the specific factors identified vary somewhat. For example, in response to mounting evidence supporting the importance of factors traditionally considered to be outside the health agenda, Health Canada adopted a new population health model in the mid-1990s. This model identified 10 social determinants as interacting with one another and with biology and genetic endowments to influence health: education,

employment/working conditions, income and social status, social environments, social support networks, personal health practices and coping skills,
health services, gender, culture, physical environments, and healthy child development (Hubka, 2003). More recently, Wilkinson and Marmot (2003) emphasized social class, stress, early life, social exclusion, work, unemployment, social
support, addiction, food, and transport. Finally, Raphael (2004), a Canadian
sociologist, draws attention to Aboriginal status, education, employment and
working conditions, food security, health-care services, housing, income and its
distribution, social safety net, social exclusion, and unemployment and
employment security.

Despite their differences, each of these models points to the importance of
social and structural factors in influencing the health of the population. Some
of the most important of these are factors that result in global and regional disparities and social class and socio-economic inequalities, as well as racial, ethnic, immigrant, gender, and other differentials.

Global Disparities

In 1800, global life expectancy averaged 28.5 years of age. A century later, it had
increased by less than four years, to 32.0 years (Riley, 2001). However, between
1950 and 1955 average life expectancy across the globe was 47.0 years, and by the
end of the century it had reached 65.4 years (United Nations, 2005).

However, global trends also hide important variations. Mortality and life
expectancy vary considerably across countries, with people living in more developed, wealthier countries generally living longer than those living in less developed, lower-income countries (CIHI, 2004a). For example, as shown in Figure
2.5, the average life expectancy of those living in more developed regions of the
globe reached 76 years by the turn of the century. Yet the vast majority (over 80
per cent) of the world's population lives in less developed regions (United
Nations, 2005). In the 50 least developed countries, life expectancy currently
stands at about 51 years of age (United Nations, 2005).

How do Canadians fare in comparison to other countries? Canada is among
the nations of the world with the highest life expectancy: 82 years for women
and 77 years for men. Only a few countries (Hong Kong, Japan, France, Spain,
and Australia) fare somewhat better (see Table 2.3). Interestingly, the United
States does somewhat worse, with life expectancy currently reaching 80 years for
women and 75 years for men. In contrast, those born in countries such as Kenya,
Afghanistan, Botswana, and Swaziland cannot expect to live much beyond the
early years of mid-life. In Kenya, for example, average life expectancy is only 46
years for women and 48 years for men. In Swaziland, women can expect to live
to only 33 years of age and men to 32 years of age (United Nations, 2005). These
differences, along with differences in fertility rates and other factors (e.g., migration), are reflected in the proportion of the population within various age
groups. In Canada, about 18 per cent of the population is under the age of 15

Figure 2.5   Life Expectancy at Birth for the World and Major Development Groups, 1950–2050

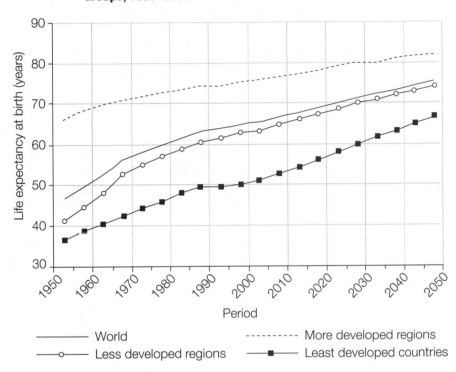

Source: Population Division of the Department of Economic and Social Affairs of the United Nations Secretariat. 2005. *World Population Prospects: The 2004 Revision. Highlights.* New York: United Nations. The United Nations is the author of the original material.

and about 13 per cent is aged 65 and older. However, in Swaziland, 43 per cent of the population is under 15 years of age and just 3 per cent is aged 65 and older (Population Reference Bureau, 2005).

One of the primary reasons for such differences between countries appears to be socio-economic. Privileged countries with higher median incomes have better health and lower illness, disability, and mortality rates than those with lower median incomes (Weitz, 1996a). According to the WHO, almost 33 per cent of the world's children are malnourished and up to 40 per cent of child deaths are due to malnutrition. The major causes of illness and death in less developed countries include communicable diseases (lower respiratory infections and diarrhea) and maternal, perinatal (low birth weight), and nutritional disorders (Murray and Lopez, 1997). In contrast, in more developed countries such as ours, illness and death from acute infectious diseases have given way to chronic illnesses and disabilities. Such diseases take many years to develop and death associated with them often occurs in the later years of life, long after the disease has been contracted.

Table 2.3   Life Expectancy at Birth and at Age 60 for Selected Countries, 2000–2005

COUNTRY	LIFE EXPECTANCY AT BIRTH		LIFE EXPECTANCY AT AGE 60	
	W	M	W	M
Hong Kong SAR	85	79	26	22
Japan	85	78	27	22
France	83	76	26	20
Spain	83	76	25	20
Australia	83	78	25	21
Canada	82	77	25	21
Israel	82	78	24	21
Sweden	82	78	24	21
Germany	81	76	24	19
United Kingdom	81	76	23	20
United States of America	80	75	24	20
Cuba	79	75	23	20
Poland	78	70	22	17
Mexico	77	72	22	21
Venezuela	76	70	22	20
China	73	70	20	17
Egypt	72	67	18	16
Iran (Islamic Republic of)	72	69	18	17
Ukraine	72	60	19	14
Russain Federation	72	59	19	14
Bolivia	66	62	19	17
India	65	62	18	16
Iraq	60	57	16	15
Ghana	57	56	18	17
Papua New Guinea	56	55	14	12
Haiti	52	51	17	16
South Africa	51	47	18	14
Kenya	46	48	18	16
Afghanistan	46	46	15	14
Botswana	37	36	18	16
Swaziland	33	32	17	15

Source: United Nations Department of Economic and Social Affairs. 2006. Available at: http://unstats.un.org/unsd/demographic/products/indwm/ww2005/tab3a.htm#src. The United Nations is the author of the original material.

Economic factors are not only important when comparing developed with less developed nations but also when looking at differences among developed nations. For example, the United States is one of the world's wealthiest nations, yet the health status of its population, as measured by life expectancy, infant mortality, and other factors, is poorer than that of people living in most other industrialized countries (Navarro et al., 2004). This disparity is widely attributed to the high levels of poverty, unemployment, and inequality evident within the country. It also suggests the greater importance of relative income inequality within a country than its overall level of economic development for determining such factors as infant mortality rates (Wennemo, 1993).

Other researchers point to the importance of a country's political structure, including the type of welfare state regime it has and whether it offers redistributive policies such as universal health care, poverty reduction strategies, and generous unemployment benefits. They argue that such factors will influence (and reduce) the impact of economic inequalities on the health of the population. Importantly, the United States is considered an example of a liberal welfare-state regime with poorer benefits than many other developed nations (Navarro and Shi, 2001).

Matters of Place: Regional Disparities

The fact that Canada fares well when compared with most other countries does not mean that inequalities in health and life expectancy are not evident here as well. Instead, it conceals very different trends among Canadian subpopulations, one of which refers to matters of place within the nation—the regions, states, or provinces within which people live.

One such subpopulation consists of those living in rural areas of Canada. Despite the absence of a clear and universally accepted definition of what rural living means, it is generally defined in relation to urban areas and refers to areas designated on the basis of indicators such as population size (smaller than in urban areas), density (lower than in urban areas) and distance (from larger urban centres) (CIHI, 2006a). Currently, about one in five Canadians lives in a rural area (Population Reference Bureau, 2005). And, although rural living is often represented by pastoral images depicting close-knit communities and stress-free, natural, and healthy lifestyles, those living in rural and remote communities are generally found to have poorer health than those living in urban areas. There is some indication that living in a rural area is associated with a lower prevalence of asthma and certain other respiratory disorders often linked to exposure to air pollutants (Iversen et al, 2005). In general, however, average life expectancies of rural residents tend to be lower and they have higher accident and disability rates. As well, rural areas tend to experience higher mortality among youth and higher mortality due to injury (including suicide and accidental causes) and some chronic diseases. Thus, greater proportions of rural people report poor or fair rather than excellent health, as well as activity limitations and long-term disability (CIHI, 2006d).

Other forms of regional variation in physical health are also evident. In Canada, population health and health care are provincial responsibilities; as a result, Canadian provinces and territories differ with respect to the health status of their populations. For example, mortality rates generally decrease from east to west and tend to be higher in the north. In 2002, life expectancy in Canada ranged from a low of 68.5 years in Nunavut to a high of 80.6 years in British Columbia (Statistics Canada, 2004a). As well, only 17 per cent of Saskatchewan residents rate their health as excellent compared to 27 per cent of those living in Quebec (Health Canada, 1999c). Similarly, while 12.4 per cent of all Canadians reported experiencing limitations to their everyday activities because of a health condition or problem, this figure was lower in Quebec (8.4 per cent) than in provinces such as Nova Scotia (17.1 per cent) (Statistics Canada, 2002c). Finally, differences in health status exist between and within cities, neighbourhoods, and rural communities. For example, people living in higher-income neighbour-hoods have longer average life expectancy than those in lower-income neigh-bourhoods, resulting in two to five years longer life among people living in wealthier urban neighbourhoods than those in the poorest urban neighbour-hoods (Wilkins, Bertholet, and Ng, 2002).

There is a little agreement regarding what characteristics of rural–urban locales, provinces, communities, or neighbourhoods matter for health. Some emphasize the importance of differences in the socio-cultural characteristics of communities, including residents' sense of belonging and pride in their commu-nity. The importance of such factors likely emerges after the bare necessities of socio-economic necessities (such as secure and safe housing, adequate nutrition, good sanitation, an ample water supply, safe transportation, and adequate income) have been met (CIHI, 2006d). In contrast, others argue that rural–urban and other locational differences likely reflect nothing more than differences in the characteristics of individuals who tend to live in particular places. In other words, living in a given neighbourhood probably has little or no effect on one's health. Instead, it is the social and economic characteristics of individuals living within the neighbourhoods that are important, that is, **compositional differ-ences** (Roos et al., 2004). And, for some reason, rural communities are more likely to be home to individuals (e.g., older adults, those with lower education and income levels) whose health status tends to be poorer than that of people living in urban areas.

However, others argue that rural–urban differences in health reflect the neg-ative impact that residence in some areas has on the social and economic factors that affect health. That is, communities differ in terms of such things as pollu-tion and environmental hazards, criminal activity, the nature and distribution of wealth, the quality of health care available, the efficiency of transportation sys-tems, safety in workplaces, social capital or cohesion, and structured social inequalities that in turn affect individual health (Veenstra, 2003). According to the Canadian Institute of Health Information (CIHI, 2006d), for example, rural

Canadians are more likely to have poor socio-economic conditions, to have lower educational attainment, and to participate in economic activities with higher health risks (such as farming, fishing, mining, and logging). For example, in 2001 almost 25 per cent of people aged 20 to 34 in rural areas had less than a high-school education compared to 14 per cent in urban communities. Income disparities are also evident, with families in rural communities having considerably lower median incomes than families living in urban communities— $49,449 compared with $56,817 (CIHI, 2006d). The impact of these factors may be further compounded in rural areas by less access to the health services required for prevention, early detection, treatment, or care.

There is mixed support for the importance of residential location for health. One Canadian study of people living in Nova Scotia found that socio-economic characteristics were not significantly related to mortality (Veugelers, Yip, and Kephart, 2001). That is, those living in lower-income neighbourhoods or neighbourhoods with high unemployment rates were no more likely to die early than those living in other less disadvantaged neighbourhoods. Similarly, a study by Roos and colleagues (2004) reported that while well-educated people with higher incomes lived longer, whether these people lived in more or less wealthy neighbourhoods was unimportant. In contrast, a number of American studies tend to support the importance of community wealth for residents' health (Yen and Kaplan, 1999). Similar differences emerge when comparing across states. For example, Lochner and colleagues (2001) found that people with similar levels of income had different mortality rates depending on whether they lived in a state that had high- or low-income inequality. Those with higher inequality also had higher mortality rates. Roos and colleagues (2004) speculated that differences in the findings across studies may reflect the fact that such differences (e.g., income inequality, access to health and social services, safety, crime rates, etc.) are more important determinants of health in the United States than in Canada and other developed countries.

Social Class and Socio-Economic Disparities

Within as well as across countries and over time, social class and the socio-economic factors associated with it are among those most strongly and consistently related to health. There is debate regarding the definition, measurement, and continuing relevance of social class as well as the relationships between social class and socio-economic status (SES) (see Annandale, 1998). Although often used interchangeably within broader literature dealing with health and health inequalities, sociologists generally consider social class and SES as distinct; while social class is frequently used to denote ownership and control over the means of economic production (i.e., a Marxist definition), SES tends to refer to one's position within hierarchies stratified on the basis of one or more of education, occupational status, or income. Some have argued that class is losing (or has already lost) its relevance in the context of shifts toward a global political economy characterized by the internationalization of capital, declines in manual labour, shifts toward a service economy, an emphasis on individualism, and the citizen as consumer rather than producer (Annandale, 1998). Yet others, such as Veenstra (2006), report findings indicating that class distinctions (such as personal autonomy at work) and SES both influenced various health outcomes.

Little Canadian research focuses directly on social class and health inequalities; most centres on socio-economic status and health (Raphael, 2006). As well, how social class and SES intersect to influence health is not clear (Veenstra, 2006). However, as Humphries and van Doorslaer (2000: 663) note, an association between socio-economic factors and health has been observed for hundreds of years regardless of the socio-economic status or the health outcome measures used. Available research supports the notion that those who are advantaged with regard to factors such as education, occupational status, income, and wealth generally live longer than those who are disadvantaged on these factors. They also tend to live a greater number of healthy years and spend a greater proportion of their overall lives healthy.

As noted above, as age increases the likelihood of illness (chronic and acute) also increases. However, those with more education seem to be able to avoid and postpone disability to a greater extent than those with less education. For example, people with a university degree often feel healthy and function well late into their sixties, seventies, and eighties, whereas those with less education do not (Ross and Wu, 1996). A recent Canadian study (Buckley et al., 2005) followed adults aged 50 and older, all of whom initially were in good health, over a three-year period. They found that the chances of remaining in good health over this period were greater among women and men in the highest educational and income groups.

With regard to occupational status, the well-known 1967 Whitehall Study (Marmot and Brunner, 2004), conducted in Britain, followed the health of more than 10,000 male civil servants, none of whom could be considered poor or deprived. Over more than two decades, men in the lowest employment levels were much more likely to die prematurely than men in the highest levels. In Canada, a recent analysis of occupational differences in health among those aged 18 to 64 shows better health among professionals and managers than other workers: only 3.9 per cent of professionals and managers rated their overall health as fair or poor, compared to 6.8 per cent of other workers. With regard to mental health, the figures were 6.3 per cent and 4.5 per cent (Muntaner et al., 2006).

Similar differences are evident in conjunction with income level, a well-established factor influencing health. It has been estimated that almost 25 per cent of premature mortality (i.e., potential years of life lost) among Canadians can be linked to income-related differences (Raphael et al., 2005). Men with the lowest 5 per cent of earnings before retirement are twice as likely to die between 65 and 70 years of age as men with the highest 5 per cent of earnings. On average, high-income earners experience about 12 more years of good health than those with lower incomes (CIAR, 1991). They also tend to see themselves in considerably better health. For example, approximately 20 per cent of Canadians in the lowest income groups rate their health as excellent compared to about 33 per cent of those in the highest income group. While about 20 per cent of those with low incomes consider their health to be fair or poor, this is the case for only 5 per cent of those at the highest income levels (Health Canada, 1999c). As well, among those with disabilities, those with low incomes also tend to be more disabled than those with higher incomes. Over 25 per cent of those in the lowest income groups report some type of long-term disability or handicap, compared to about 14 per cent of those in the highest income groups (Health Canada, 1999c).

It is important to acknowledge that despite consistent educational, occupational, and income disparities in health, not all diseases and causes of death are related to such factors in the predicted way. On the one hand, those with the lowest incomes are more than three times as likely to experience arthritis and almost nine times as likely to experience emotional difficulties as those in the highest income groups. However, some diseases, such as breast and prostate cancer, increase in prevalence as social class or SES increases (Gorey et al., 1998).

It is also important to note that relationships between income or other aspects of SES and health are not just about poverty. Instead, every increase in income appears to be associated with an increase in health; even the very rich report better health than the not quite so rich. In other words, lower SES and social-class standing is associated with poorer health, with a graded rather than a threshold effect—poor health does not disappear when a certain level of income is obtained. Yet it is also the case that the average difference in health status between those near the bottom of the income ladder and those just a few steps up is more pronounced than it is among steps nearer the top (Veenstra, 2003).

The relationship between social and economic disparities and health status differences appears to hold at all ages and in all race/ethnic groups, although it is weaker among older adults than among those of working age. Similarly, average neighbourhood income and household income are directly related to life expectancy, health, and illness for both men and women. However, while those in the lowest income groups are more likely to report health problems than those in the higher income groups, evidence suggests that this difference may be due primarily to differences among women rather than men. Statistics Canada (1994) reports finding that women in the lowest income group were considerably more likely to report health problems compared to women in the highest income group. Among men, however, there was little difference evident between those in the lowest and highest income groups.

Why do those in lower social class and SES groups have poorer health? Some argue **social selection**, that those who are healthy are more likely to succeed and achieve higher social class or SES while those who are not healthy are impeded from educational, occupational, or income attainment. Others favour a **social causation** argument, contending that higher social-class position leads to better opportunities, living situations, and access to resources that also lead to better health and well-being. While it is likely that prolonged or serious illness results in declines in class, income, or occupational standing (i.e., downward mobility) for some, research indicates that social causation is, by far, the more important component.

How then do social class and socio-economic inequalities lead to poorer health? Those who are not familiar with a sociological perspective often assume that those who differ in social class or socio-economic standing also differ in their individual lifestyle preferences and associated behaviours, which, in turn, influence health (i.e., a cultural/behavioural explanation). These activities include such things as the consumption of harmful commodities (i.e., high fat and refined foods, tobacco, alcohol, other drugs), lack of adequate exercise, and the failure to make use of preventive health measures (such as contraception and vaccination). For example, a recent public opinion survey (CPHI, 2005) reports that when Canadians were asked what the major determinants of health were, the most common responses referred to individual behaviour and lifestyle factors including smoking (80 per cent), diet (72 per cent), obesity (71 per cent), stress (68 per cent), and physical activity (65 per cent). From this perspective, such behaviours reflect socially-situated individual decisions and consequently, if people's dietary, smoking, and other health practices improve, socio-economic inequalities in health will disappear.

From a sociological perspective, individual decision-making and behaviour must be seen in the context of the social structure and the constraints and facilitators that either impede or encourage the behaviours of people situated within it. According to Link and Phelan (2000), for example, the problem with focusing on smoking, exercise, diet, and other individual behaviours as risk factors is that they cannot account for the persistence of SES or class inequalities in disease and mortality over time. They note that, historically, there have been dramatic changes in people's social and health conditions, in life expectancy, in the diseases affecting people's health, and in the health care available to the population. In the past, the major health problems were diseases such as cholera and tuberculosis, whereas current problems include cardiovascular disease and cancer. Despite the different risk factors for past and present diseases, the relationship between social class or SES and health status persists.

To try and account for this situation, Link and Phelan propose a **fundamental cause explanation**. This approach suggests that social class and socio-economic inequalities represent fundamental social causes of disease or 'social conditions whose association with health persists even when profiles of risk and protective factors change radically' (2000: 39). They argue that the major reason that socio-economic inequalities are consistently related to disease is that they embody various resources (including knowledge, money, power, and prestige) that can be used to avoid risks and protect against disease 'no matter what the protective factors happen to be at a given point in time'. Consequently,

[w]hen new risk factors (such as chemical pollutants) arise, when new knowledge about risk factors (such as smoking) emerges, or even when new treatment
technologies ... develop, those who command the most resources are best able
to avoid the risks and take advantage of the protective actors, resulting in the
emergence of an SES gradient in these factors. (Link and Phelan, 2000: 39)

Link and Phelan's fundamental cause explanation exemplifies a 'materialist'
approach. Recently, Raphael (2006) identified three dominant social causation
explanations: (1) materialist, (2) neo-materialist, and (3) psychosocial comparison. A **materialist approach** draws attention to the role of the material/living
conditions experienced over the life course. From this perspective, the material
conditions of life determine health by influencing such things as the quality of
individual development, family life and interaction, and community environments. Without adequate access to nutritious food, clean drinking water, quality housing, safe working conditions, transportation, and other resources, health
is compromised and challenged. A **neo-materialist approach**, in contrast,
directs attention not only to the effects of living conditions on individuals'
health but also to the societal factors that determine the quality of the social
determinants of health. It also considers how a society decides to distribute
resources among its citizens—that is, the social infrastructure (e.g., health, education, and social services) as determinants of health.

Finally, some argue that while low incomes and other objective disadvantages may be important, one's perceived position in the social structure matters
just as much, if not more. In other words, while access to income and other
resources will be related to one's standing in a hierarchically ordered structure,
it is this supposed relative inequity rather than the objective conditions themselves that results in poorer health (Wilkinson and Marmot, 2003). This **psychosocial comparison approach** draws attention to the impact of citizens'
perceptions of their standing in the social hierarchy and the implications of negative comparisons (i.e., perceived relative deprivation compared to others) on
psychosocial stress (at the individual level) and social cohesion (at the commu-
nal level). From this perspective, the stress associated with seeing oneself as
occupying a lower position in the social hierarchy and also perceiving this as
unfair or inequitable can have a negative impact on health both directly and
indirectly. In other words, not only can stress itself cause poorer health, but it
can also lead people to smoke, consume too much alcohol, eat too much or too
little, or sleep too little, all of which can have a negative impact on health (Link
and Phelan, 2000). Others operating from this perspective draw attention to the
importance of hierarchical position for people's view of power and control
rather than perceived deprivation compared to others. They argue that perceptions of power and control have health benefits, while perceptions of lack of
power or control over one's life are stressful and can have negative implications
for people's health (Link and Phelan, 2000).

Race, Ethnic, and Immigrant Inequalities

Racial, ethnic, and immigrant inequalities in health are also widely reported. Much of the research in this area focuses on the impact of racial inequalities in the United States, where African-, Hispanic-, and Native-American adults are consistently found to have poorer health and longevity than Caucasians, no matter what aspect of health status is considered. An exception involves African Americans aged about 75 years, who at this point begin to outlive their Caucasian counterparts. Some researchers also report similar findings with regard to differences in disability (Kelley-Moore and Ferraro, 2004). However, this occurrence does not mean that the health of African Americans improves in the last years of life. Instead, it probably reflects the fact that African Americans are much more likely to die at younger ages and that those who live to advanced old age are a very select group of *survivors*.

In contrast with the situation in the United States, health differences among racial groups in Canada are evident but less pronounced, except among First Nations peoples (McMullin, 2004). To some extent, this may reflect a lack of research rather than confirmation that such differences do not exist. However, the health of Aboriginal peoples in Canada (including First Nations, Inuit, and Métis people) is known to be poorer than that of the overall Canadian population on virtually every health-status measure (CIHI, 2004a; Waldram, Herring and Young; 2006). For example, the average lifespan of Inuit women is 14 years less than the average for other Canadian women (68 *v.* 82 years); for men the difference is six years (70 *v.* 76 years) (CIHI, 2004a). Despite long-term declines in national mortality rates, Aboriginal infant mortality rates remain approximately 22 per cent higher than those for Canada as a whole (Health Canada, 2005b). It is important to note, however, that variation also exists within the Aboriginal population. For example, among Aboriginal women, life expectancy is shortest among Inuit women, followed by First Nations and then Métis people. Aboriginal people in Canada face higher rates of infectious as well as chronic disease than the general Canadian population. Death rates from infectious and parasitic diseases (associated with inadequate housing, unsanitary conditions, and so on) are well above average national levels. Tuberculosis rates are approximately 10 times higher among First Nations and Inuit than other Canadians, and Aboriginal people are also over-represented among those with HIV. Aboriginal people represent 3.3 per cent of the Canadian population, but 5 to 8 per cent of those currently living with HIV in Canada and 6 to 12 per cent of new infections (Health Canada, 2006a). Finally, while HIV rates have declined in recent years for the Canadian population as a whole, it appears that they have been steadily increasing in First Nations and Inuit populations (Health Canada, 2006a).

With regard to chronic diseases, Type II diabetes rates are three to five times higher among First Nations and Métis people (Health Canada, 2004). According to Wister and Moore (1998), two-thirds of all First Nations elders reported disabilities compared to just over one-third of non-First Nations people of the same age. As well, the number of deaths associated with heart disease are 20 per cent higher than the overall Canadian rate and with stroke almost twice as high (Health Canada, 2005b). Interestingly, however, First Nations cancer mortality rates, with the exception of prostate cancer, are lower than those for the Canadian population as a whole (Health Canada, 2005b).

The largest cause of premature death within the Aboriginal population on reserve is injuries. For Aboriginal people under the age of 45, the leading causes of death due to injuries are motor vehicle accidents, suicide, drowning, and fire (CIHI, 2004a). Unintentional injuries are approximately four and a half times higher than the overall Canadian rate (Health Canada, 2005b). Among youth, suicide rates are five to six times higher than the national average, with suicide being the most frequent cause of injury-related death among Aboriginal people (Health Canada, 2004). First Nations people living on reserve have suicide rates twice that for the Canadian population as a whole. In 2000, suicides accounted for three times as many **potential years of life lost** (PYLL) among Aboriginal people than the overall Canadian population (Health Canada, 2005b). This quantitative estimate refers to the number of years of potential life that are lost when a person dies prematurely, generally defined as dying before the age of 75. For example, a person who dies at age 25 is considered to have lost 50 potential years of life.

Why is the objective health status of Canadian Aboriginal populations so poor? Racial and ethnic differences often tend to be seen as biologically and genetically determined rather than socially constructed. Consequently, explanations of racial/ethnic disparities in health often do not consider the effects of racism (Krieger, 2003). Yet it has been noted that Aboriginal populations share a common history, one characterized by prejudice and discrimination that continues to have a profound effect on their health and well-being (Trovato, 2001). Significant factors to be considered include the effects of colonialism—the extension of Canadian sovereignty over Native lands and the displacement of indigenous populations. The health effects are direct as well as indirect and include smallpox, measles, and tuberculosis epidemics, as well as cultural loss, discrimination, unemployment, and poverty (McCormick et al., 1997). Continuing inequalities in income, education, employment, and housing are a fundamental contribution to the poorer health of Aboriginal peoples in Canada (Waldram, Herring, and Young, 2006). Aboriginal communities often lack adequate water and sanitation facilities. Housing is frequently characterized by inadequate heating, lack of proper ventilation, and susceptibility to fire hazards. The leading causes of death among Aboriginal people often reflect these living conditions as well as lack of access to appropriate health care (Segall and Chappell, 2000).

Immigrant groups show a pattern of health status over time that differs from both Aboriginal peoples and from other non-immigrant Canadians. In 2001, almost one-fifth of Canada's population was born outside of Canada

(Ng et al., 2005). Although immigrants tend to report poorer health status than non-immigrants, this does not seem to apply to recent arrivals. One study found that six months after their arrival in Canada, 97 per cent of immigrants rated their health as good to excellent compared to 88 per cent of the general Canadian population (Chui, 2003). In the first few years following immigration, morbidity and mortality tend to be lower among immigrants than the Canadian-born population (Newbold and Danforth, 2003). This pattern has been observed to varying degrees for health outcomes such as chronic diseases, disability, dependency, life expectancy, and disability-free life expectancy (Chen, Ng, and Wilkins, 1996) as well as mental health status (Ali, 2002).

One possible explanation for the finding that recent immigrants tend to have better health than non-immigrant Canadians is that it reflects a **social selection effect**, whereby those entering the country tend to be better off financially and in terms of health than the Canadian-born population. Immigrants are selected for entry based on a 'points program' whereby potential immigrants are scored based on their language abilities, skills, education, age, and ability to invest in the country (Newbold and Danforth, 2003). The Canadian government also requires potential immigrants to meet a minimum standard of health before they will be admitted; therefore, healthier people are more likely to immigrate.

Although immigrants are generally healthy at the time of arrival and indeed have better health than non-immigrants, their health status eventually converges downward toward the Canadian average. In other words, it seems that this **healthy immigrant effect** tends to dissipate over time and disappears altogether after about 10 years (Chen et al., 1996; Wister, 2005a). Perez (2002), for example, notes that the likelihood of reporting any chronic condition increases with time spent in Canada, despite initially superior health relative to the Canadian born. Yet this convergence also hides important variations within the immigrant population as a result of differences in factors such as socio-economic standing. For example, the declines in health that take place following immigration are more likely to occur in some groups than others. Those from non-European countries appear twice as likely to report a decline in their health as Canadian-born individuals (Ng et al., 2005; Noh and Kaspar, 2003). Kopec and colleagues (2001) report that non-English speaking European and Asian immigrants fared worse in terms of health than did English Canadians, a finding not explainable by differences in SES. Importantly, during the 1980s and 1990s, the vast majority of immigrants were from non-English speaking countries within Asia, Africa, and South America. As well, 75 per cent of recent immigrants were members of racialized groups (Pederson and Raphael, 2006).

A recent study conducted in Ontario by Sword, Watt, and Krueger (2006) gives further evidence to the declining health of immigrants. This study compared Canadian-born and foreign-born women's experiences in the first four weeks after giving birth and found that immigrant women reported poorer overall health and greater postpartum depression than did women born in Canada. These researchers refer to the greater social isolation and low levels of support often available to immigrant women as explanations for these results. Others attribute it to the socio-economic disadvantages that immigrants face following entry into the country. For example, Dunn and Dyck (2000) point out that recent immigrants tend to have lower incomes than non-immigrants. Galabuzi (2004, 2006) reports a 30 per cent income gap between racialized and non-racialized groups in Canada, higher than average unemployment, deepening levels of poverty, over-representation in low-pay and low-status jobs, differential access to housing, and increasing racial and economic concentration in Canadian urban areas.

Statistics Canada data indicates that the low income rates among immigrants have been rising during the 1990s while falling for the Canadian born (Picot, 2004). Others argue that the SES of foreign-born individuals does not tend to decline with duration of residence and that **acculturation**, including the notion that foreign-born individuals gradually adopt the cultural beliefs and practices of the host society (e.g., health-related lifestyle factors such as smoking, drinking, diet, and exercise) are important to consider (Wister, 2005a). Others point to the importance of all of these factors (Newbold and Danforth, 2003).

Gender Inequalities

Biological, physiological, and anatomical factors differentiate males and females in terms of health. However, these sex-related differences also overlap with, and therefore are difficult to distinguish from, social- or gender-related differences when addressing health variations associated with being male or female.

Gender-based inequalities in health are widely reported (Denton, Prus, and Walters, 2004). Globally, for example, women's health tends to be poorer than that of men, particularly in developing countries, where women frequently die in childbirth. Women's lowered life expectancy in these countries has been attributed to a combination of adverse social and economic circumstances that have led to female infanticide, early deaths due to the complications of frequent child-bearing and sexually transmitted diseases, inadequate diets, infections and hemorrhages following genital mutilation, and restricted access to health services (Annandale, 1998; Lorber, 2005).

In Canada as well as other more developed, industrialized countries, women's life expectancy is often greater and mortality rates somewhat lower than those of men. This was not always the case. Before industrial capitalism, the mortality rates for women were often higher than male rates due to high rates of maternal mortality. Women were also more susceptible to such problems as malnutrition and acute infectious diseases such as tuberculosis (Annandale, 1998). However, while life expectancy increased steadily for both men and women over the course of the past century or two, it did so more rapidly for women. This shift was due largely to reductions in mortality associated with

childbirth. As a result, by the 1920s, Canadian men could expect to live an average of 59 years while Canadian women could expect to live 61 years (Statistics
Canada, 2005). As previously stated, Canadian women currently live over five
years longer than men (Statistics Canada, 2005).

The fact that men have higher mortality rates and lower life expectancies
than women might lead us to expect that women will be healthier than men
throughout life. However, the pattern is more complicated. For example,
women, particularly those in older age groups, are more likely than men to
report multiple health problems associated with chronic conditions such as
arthritis and rheumatism, high blood pressure, back problems, and allergies
(Chappell et al., 2003). Older women are also more likely to report one or
more chronic conditions than are older men. The likelihood of disability
increases with age for both men and women. However, across all age groups
except for children aged 0 to 14, women are more likely to experience limitations in activities of daily living or disability (Statistics Canada, 2001b).
Women also report more severe disability than men—although men have
lower life expectancy, a greater proportion of their lives are lived without disabling conditions.

Given the gender differences evident in physical health, we might expect
women to evaluate their health more poorly than men do. Yet the differences
appear slight. In general, about two-thirds of Canadian women and men rate
their health as excellent or very good. The percentage of females (73.2 per cent)
and males (73.4 per cent) reporting excellent or very good mental health are also
very similar (Health Canada, 2006b). Yet women report higher levels of depression and distress than men (Denton, Prus, and Walters, 2004). They are nearly
twice as likely as men to be diagnosed as being depressed or as having anxiety
disorders, while men tend to be more frequently diagnosed as being schizophrenic, having various personality disorders, or as having substance abuse
problems (Pederson and Raphael, 2006).

Lorber summarizes these differences by asserting 'women get sicker, but
men die quicker' (2005: 164). A number of explanations have been proposed to
account for this paradox. Some argue that the difference is more apparent than
real; women simply are more likely to be perceived, diagnosed, and treated by
others (including physicians) as having poorer health. Those who hold this perspective argue that men in fact have poorer health than women. In contrast,
those who suggest that the differences are accurate and that women's health
tends to be worse than men's argue that women report higher levels of health
problems because of their reduced access to the material and social conditions
of life that foster health as well as from the greater stress associated with their
gender and marital roles (a **differential exposure hypothesis**; see Denton et al.,
2004). For example, women are less likely than men to be employed but more
likely to have lower incomes and to be single parents. Others suggest that women
report higher levels of health problems because they react differently than men

to the material, behavioural, and psychosocial conditions that foster health (**a differential vulnerability hypothesis**). Support for this perspective is provided by evidence indicating that high incomes, working full-time, and having access to sources of support are more important in bringing about good health for women than they are for men (Denton et al., 2004).

The proportion of the older adult population that is female is increasing over time. To the extent that older women experience greater illness and disability than older men, this **feminization of aging** likely means that the overall health status of the older population will decline and the need for services will increase. Also, given the tendency of older women to have fewer resources than older men, it is likely that needs for care will increase. However, there is also evidence such feminization will not occur, but that gender differences in longevity may be declining in industrialized societies due to improvements in the life expectancy of men (Trovato and Lalu, 1996). (See Chapter 3 for other potential changes in gender roles in old age.)

Age Inequalities
While sociologists tend to acknowledge gender and race/ethnicity as both biological and social constructs in relation to health, age is often regarded as exclusively biological, with its social components less often acknowledged. Yet age is also both a social and biological determinant of health.

When we think about the relationship between age and health, we tend to associate childhood and youth with health and old age with health decline. After all, death rates increase steadily with age and in Canada as well as other Western societies, death is heavily concentrated among those who are older. Age is the factor most strongly related to health and illness, primarily evident with regard to physical health. Physical changes gradually occur and accumulate over the course of our lives; for example, our eyesight generally begins to deteriorate in the middle years of life. Chronic diseases also tend to be concentrated among older adults. However, unless something severe happens, such as a major heart attack or a diagnosis of Alzheimer's disease, older adults generally adapt well as their health slowly changes.

Activity limitations are among the most common implications of health-related problems encountered in later life. According to the *2001 Participation and Activity Limitation Survey* (Statistics Canada, 2002c), while 12.4 per cent of Canadians of all ages reported experiencing activity limitations (including everyday activities such as work, school, or housework), this increased from a low of 3.3 per cent among children aged 0 to 14, to 9.9 per cent of those aged 15 to 64, and to 40.5 per cent of those aged 65 and older. Of those aged 75 and older, 53.3 per cent reported such a disability. Among younger children, the most common disability is that related to a chronic health condition (e.g., asthma or severe allergies, cerebral palsy, migraines, autism, heart conditions). Among working-age adults (aged 15 to 64), the most common source of activity limitations is pain or discomfort. Among older adults, in contrast, mobility problems are the most frequently reported type of disability, followed by chronic pain, agility limitations, and hearing problems (Statistics Canada, 2002a). It is widely assumed that the prevalence of any form of disability increases with age. While this notion is true for disabilities related to mobility, agility, hearing, vision, and pain, it is not the case in all areas (Statistics Canada, 2002a). For example, when it comes to limitations associated with emotional, psychological, or psychiatric conditions, those aged 45 to 64 have higher rates. According to the *Canadian Community Health Survey* (*CCHS*) (Statistics Canada, 2003), mental disorders are present throughout life, but there are differences among age groups. Teenagers and young adults (aged 15 to 24) are most likely to suffer from various mental health problems (including major depression, mania disorder, panic disorder, social phobia, and agoraphobia) and substance dependence problems (18 per cent).

Despite the fact that our physical health deteriorates as we age, most (73.3 per cent) older adults tend to view their general health as good, very good, or excellent (Statistics Canada, 2003). The same positive picture is evident with regard to psychological health or well-being. Those aged 75 and older are three times more likely than 18- and 19-year-olds to score high on a sense of coherence (that is, a perception that life is meaningful, events are comprehensible, and challenges are manageable). Self-esteem and mastery also improve with age, peaking in middle age followed by only modest declines in later life (Statistics Canada, 2001c; 2002g). Finally, according to results obtained by the CCHS (Statistics Canada 2002d), younger adults are somewhat less likely to say they are very satisfied with their lives than are those aged 65 and older. Overall, 83.6 per cent of those aged 15 to 24 report being satisfied to very satisfied with their lives compared with 84.8 per cent of those aged 25 to 64 and 89.4 per cent of those aged 65 and older (Statistics Canada, 2002c).

The reasons why older adults often report and indeed exhibit such good psychological well-being, even though their physical health is often worse than younger adults, is unknown. Perhaps life itself becomes more important as people age. Alternatively, it may be that those with better psychological well-being tend to live longer. Others point to the importance of taking social factors into account. While it is a biological fact that as people age their bodies tend to degenerate gradually, there are also social causes of age differences in health, including distinctions in life experiences. People of different ages or generations have lived through different historical and political-economic circumstances. Today's older adults have lived though specific major world events such as war and economic depression that may, in comparison, help them view their current situations with favour. Although they now benefit from Medicare, most can remember a time when such services were not available. It is often speculated that older adults compare themselves with the situations of their peers who are worse off or deceased.

Multiple Jeopardy and Intersectionality

When we think about age, gender, class, ethnic, or other inequalities, we tend to think about each on its own. If we do consider them together, it is often to ask which dimension is the most important. For example, are racial, ethnic, or immigrant inequalities really about social class and socio-economic inequalities? What about gender differences, given that poverty is often concentrated among women? Alternatively, we may wonder about the implications of adding one type of inequality to another. For example, are the health consequences of being older as well as female worse than those associated with being older but male? What happens when we add ethnic or racial minority group status to the mix?

Some sociologists argue that each dimension has an impact and that experiencing more than one source of inequality will make the situation that much worse, an idea known as **multiple jeopardy**. Others suggest that they cannot simply be added together. Instead, factors such as gender and race or age intersect so that one cannot be understood apart from the other. What this means in terms of health inequalities is that women may respond differently than men to economic or other factors that influence health (e.g., health behaviours, stressors). For example, women's health is more adversely affected by living in poverty than is the health of men (Prus and Gee, 2002). As a result, the greatest differences in life expectancy between men and women have been observed among those living in the most disadvantaged areas (DesMeules et al., 2004). Providing care to other family members also seems to be more important to the health of older women than men, while there are indications that smoking and alcohol consumption may have a greater impact on the health of older men (Denton and Walters, 1999).

EXPERIENCING HEALTH AND ILLNESS: OPPORTUNITIES FOR AGENCY

While health and illness are strongly associated with social-structural location, this understanding tells us little about the interpretive experience of people within different locations. Does this mean that little or no opportunity exists to act on the basis of these understandings? As noted in Chapter 1, recent theorizing in the areas of health and illness suggests that it is through our interpretive practices and associated behaviours that we can modify social structures (Hendricks, 2003). In this section we talk about both the experience of health and illness with examples of agency.

Sociologists working in the areas of health and illness have long argued that meanings of health and illness are subjectively rather than objectively defined. They often draw a distinction between disease, illness, and sickness. Diseases are physiological in nature and refer to disorders in the structure or functioning of bodily organs or systems. As such, they are relatively objective and medically defined, typically diagnosed and treated by physicians. Health is often thought of simply as the absence of disease. However, in reality, health and illness are not objectively defined but are situated in individual experiences. As noted earlier, according to the WHO, health incorporates not just physical but also mental and social well-being. **Illness**, in contrast, refers to the personal or subjective experience of the individual who has a disease or does not feel well—how she or he perceives, lives with, and responds to symptoms and disabilities (Eisenberg, 1977). Not everyone will experience symptoms in the same way. Finally, **sickness** is a social phenomenon that refers to the socially defined actions (such as the rights and duties defined by Parson's sick role; see Chapter 1) taken by a person as a result of illness or disease (e.g., taking medication, visiting the doctor, resting in bed, or staying away from work). Consequently, physicians diagnose and treat disease, while patients perceive illness and enact sickness (Twaddle, 1994; Hofmann, 2002). Although a disease is typically considered to lead to illness (perceived as symptoms) that then leads to sickness (behaviours undertaken in order to respond to illness), the three may or may not be related—for example, one can experience illness and enact sickness but be told by a physician that there is no evidence of disease.

People's experiences of health do indeed reflect more than the mere absence of disease. In fact, even among those who are supposedly healthy, almost everyone experiences some symptoms of disease. This suggests that we may to some degree be diseased every day of our lives (Zola, 1973). Yet most of the symptoms we experience are minor and, when asked, people will generally say that they are in good to excellent health. As discussed in the section on age, this finding is especially the case among older adults. If they do not define themselves as healthy based on symptoms or on severity of disease, what standards do they use? One study of older persons living in Scotland found that the main dimensions of health included an absence of illness, a reserve of strength, and a feeling of being generally fit or capable of accomplishing daily tasks (Williams, 1990). Similar results were found among middle-aged French subjects, who described health in terms of absence of illness, equilibrium in daily life, and a capacity to work (Herzlich, 1973; Herzlich and Pierret, 1987).

Interestingly, however, we know much more about how people experience illness and particularly major and chronic illnesses and disabilities, than about how they experience health. Early research focused on illness experiences from the outside—as defined and viewed by sources other than the person directly involved—and was later widely criticized for doing so. For example, Parsons (1951) conceptualized people's experiences as being normatively defined in accordance with a socially defined role—the sick role. From this perspective, a person is required to act according to the normative expectations associated with the role, including the obligation to seek and comply with medical treatment. Critics of this approach argue that it reduces the ill person to being a patient and restricts her or his agency to compliance. The physician, not the patient, is the active agent in the illness process (Frank, 1997).

Research that followed began to take an **insider perspective** and to focus directly on people's subjective experiences, living with and in spite of illness, within the contexts of their everyday lives (Lawton, 2003). It addressed issues such as the meaning of illness to the person experiencing it as well as to her or his family and friends, the social organization of the sufferer's world, and the strategies used to cope with illnesses, as well as the negative experiences some-times associated with them. It has been widely noted that those who are ill often have to deal with a variety of issues as part of their illness experience. These include issues of loss (e.g., loss of body parts, of bodily functions, of current and future capacities and roles); issues of time (including scheduling life activities around one's illness and the reassessment of one's future); issues of symptom management (e.g., what therapies to use, concealing symptoms from others); issues of social relationships (e.g., loss of independence, social isolation); and issues of social marginality (including stigma) (see Freund and McGuire, 1999). According to Weitz (1996b), for example, the experience of living with AIDS involves developing strategies to make living with the disease more manageable, including how to cope with the fear and reality of stigma, changes in social rela-tionships, the impact of illness on their bodies, and impending death. She notes that some manage to do this while others remain overwhelmed until they die.

Early works on the meanings of the illness experience focused on concepts such as stigma, biographical disruption, and loss of self. For example, Strauss and Glaser (1975) and others pointed out that chronic illness is often accompa-nied by **stigma** (an attribution that discredits the value of a person; see Goffman, 1963) that can affect personal identity as well as relationships with others (see, for example, Box 2.3). Others turned their attention to how illness interrupts a person's assumptions about himself or herself. For example, Bury (1982) interviewed relatively young and recently diagnosed people suffering from rheumatoid arthritis and concluded that the onset of chronic illness can be seen as a major disruptive experience—or what he refers to as a **biographical disruption**—in people's lives. This disruption can take place on various levels, including personal relationships, material and practical affairs, and structures of meaning. For example, it can disrupt assumptions about everyday life and the future as well as of the explanatory frameworks that people use to make sense of their experiences. It can be reflected in questions such as 'Why me?' or 'Why now?' It can also involve confronting pain and the possibility of death, usually seen as remote possibilities rather than imminent realities within everyday lives.

Bury suggests that this disruption requires a fundamental rethinking of one's biography and one's self-concept. Coping is therefore seen as a cognitive (mental) process through which the individual learns how to tolerate the effects of chronic illness. 'Normalization' of an illness or its effects is a form of coping that minimizes the potentially negative impact of illness on self-identity. For instance, older adults may consider chronic illness a normal part of aging rather than a profound disruption. Sanders, Donovan, and Dieppe (2002) conducted in-depth interviews with men and women (aged 51 to 91) with arthritis. They found that these people portrayed their symptoms as normal and an integral

Box 2.3
My Weight Loss Story

As I stepped down from the podium at the International Congress of Nursing in London, England, in 2000, an event occurred that changed my life forever. A woman approached me and said, 'Hi, Elaine. Remember me from our days at Duke University?' I did not recognize her and she said, 'It's me, Liz. I have lost over 100 pounds and I want to tell you about it. It has been like a miracle.' And so my miracle began. My friend had had a lap-band put in place in Israel and as the months ensued and I conducted research on the procedure, I soon knew it was the answer to my prayers and the first sign of hope that I did not have to live out the rest of my compromised life as a yo-yo dieter, or worse still, as a person who had given up all hope of ever weighing less than the current 360 pounds.

The 10 years I lived in that body were like a nightmare. I knew I was in there somewhere, but suffered in silence the stares and laughter of a busload of tourists, the jeers of young children at a waterslide park, the anxious look of airline passengers as I moved down the aisle in their direction. As the pounds slowly melted away—all 200 of them—I still felt like I was in a surreal dream. But this time it was like a flying dream, a freedom trip that let me eat a meal slowly, enjoyably, without the gnawing feeling that this may be my last. Each trip to the consignment store brought the joys of a size or two smaller clothing. Stabilized now at a normal weight for over two years, I mostly enjoy being anonymous in a crowd, not standing out, not searching desperately for a chair without arms at every occasion, and not worrying that when I found that chair and sat in it, it would collapse. They often did.

Source: Anonymous.

part of their biographies but also talked about the highly disruptive impact on their daily lives. Ciambrone (2001) interviewed 37 women with HIV and found that, despite initial disruption, other events in these women's lives such as drug use and mother–child separations were often considered more disruptive than the onset of HIV.

Along similar lines, Charmaz suggested that people's experiences with chronic illness often reflect a loss of self that takes place as 'former self-images crumbl[e] away without a simultaneous development of equally-valued new ones' (1983: 168). She sees their experiences as leading to social isolation, shame by self and others, and the humiliation of being a burden on others. However, she also notes that, as people live with the ambiguities and uncertainties associated with chronic illness, they also tend to choose among various preferred identities in an attempt to attain, maintain, or recreate valued selves (Charmaz, 1987, 1991, 1994). These range hierarchically from a **supernormal social identity** (an identity founded on extraordinary achievement and therefore on trying to do everything better than those who are not ill) to a **salvaged self** (wherein people try to retain a past identity associated with their previously healthy selves) (Charmaz, 1987).

Over the past decade, researchers have also begun to shift their attention away from the negative aspects of the illness experience (including notions of stigma, loss of self, and biographical disruption and the need to cope with the personal and social challenges posed by chronic illness) toward a more optimistic view that emphasizes self-development and personal liberation. From this perspective, the pain and tragedy of illness also allow one the opportunity to reflectively reconstitute one's self and social relationships. For example, Williams (1984) focuses on the narrative reconstruction that occurs as those with long-term chronic illnesses try to create a sense of coherence, stability, and order in the aftermath of a biographically disruptive illness onset (Lawton, 2003). He notes that narrative reconstruction can be used to 'reconstitute and repair ruptures between body, self, and world by linking and interpreting different aspects of biography in order to realign present and past and self and society' (Williams, 1984: 197).

Along similar lines, Frank (1993, 1997), a Canadian sociologist who survived a heart attack and cancer in his late thirties, draws on narratives written by critical and chronic illness survivors in order to examine how those who are ill try to maintain or recover a sense of personhood. He notes that those whose lives are most affected by illness typically have little choice but to try and 'rise to the occasion' (1997). Yet illness also presents an opportunity for self-reflection and self-change and allows people to discover and mobilize personal resources to meet the crises it creates. As noted by Zaner (1994: 235), 'while clearly "disabling", illness or distress is at the same time among the most powerful and morally "enabling" of our experiences . . .'. Frank suggests that in the end it may even be possible to shift our attention away from the undesirability of illness to being 'successfully ill', a process in which people with illnesses succeed in living with them creatively and meaningfully (1997: 136). Not everyone accomplishes this goal; however, Frank (1993) proposes three typical change narratives that illness can bring about: (1) the rediscovery of the self who has always been; (2) the entirely new self who is in the process of becoming through the epiphany of illness; and (3) cumulative epiphanies involving a slow but constantly changing self constructed as people live with lifelong or very long-term illnesses. All three involve the creation of something new. This can be the discovery that one already had the resources necessary to deal with the life crises posed by serious illness. Frank refers to Robert F. Murphy's (1987) book entitled *The Body Silent*, which describes his experience of illness associated with the growth of a benign tumour in his spine as an example. While the illness brought about major changes in Murphy's life (including a transition from a position of academic power as chair of the anthropology department at Columbia University to one of complete physical dependence), at the same time, he was able to establish his identity by applying his academic and research skills to his own illness experience: 'This book was conceived in the realization that my long illness . . . has been a kind of extended anthropological trip . . .' (1987, ix; cited in Frank, 1993: 43). According to Frank, over the course of his illness, Murphy does not become a new self, but refines what he always was: '[u]nable to do "outside" research, the anthropologist journeys within' . . . (Frank, 1993: 44).

Finally, Bury (2000) suggests that in the past those with chronic illness and disabilities were perceived as passive and treated with a mixture of social control and care. Yet he contends that this has changed in recent times and that new, more active images now prevail. One such image of chronic illness and disability prevailing in contemporary times is referred to as 'the wounded storyteller'—someone who is no longer portrayed as a victim but as someone who finds strategies to deal with the effects of illness and disability, adopting lifestyles that refuse to accept these states as defeats. Another contemporary image is more political in nature and portrays the disabled individual as an activist, involved with others in collective action to maximize the integration of those who are chronically ill or disabled into mainstream society. For example, the disability movement has criticized the personal tragedy view of illness and disability adopted by medical sociologists. The main tenet of the movement is that disability is not really a characteristic of individuals but instead represents a product of social organization (Sanders, Donovan, and Dieppe, 2002).

However, the view that the illness experience is subjectively defined, that those who experience illness are actively involved in giving meaning to their experiences and in shaping their personal identities and sense of self, and that their illness experiences can be positive and liberating in nature has also been criticized as inadequate. Critics charge that it, like the objectivist view that preceded it, is one-dimensional:

> In contemporary writings on illness and disability . . ., even conflict perspectives are downplayed, as attention increasingly focuses on individual and collective action . . . Expert discourse is now replaced by the moral career and personal narratives of the sufferer, and patienthood is replaced by the rights of personhood. (Bury, 2000: 174)

Yet illness is a multi-dimensional experience and therefore requires that attention be paid to multiple levels of analysis (Kelly and Field, 1996).

Researchers also acknowledge that our interpretive understandings and opportunities for agency do not take place in a social vacuum but are also constrained and facilitated by structure and are consequently differentially accessible to those with varied social and economic circumstances. As Frank (1997) notes, individuals must decide how to live as an ill person—to sort out/construct their own version of an inter-subjective reality within organizational and cultural parameters. To address this issue, attention has been directed towards the ways in which social class, race/ethnicity, and other factors also serve to shape people's health and illness experiences. Wainwright and Forbes (2000) point to a number of studies that make useful contributions to our understanding of the inner world of health inequalities by providing interpretive accounts of how and why people within different social groups rationalize and explain their views on health. For example, while both working- and middle-class individuals tend to think of health as referring to an absence of illness, working-class persons often characterize health as a resource in their everyday lives, one that enables them to carry out their work and family responsibilities. Middle-class individuals, in contrast, appear more likely to refer to health using broader notions such as energy, positive attitudes, and an ability to cope well and to be in control of one's life (Calnan, 1987; Blaxter and Paterson, 1982). One author suggests that the sense of being in control may be particularly important to middle-class individuals insofar as it is consistent with their experiences of making decisions and being able to have some control over their work and daily lives. In contrast, working-class persons are likely to have somewhat less control over their lives and, as a result, this value may be less familiar to them (Freund and McGuire, 1999).

Along similar lines, Calnan (1987) points to social class differences in individuals' perceived abilities to prevent illness. While middle-class women believed they could prevent illness from taking hold, working-class women were more likely to view the experience of illness as a matter of fate or luck and therefore something over which they had minimal influence. Similarly, Mirowsky and Ross (1998) draw on the concept of human capital and suggest that education improves health because it increases individuals' abilities to exercise effective agency, arguing that health is not just a fortunate but accidental consequence of the economic prosperity that results from education. Education itself also enables people to perceive and exercise effective control over health and other outcomes in their lives. This in turn leads to better health through health enhancing behaviours.

Much less attention has been devoted to perceptions of health, other than the persistent finding that they tend to be positive, even when objective measures of disease and disability demonstrate the individual could be considered sick, even very sick. We do not know why this is the case. In response to satisfaction surveys, most people say they are satisfied or very satisfied with various aspects of their lives, even with housing that has been officially condemned! Are we so adaptable that what 'is' becomes normal and we are accepting of it? Are many objective diseases and conditions not particularly difficult to adjust to and live with?

On the other hand, we also know that most people define health in terms of physical criteria and often as the absence of disease and illness (Litva and Eyles, 1994; Simon et al., 2005). Interestingly though, when people are asked to talk about the personal meaning of being healthy, they answer differently. Litva and Eyles (1994) found that people often refer to the quality of life and psychological well-being when talking about being healthy. At the personal level, being healthy seems to refer to something more holistic than does health per se; it refers to something subjective. Other concepts such as wellness and level of fitness (including physical, mental, and social fitness) are sometimes used to convey this broader sense of well-being. This evidence leads to the possible conclusion that people refer to this broader sense of being healthy when conveying their perceptions of their own health.

HEALTH AND ILLNESS OVER THE LIFE COURSE

As noted in Chapter 1, we tend to focus on the here and now, forgetting that current and future circumstances are informed by the past and that such circumstances may or may not change in the future. Yet there is increasing recognition of the importance of such factors, particularly of the impact of inequality experiences in early years of life, for subsequent health problems. Early setbacks and deprivations can delay development and result in a sequence of negative outcomes in the future. Poor early childhood development can limit brain development, reduce language development, restrict capacity for communication and literacy, and result in poorer physical and mental health throughout life (CIHI, 2004a). Consistent with this view are associations between low birth weight and lower cognitive development at ages 7, 11, and 16 (Jefferis, Power, and Hertzman, 2002).

There are also indications that the negative effects of social deprivations and inequalities experienced early in life may in fact increase over time. Poorer people are less able to buy healthy foods, to afford adequate housing, to have access to efficient transportation, to live and work in environmentally 'friendly' places, and to have all the other basic requirements of living. This problem is compounded for children, whose life chances are compromised because they are more likely to have been born at low birth weight and are less likely to have food provided to them that is adequate for their health and growth. Such early deprivation multiplies. The effects of poverty on children increase as they age; this is exacerbated as they have less access to quality education, health care, and a myriad of other social circumstances associated with high morbidity and mortality.

Perhaps as a result, some factors seem to become more important in middle or later life and to result in greater gaps or inequalities in health over time. The gap in health appears to increase in size as people reach their middle years (forties to sixties), and then declines in old age (Martel et al., 2005). In Australia, Mishra and colleagues (2004) studied changes in the health of middle-aged and older women over time. They found clear SES differences in health for both cohorts. However, they also found greater declines across SES groups in middle-aged than older women. That is, greater declines in health (physical functioning, perceived health) were evident in the lower SES than in the higher SES group; there was less difference across SES groups within the older age cohort.

When we talk about those who experience poverty and inequality, we tend to assume stability of people's economic standing throughout their lives.

However, it is important to keep in mind that people experiencing low income are not necessarily the same people from month to month or year to year. Between 1993 and 1998, only 8 per cent of Canadians aged 16 to 59 were consistently in low-income households. Particular population groups tend to have high rates of persistent poverty; they include lone parents with at least one child under 18, people with a long-term disability, and off-reserve Aboriginal people (CIHI, 2004a).

Is persistent poverty worse for health than temporary setbacks? Alternatively, is newly experienced or intermittent poverty worse? These are complicated questions, for which we do not yet have adequate answers. A recent American study by McDonough and Berglund (2003) points to the greater importance of a persistent history of poverty for people's health but notes that falling incomes also had an impact. In an earlier study, McDonough et al. (1997) report finding that those who experienced an income loss of more than 50 per cent over a period of five years were 30 per cent more likely to die during this period than those who did not experience such a loss. The negative impact of income loss was particularly evident among those in the middle income group and increased their risk to a level similar to that of individuals with low incomes. In another study, conducted in the Netherlands, four groups of older adults were compared—those with lifetime low SES (measured using parent and own education), those with downward or upward mobility in SES, and those with lifetime high SES. The findings revealed that those with high SES or who were upwardly mobile were at lower risk of chronic diseases (men only), functional limitations, mortality, depression, and loneliness compared to those with a lifetime of low SES. However, few differences were found when comparing those with a lifetime of low SES and those who experienced downward mobility (Broese van Groneau, 2003).

CONCLUSIONS

Evidence that mortality and disability rates are declining and life expectancy is increasing in Canadian society suggests that our population's physical health may be improving. Since the 1950s, Fries (2000) has argued that population health status will improve in the future as public health improves and as people's lifestyles (including dietary and exercise patterns) improve. As a result, the period of morbidity or illness experienced prior to death would be compressed or shortened and, increasingly, people would live a relatively healthy life until they died, usually in very old age. This argument, known as the **compression of morbidity** hypothesis, continues to be debated today. On the one hand, there are repeated claims that baby boomers and younger adults are better educated and wealthier than older cohorts and consequently should have better health practices and better health. However, critics of this idea charge that we have added years to life but have been somewhat less successful in adding life (thus, health) to years, particularly among disadvantaged groups. We may be increasing the years that people live, but these added years are fraught with chronic illness and disability.

Others, focusing on the impact of structural inequalities on health, offer a considerably less optimistic scenario. They argue that while the incomes of Canadians are increasing on average, poverty and inequality are also increasing in Canada as well as in other developed nations. For example, inequality in the distribution of income increased in Canada from 1980 to 2001, including such areas as market income inequality (income from employment and investments), total income inequality (market income plus government transfers), and disposable income inequality (total income after taxes). The distribution of wealth (i.e., net worth) appears even more unequal. Over the past 30 years, the wealthiest 10 per cent of Canadian households increased their wealth by more than half a million dollars while the poorest 10 per cent experienced a reduction in overall wealth (CIHI, 2004a). To the extent that societies with greater class and socio-economic inequalities tend to have poorer health, the implications may include increasing inequalities in health. In the future some groups may experience improved health, while others may experience worse health than at the present time.

Questions for Critical Thought ───────────────────────────────

1. Outline the various ways that health has been defined. What are the implications of each of these views?
2. How does the health of Canadians compare to that of those living in other developed countries (such as Japan and the United States) and those living in less developed countries (such as Kenya and Afghanistan)?
3. Compare and contrast structural and cultural explanations of rural–urban and social class differences in health.
4. It has been observed that while women tend to be less healthy than men in their daily lives, they tend to live longer. How can this apparent paradox be explained?
5. Discuss biographical disruption as a result of illness.
6. Suggest some ways that illness experiences can be considered positive and liberating.

Suggestions for Further Reading ───────────────────────────

Bury, M. 1982. 'Chronic Illness as Biographical Disruption', *Sociology of Health & Illness* 4, 2: 167–82.

Clarke, J.N. 2008. *Health, Illness, and Medicine in Canada*, 5th edn. Don Mills, ON: Oxford University Press.

Frank, A. 1993. 'The Rhetoric of Self-Change: Illness Experience as Narrative', *Sociological Quarterly* 32, 1: 39–52.

McKinlay, J.B., and S.M. McKinlay. 1987. 'Medical Measures and the Decline of Mortality', in H.D. Schwartz, ed, *Dominant Issues in Medical Sociology*, 2nd edn., New York: Random House.

Raphael, D. 2006. 'Social Determinants of Health: An Overview of Concepts and

Issues', in D. Raphael, T. Bryant, and M. Rioux, eds, *Staying Alive: Critical Perspectives on Health, Illness and Health Care*. Toronto: Canadian Scholars' Press, 115–38.

Whittle, K.L., and K.L. Inhorn. 2001. 'Rethinking Difference: A Feminist Reframing of Gender/Race/Class for the Improvement of Women's Health Research', *International Journal of Health Services* 31, 1: 147–65.

Chapter 3

Self- and Informal Care

Learning Objectives:
In this chapter, you will learn that:

- We all engage in various forms of self-care, both in health and in illness.
- The personal determinants of health consist of both health beliefs and behaviours, including positive health behaviours, risk avoidance, maintenance, and prevention.
- Health beliefs and behaviours vary by social class, gender, race, or ethnic group but do not easily cluster into a 'healthy lifestyle' despite the popularity of the notion.
- Health beliefs and health practices are related in complex ways.
- Informal care is much more prominent than formal care when we are ill.
- Self- and informal care during illness are socially constructed and vary by structural factors, sometimes in unexpected ways.
- The current trend toward economic globalization is increasing demands on informal caregivers.

INTRODUCTION

The discussion of caring for ourselves, or self-care, typically focuses on illness and the formal health-care system. Although less attention is paid to care when we are healthy, we engage in self-care at all times. Even when we are ill, we often continue caring for ourselves and usually involve our family and friends in our care both prior to and while obtaining services from the formal health-care system. In this chapter, we focus on self-care in health and in illness, as well as on informal care (received from family members and friends) when our health fails.

Once again, we examine self- and informal care from social psychological perspectives and then from structural perspectives. As Walker (1996) notes though, one effect of the dichotomous scientific construction of the social world, in this instance of social psychological and of structural approaches, is to imply less interaction between them than is found in reality. We must therefore be mindful of how both levels interact with one another as well as their relationships with the meso level of social interaction. Examples of these interconnections are provided throughout. We begin with an understanding of self-care, what it consists of, and what we do to care for ourselves.

SELF-CARE WHEN HEALTHY

Although self-care is a term commonly used in everyday parlance, it is elusive to define. In fact, researchers have been unable to agree upon a definition. A panel of 15 experts who were asked to develop a consensual definition of the term, failed to do so. Gantz (1990) reports that they listed 80 descriptors of self-care and 56 barriers. They did specify four characteristics that all panel members from different disciplines agreed described the concept: situational and cultural specificity; individual agency; affects of knowledge, skills, values, motivation, locus of control, and efficacy; and inclusion of only aspects of health care for which the individual has some control. Generally, **self-care** refers to any form of caring behaviour that we ourselves initiate. Another person, such as a heath-care provider, does not instruct us to do it. To some researchers self-care also includes making personal decisions about what behaviours to engage in and about the management of health-care resources. The essence of self-care is control by individuals themselves, not by others (Segall and Goldstein, 1989). Dean (1981) and Levin and Idler (1983) noted that self-care is the basic, primary, and dominant form of health care among the many informal and formal resources an individual might access concerning his or her own health. The notion of self-care draws attention to the fact that we are all health-care providers, health-care consumers, and health producers. It includes decisions and actions taken to promote and maintain our health (positive health behaviours) and to prevent illness, as well as the evaluation of symptoms, decisions about action to take or not to take when evaluating those symptoms, and treatment practices.

Self-care includes risk avoidance behaviours such as wearing seatbelts, not smoking, and not drinking alcohol to excess; preventive behaviours such as dental check ups and immunizations; and positive health behaviours such as eating nutritionally, exercising regularly, and getting enough rest (these can also be viewed as preventive behaviours). A decision not to engage in a particular behaviour (e.g., smoking) also constitutes self-care. The actions we take may not actually maintain or promote our health, but if we engage in them because we believe they do, they are considered self-care. It is our motivation for engaging in them rather than resulting effects on our health that is important.

The concept of self-care is relevant throughout the life course. In addition to immediate impact (such as a deadly car crash after excessive alcohol consumption), our health behaviours have medium- and long-term influences.

Those who engage in healthy lifestyles are less likely to lose their good health, even in advancing age (Martel et al., 2005).

Self-care typically includes an interest in **personal determinants of health**, primarily our health beliefs and our personal health behaviours. Examples of self-care are readily available from national data collected regularly by Health Canada. Their *National Population Health Survey* conducted in 1994–95 (Health Canada, 1997) reveals that 77 per cent of middle-aged Canadians (aged between 45 and 64 years) are more concerned with the amount of fat they consume than any other age group (see Table 3.1). The majority of those who believe that they are consuming too much fat (86 per cent) are taking action to reduce that intake, such as eating fewer fried or deep-fried foods, using fewer high-fat milk products, and so on. Interestingly, the proportion of those doing something about their concern increases as age increases—86 per cent of 20- to 24-year-olds are taking action while 92 per cent of those 65 and older are doing so.

In the same survey, 44 per cent of Canadians say they are concerned about having enough starch and fibre in their diets. Those aged 20 to 24 are less concerned than those aged 65 and older. Again, most of those who believe they should eat more starch and fibre are taking action: 60 per cent are eating fruits and vegetables at most meals, eating whole-grain products, eating less meat, choosing foods high in fibre, or taking other similar actions to increase their intake. As age increases so too does the tendency to take action on this front: 59 per cent of those aged 20 to 24 are doing something about their concern, while 65 per cent of those aged 45 to 64 are.

Sociologists are interested in health beliefs because it is thought that they are related to our behaviours. **Personal health behaviours** include a wide range of activities undertaken in an effort to maintain good health. We select certain foods to eat, engage in exercise, ensure rest, and avoid or limit smoking and alcohol consumption. We wash our hands (especially after the SARS scare); we install smoke detectors and air filters in our homes, and cross the street at crosswalks, all in order to try to ensure our health and safety. Canadians are well aware of the importance of personal health practices. Eyles and colleagues (2001) asked Prince Edward Islanders about the factors they believe affect our health. Members of the public, family physicians, health-service providers, support staff, program managers, senior managers, and board members were asked to rank personal health practices, employment, formal health care, education, healthy child development, income, social support, or the physical environment as important factors that influence health. They ranked personal health practices first, ahead of all the other factors.

Considerable information on individual behaviours is available. In 1996–97, only 21 per cent of Canadians aged 12 and older were physically active (defined in terms of total energy expenditure for all leisure-time physical activities; greater than or equal to 3.0 cal/kg/day), dropping until age 24, then showing stability thereafter; 23 per cent were moderately active and 57 per cent

Table 3.1   Canadian's Concerns with Healthy Eating

	AGE				
	12–19	20–24	25–44	45–64	65+
Concerned with:					
Amount of fat consumed	45%	63%	N/A	77%	73%
Sufficient starch and fibre	N/A	36%	N/A	N/A	55%

Source: Health Canada. 1997. *Canadians and Healthy Eating: How Are We Doing?* Reproduced with the Permission of the Minister of Public Works and Government Services Canada, 2008.

inactive. Among young adults and youth (those aged 12 to 24), 35 per cent are optimally active, 24 per cent moderately active, and 40 per cent inactive (Health Canada, 1999c). (See Box 3.1 on obesity.)

In terms of drinking alcohol and smoking, three-quarters of Canadians had a drink over the past 12 months, but among those who consumed alcohol, the figure drops to just over a third who do so at least once a week. Men consume more than women (48 per cent of men compared with 25 per cent of women

Box 3.1
Obesity

As in other countries, rates of obesity are rising in Canada. A third of Canadians who were of normal weight in 1994–95 became overweight by 2002–03; almost a quarter of those who had been overweight became obese. In 2000–01, an estimated 3 million Canadians were obese (15 per cent of the population) and an estimated 6 million were overweight. However, at the present time, our rates lag behind those found in the United States, where 1 in 5 adults is obese (21 per cent).

The relationship between weight gain and selected personal health behaviours is complex. Among overweight women, those who drink occasionally are 50 per cent less likely to become obese than overweight women who never drink. A similar pattern was less strong among men. Several factors might explain this finding. It is speculated that alcohol increases the metabolic rate, burning more calories. Those who drink occasionally may also engage in healthy eating habits. Overweight individuals are often restricted in their physical activity, which leads to obesity. Physical activity seems to be protection against becoming obese for women but not for men. Overweight men who smoke are more at risk of becoming obese.

Source: LePetit and Berthelot. 2005. Based on National Population Health Surveys conducted between 1994–95 and 2002–03.

drink at least once a week). Fewer Canadians smoke—a quarter do so on a daily basis. Men are only somewhat more likely to smoke than are women (26 per cent v. 21 per cent) (Health Reports, 2001).

The Individual and Self-Care

There is much research in this area conducted from a social psychological perspective. We all hold beliefs about what makes us healthy and what makes us sick. Our beliefs provide meaning to our experiences by offering interpretive frameworks explaining health and illness; they can influence the behaviours we engage in and have important implications for our health. For example, older adults tend to interpret common health concerns (also known as **general symptomatology**) as simply part of aging. That is, they normalize symptoms such as weakness, aches, and pains, tending not to view them as warning signs of specific illnesses (Leventhal and Prohaska, 1986). This has obvious implications in terms of early detection for certain illnesses. Interestingly though, Simon and colleagues (2005) report that those who normalize age-related physical and functional decline are less bothered by the accompanying symptoms.

An important factor in good health is a sense of coherence, which helps shape our beliefs and decisions about our health. For Antonovsky (1979), a sense of coherence is a general orientation that reveals itself in a pervasive and enduring feeling of confidence that our internal and external environments are predictable. Coherence and predictability are the key ideas within this concept. Later, Antonovsky (1987) posited the three core components of a **sense of coherence** as comprehensibility (a belief that the world is ordered, consistent, and predictable), manageability (a sense of confidence in our ability to cope with life's problems), and meaningfulness (a belief that areas of life make sense to us emotionally and are worth commitment).

The **Health Belief Model** (Rosenstock, 1974) focuses on the subjective experience of decision-making to engage or not engage in health behaviours, positing that people are motivated to act if they perceive the severity of the disease and their susceptibility to getting sick as greater than their risk if they do not take a particular action. Both perceived barriers and perceived benefits of behavioural adoption also influence the decision. The person's perception of their ability to adopt the behaviour and the influence of external cues promoting it were later acknowledged. Proposed in the early 1970s, when there was little focus on health promotion and disease prevention and the importance of social factors were only beginning to be recognized, the Health Belief Model has been popular among researchers who have drawn upon it to explain, for example, how individuals decide to conduct breast self-examinations, to comply with chronic disease regimens, to receive vaccinations, and to quit smoking (Weiss and Lonnquist, 1997). The model has, however, been criticized as being disease specific, not considering general health promotion or disease prevention, and assuming rational and purposive action when determining health behaviour

(Pescosolido et al., 2001; Young, 2004), thereby ignoring the social factors that may influence choices. Such criticisms are justified and demonstrate the evolving nature of our thinking in the areas of medical sociology and the sociology of health and health care.

Many kinds of health-related beliefs can be studied—the controllability of our health or a particular illness, our susceptibility, and the seriousness and severity of a particular problem, among others. Within this area, there tends to be an assumption, adopted from a biomedical model of ill health, that each disease has a specific cause. However, some researchers argue that this approach is erroneous (Evans and Stoddart, 1990). They posit that we should be examining the individual's **host response** or **general susceptibility** to ill health. In essence, they argue that we each have a general susceptibility to illness per se rather than to one particular illness—if we found a cure for cancer, the individual who would have contracted cancer may now become ill with another serious disease. Although there is no consensus on this issue, if it is true, it has important implications for preventive health care at both the individual and structural levels.

As already noted, interest in beliefs is rooted in their relationship to behaviours. Personal health behaviours are part of our lifestyle or general orientation toward life (Wister, 2005a and 2005b), as are our beliefs and values. We often talk about healthy or unhealthy lifestyles. Over 25 years ago, Harris and Guten (1979) identified three dominant positive health behaviours: what we eat, how much we sleep or rest, and how much we exercise. However, despite the intuitive appeal and general usage of the term, most research has failed to confirm the existence of a clustering of our personal health behaviours; that is, those who have good nutritional practices are not necessarily also physically fit, tend not to smoke or drink, and so forth. The exception seems to be a moderate association between smoking and drinking (Krick and Sobal, 1990). In terms of other behaviours, however, we seem to eat both healthy and unhealthy foods, perhaps have a spinach salad with our dinner but have cheesecake for dessert. Alternatively, we may exercise well during the week without any alcohol consumption but not exercise and drink a lot on the weekends. The complexity of the area is reflected in the lack of clarity of the concept of **lifestyle**. There is no consensus in theory or practice as to what constitutes a healthy lifestyle. Added complications arise from the difficulty of collecting valid data in this area and from inconclusive knowledge. For example, it is difficult to document actual nutritional intake of a variety of foods knowing that nutritional content may vary within foods—one apple may contain a different nutrient density than another apple even of the same type. Similarly, although we used to be told that oat bran was exceptionally good for us and that jogging was better than walking, both claims have since fallen from favour.

Research tends not to distinguish between routine and spontaneous activity; it looks for logically consistent behaviour patterns. Perhaps most of us most of the time engage in health behaviours in complex and illogical ways, trading off positive and negative behaviours to balance overall health (or to balance what are perceived as beneficial versus 'fun' behaviours) (Backett, Davison, and Mullen, 1994). Part of the appeal of the concept, however, is its suggestion that good health is within our control and therefore can potentially help us obtain healthier lives.

We also know little about the cumulative effects of engaging in several negative behaviours. In some instances they would appear to be additive. For example, some research suggests that the more risky behaviours adolescents engage in, the more likely they are to sustain injury. Pickett and colleagues (2002) show that, among Canadians aged 11 to 15, those engaged in multiple high-risk behaviours (seven or more) experience rates of injury over four times higher than those who reported no high-risk behaviours. The relationship was especially strong in relation to severe and multiple injuries.

Whether and the extent to which beliefs lead to certain behaviours is of great interest. In situations where they are not related, there is little point expending resources to convince people to change their beliefs. If those with diabetes know that nutritional intake is key to self-management but cannot act on this belief, educational sessions will not be effective. In many areas, we know there is a relationship between the two. For example, beliefs about the negative health effects of smoking are part of the explanation as to why some young people do not smoke. Why then do some teenagers continue to smoke? Although a minority, some people still deny the health risks of smoking. In 2001, for example, 18 per cent of the US population said that we do not know for sure if smoking is a major cause of lung cancer. Another US survey found that 12 per cent said 'no' or 'don't know' when asked whether they believe smoking increases their risk of getting lung cancer. Interestingly, smokers perceive that they are more likely than non-smokers to experience a wide range of physical conditions, including some that are unrelated to smoking, such as getting the flu, having an accident, becoming sterile, or developing cirrhosis of the liver (Krosnick et al., 2006). This appears consistent with their belief in a generalized susceptibility or host response, as discussed earlier. Among smokers, advertising-based beliefs about smoking addictiveness and the dangers of environmental tobacco smoke are related to considerations of quitting, as are beliefs about the deceptive advertising practices engaged in by the tobacco industry (Netmeyer, Andrews, and Burton, 2005).

The extent to which we believe there are health risks seems to vary depending on the type of risk involved. Based on discussion groups conducted with a range of people 'off the street', Petts (2004) reports little awareness of the health impacts of air pollution. When asked about risks to health, respondents did not mention air pollution unless prompted. When raised, a link between air pollution and increasing traffic was recognized but not seen as a serious health concern, even among those who had bronchial, lung, or heart diseases. Older people saw air pollution as something that had occurred in the past ('pea souper' smog of the 1950s), and teenagers had difficulty believing it caused serious health problems, even among those with asthma.

In contrast, knowledge and concern about immunization was evident. Parents in Petts's group believed immunization was good and many had had older children immunized. New concerns about side effects (such as a link with autism) elicited fear, stress, and anger that a previously accepted and even habitual behaviour (they would have their children immunized without having to think about it) may not be safe. Women explained their beliefs in terms of enhanced concerns about their children's health and their responsibility for making correct decisions that would protect their children. This is in contrast to air pollution, where respondents either passively distanced responsibility to others in society or actively transferred responsibility to government and industry. That is, additional information did not translate into empowerment—instead, people began to stay indoors or to adapt medication for better relief on days when pollution levels were high.

An emphasis on personal health beliefs and behaviours recognizes the role of human agency in the health of the individual. However, an exclusive focus on beliefs and behaviours has been criticized as inevitably leading towards **blaming the victim**. That is, if someone experiences health problems, it is considered his or her 'fault' for engaging in negative health behaviours or not engaging in sufficient or appropriate positive health behaviours. While available research demonstrates that our health behaviours are important for health outcomes, the relative importance of individual health behaviours compared with other social structural factors such as structured inequality, is the subject of debate (Lantz et al., 1998; Williamson, 2000). In addition, the beliefs and behaviours that we choose are themselves influenced by our position within the structured inequalities of society. As becomes evident in the next section, sociology is uniquely equipped to understand these more macro forces that help shape our beliefs and actions regarding health and that have their own independent impact on our health.

Structural Determinants of Self-Care

As already noted, the social determinants of health approach highlights the impact of differences in access to material living conditions and resources for health. People vary in terms of the quantity and quality of physical, social, and personal resources, including income, food, housing, employment, health, and social services, that are available to them (Raphael, 2006). Structural determinants are also related to self-care.

Socio-economic status, for example, is related to our health beliefs and behaviours. Those in lower-income groups tend to believe in the value and practice of preventive behaviours less than those in higher-income groups (D'Arcy, 1998). Martel and colleagues (2005) analyzed Canada's *National Population Health Survey* (*NPHS*) for the years 1994–2003 for adults aged 45 and older. They reported that education level is significantly associated with maintaining good health from middle to older age, arguing that better-educated individuals are more likely to be aware of health risks, to adopt healthy behaviours, and to use medical services more effectively than those with less formal education (see also Public Health Agency of Canada, 2002). Others note that adult smokers from higher social classes are more likely to quit than those from lower social classes, probably due to their access to and use of effective resources for quitting as well as more restrictive home environments (Honjo et al., 2006). Such factors may assume lesser importance for those in lower social classes, given the broader conditions of their lives.

Social inequality is not the only influence on health behaviours. Pickett and colleagues (2002), referred to above, reported that injuries increase in number and severity with the number of risky behaviours engaged in for those of lower as well as higher socio-economic status. Yong, Borland, and Siahpush (2005) found that older smokers (aged 60 and older) perceived themselves as less vulnerable to the harmful effects of smoking and were less concerned about the health effects, less confident they could quit, less likely to perceive any health benefits from quitting, and less willing to quit, despite social class level. These examples suggest that we still have much to learn about the influence of socio-economic status and class relations.

Women and men experience social class positions differently. Even today, opportunities are structured differently in Canadian society depending on whether one is male or female. Women are excluded from certain labour force opportunities and still earn less than men. Women tend to have more friends and to establish and maintain family and friend networks throughout their lives (Chappell, 1992; Moore and Rosenberg, 1994). They continue to be the main caregivers (see below), both when raising children and when caring for those who are ill or disabled. Furthermore, as noted in Chapter 2, even women and men in similar positions may experience them differently. For example, women are more likely to carry both labour force and domestic responsibilities and consequently to experience more home-to-work spillover (Flack, 2000). In past years, unemployment might have been less significant for women because, until recently, men were expected to be employed while women were not necessarily so. Differential health beliefs, health behaviours, and ultimately health implications may result.

There are other gender differences as well. As we saw in Chapter 2, women tend to report more illness than men, yet they tend to live longer and, as will become evident in Chapter 4, also use more medical services. Women tend to use more medications (both over-the-counter and prescription) than men, which is partly explained by their greater symptomatology. Women are generally the communicators within the family when it comes to the subject of health and therapies. Mothers monitor their own and other family members' well-being and tend to be more knowledgeable than other family members about health matters. These findings are consistent across several Western countries (Obermeyer et al., 2004).

In terms of self-care in health, women are more willing to use preventive services, to seek help when ill, and to adopt illness behaviours (Cecile et al., 1999). With this as their point of departure, Green and Pope (1999) analyzed data from a large US household survey and found that gender predicts utilization of health services (including preventive services) even when controlling for self-reported health, symptom level, and psychosocial and behavioural factors (women used more services). Furthermore, gender (along with age) predicts utilization over the long term, becoming more important over longer time periods. Whether gender becomes a better proxy of changing social factors over time or gender differences in morbidities become more important as we age, or both, is unknown. Importantly, health knowledge does not predict a decision to seek formal services, but attitudinal and behavioural measures do. This suggests that media strategies aimed at transmitting information and educating people about certain illnesses may not be effective in influencing their use of various services.

Gender differences, though, are not always straightforward. For example, the belief that smoking is less damaging to your health than suggested allows a young person (sixth- to twelfth-graders in one United States study) to begin the habit more readily, but this belief operates differently among boys than girls. Beliefs about the health effects of smoking insulate girls from doing so only when they also highly value their health. If they do not, such beliefs do not inhibit the behaviour. Among boys, beliefs about health risks due to smoking are an insulating factor irrespective of the value they place on their health (Krosnick et al., 2006).

Men and women respond differently when it comes to health messages, at least in some areas. Humpel and colleagues (2004) studied changes in moderately intense walking activity in association with perceptions of change in the local environment. Both men and women were more than twice as likely to increase their walking after perceiving greater convenience within the neighbourhood. However, in response to lessened traffic, men were 61 per cent *less* likely to have increased their walking whereas women were 76 per cent *more* likely to have done so. Gender differences extend to proactive health beliefs in terms of the protective effects of marriage for men but not necessarily for women; recent research (Markey et al., 2005) finds that married men are more likely to adopt proactive health beliefs than those who are not married—the same is not the case for married women.

Racial and ethnic status is also related to self-care. As we learned in Chapter 2, many Aboriginal and ethnic minority people in Canada live in conditions that are not conducive to good health. Reviewing 118 countries, Zong and Li (1994) conclude that economic conditions and not cultural influences are responsible for differences in life expectancy and infant mortality rates. Furthermore, it is not clear that people living in these conditions hold more negative health beliefs than others. For example, McKinnon and colleagues (1991) find that Native youth in Alberta are more knowledgeable about dental health, fire safety, and the effects of smoking, alcohol, and drugs than their non-Native counterparts. On the other hand, they know less than non-Native youth about first aid for burns, nutrition, communicable diseases, and personal health.

Both Chinese and Indian societies have traditional holistic notions of health that combine body, mind, and spirituality, encompassing all of life. Asian cultures generally embrace a collectivism that contrasts with North American individualism. Decision-making is often a family rather than an individual undertaking and, in the case of older adults, may be assigned to other family members, such as the eldest son (McLaughlin and Braun, 1998). The welfare of the social unit, usually the family, comes before that of the individual. Preserving harmony is especially important to Asians, who are often reluctant to share bad news concerning health. Health care is often not accessed until very late in the disease process but once it is, great respect and unquestioning acceptance of care providers is the norm (Chappell and Kusch, 2007; Whyte, 2004).

In addition, the high value placed on cognitive function and reason in the West differs significantly from the value that the Chinese place on affectivity as prior to and more authentic than reason. In this concept, both heart and mind encompass a dual concept of the self, reflected in beliefs about balance and nurturing of both aspects for good health. Especially in the early stages of mental illness, this translates into an acceptance that the person is still 'there', and an acceptance as part of the group with rights to participation in social interaction. In terms of dementia-specific beliefs, we know that in both China (Ikels, 2002) and the United States (Hicks and Lam, 1999; Hinton, Fox, and Levkoff, 1999), the Chinese view dementia largely as a part of normal aging. Chinese families will often not consider it very salient in terms of their interaction with or judgment of the older adult (Ikels, 1998; 2002).

It might be expected that age would be related to health consciousness. Indeed, Lawton (2002) finds that older participants in her study are more health conscious than younger age groups, a relationship that is stronger than gender or class variations. Older people are more likely to perceive the certainty of ill health and good health in their futures, while younger persons are more likely to see them only as possibilities. However, the threats of morbidity and mortality are related to embodied ill-health rather than chronological age per se; the fact that older people are more likely to experience morbidity translates into more older people being health conscious. However, older people who do not experience ill-health are not more health conscious. Changes in lifestyle are motivated reactively by ill-health experiences. These findings are important because they suggest that the embodied experience of ill-health is a prerequisite for perceiving the need to take action, at least a partial explanation for why it is so difficult to motivate younger adults to change their health behaviours.

While research has delved into the health beliefs and practices in many areas, there are others that we still know little about. Gay and lesbian health beliefs and practices is one such area, although Coleman and colleagues (1993) report that lesbian mothers believe their own and their children's social and psychological needs are best met through informal means. These include self-help groups, support groups, and parenting classes. They want health-care professionals who are sensitive to their needs. We also know little about the effect of the media on health beliefs and practices. However, excessive television viewing has been linked to obesity development, increased energy consumption, reduced energy expenditure, negative body-image development, and reduced concern with self-care (Wadsworth and Thompson, 2005). The effects on children and youth are of particular concern, both in terms of their vulnerability to the messages that are provided and also the potential for long-term damage to their health. This is another area where we have much to learn.

Social Interaction

Sociological interest in the area of social interaction is twofold: interaction as a social determinant and as a major care system in its own right. Family and friends constitute the dominant care system within all societies. In other words, it is informal care and not the formal care system that provides the vast majority of care when our health fails. When we are healthy, social interactions, including both supportive and negative interactions, are a part of our daily lives. We are all embedded in networks of family, friends, acquaintances, and strangers. When we become ill we draw on these networks of informal care. In health and in illness, social networks serve as the venue for the exchange of opinions, information, and affection and they constitute our social worlds where meaning is constructed, reconstituted, and negotiated, providing an approach to the study of health and illness that is the middle ground between micro and macro sociological perspectives (Pescosolido, 1992; Young, 2004).

Demographic data reveal that the composition of families is changing. We are living longer and, for the first time in history, virtually everyone in our society can expect to live to old age, barring accidental death, war, and suicide. Although we are living longer, fertility is decreasing. This, together with increased longevity, means that there can be several generations of one family alive at one time (**vertical extension**), but that each generation has fewer members (**horizontal shrinkage**). Beanpole families—those with four and even five generations still alive (Qualls, 1993)—have increased but are not common and never will be, partly because of the increased age of child-bearing (Rosenthal, 2000). When women are in their thirties before having their first child, it limits the number of generations who can be alive at one time, unless longevity increases as well.

Change in family forms is occurring within other societal changes. Fewer families take the nuclear family form of mother, father, and child(ren); more alternative family forms are apparent, including gay and lesbian unions, lone-parent families, and reconstituted or blended families. Multi-generational families living together are not popular in Western societies, although this family form is more evident among certain ethnic groups. Among Chinese Canadian families, for example, it is not uncommon for elderly parents to live with one of their children and his or her family, even when both parents are still living. Among non-ethnic North Americans, older parents seldom live with a child, even in severe frailty, as long as they are both alive to look after one another (Chappell and Kusch, 2007). Attitudes about multi-generational living are linked to past living arrangements; those who grew up in a multi-generational houschold or who lived with their parents as adults before they married have more positive attitudes towards living with their parents as their parents age (Goldscheider and Lawton, 1998). Living in multi-generational households when young predisposes people to view multi-generational living positively and to bring aging parents into their homes (Szinovacz, 1997).

Even though multi-generational living is not strong among non-ethnic groups in Canada, we see a prolonged period before children leave the parental home. Recent statistics show 41 per cent of those aged 20 to 29 lived with their parents in 2001. Among this group, the figure is 19 per cent for women and 29 per cent for men (Statistics Canada, 2004a). Using national data, Mitchell, Wister, and Gee (2002) report that the strongest predictor of Canadian adults aged 25 to 34 living at home is emotional closeness to the mother when growing up. We also see children returning to the parental home after they have left—the **boomerang kids**. In 2001, about 33 per cent of men and 28 per cent of women aged 20 to 29 returned home at least once after initially leaving (Statistics Canada, 2004a).

These children are not failures who have been unable to attain full adult status (Mitchell, 2000; Gee, Mitchell, and Wister, 1995). Approximately 25 per cent returned home for reasons of financial difficulty and another 19 per cent to save money (many indicated that they could afford to live on their own). Diminished opportunity structures in the labour market and a welcoming family are important factors, pointing to a source of inequality among today's young adults; those who are able to return home have social and economic advantages that others may lack (Mitchell and Gee, 1996).

The examples of multi-generational families and boomerang children demonstrate how families help one another throughout their lives and not only when illness strikes. Intergenerational exchanges vary by age and life course stage (Stone, Rosenthal, and Connidis, 1998), in sync with changing needs of each generation over time. Parents receive the most help when they are at advanced ages; children receive the most help from parents when they are young and when they are raising their own children. The help that children receive from their parents is instrumental, largely in the form of child care and financial assistance. Soldo and Hill (1995) also report substantial amounts of money transfers from older parents to children. Limited research on aging gays and lesbians suggests that they have fewer intergenerational supports, largely due to intrafamilial discrimination (Blando, 2001; Cahill, South, and Spade, 2000).

Within the family, siblings hold a special place. The sibling relationship often lasts longer than any other family tie and siblings almost always share a common cultural background, genetic pool, and early life experiences. They tend to keep in touch throughout their lives; they have been characterized as 'standing ready' should help be needed. Older adults report feeling closer to siblings than to any other relatives except their own children and perhaps their spouses. Siblings are especially important to the never-married, the childless, the divorced, and the widowed (Connidis, 2001). Among today's seniors, approximately 80 to 85 per cent have at least one living sibling. This figure will change as the reduced fertility rates of recent times move along the demographic journey; when today's university students reach old age, many more will have no siblings. An extreme case is found in present-day China, where the success of the one-child policy in urban areas means that these cohorts are journeying throughout life without siblings.

Social networks such as families encourage healthy lifestyles and promote preventive health-care use. Berkman and Syme's classic study (1979) demonstrated that those who had more contacts with friends and relatives, who were married, and who were involved in groups including church membership (formed into an index that refers to **social connectedness**) adopt more positive health behaviours. The complex ways in which different groups affect our health beliefs and behaviours are well illustrated in research on smoking. Krosnick and colleagues (2006) report that peers, by their behaviours and their subjective norms, are the most powerful influence on smoking onset among sixth to twelfth graders. Parents' behaviour, including whether they smoked themselves, but not their attitude towards their children's smoking, is also influential. However, parents' behaviour appears less important than that of their children's peers. Furthermore, parents' behaviour is influential only for those children who wish to comply with their parents' wishes. For children who are not so motivated, parents' behaviour has no effect. Siblings also influence smoking behaviour, but only for same-sex siblings. That is, if older sisters smoke, then younger sisters are more likely to begin and if older brothers smoke, younger brothers are more likely to begin.

Social interaction, though, can also be negative. Indeed, much interaction includes both positive and negative elements, despite an assumption evident in much of the early research in this area that interaction is necessarily supportive; measures typically identified interaction without assessing its supportiveness. Categorizations of types of social support often incorporate negative interaction, but supportiveness is assumed in measurement. One example is Cohen and Syme's (1985) three-fold classification schema that includes the following: (1) emotional support; (2) information that may or may not lead to confirmation or heightening of self-esteem; and (3) tangible support, such as assistance with activities of daily living. House and Kahn's (1985) categorization distinguishes between social networks, social support, and social integration. Social networks are relationships described in terms of their structure, using such terms as their density or homogeneity; **social support** refers only to the functional content of social relationships, such as emotional concern, instrumentality, and information; and **social integration** and **isolation** refer to the existence or quantity of relationships.

There is increasing research on negative interaction with others or interaction that includes elements of both the positive and negative. However, the overwhelming majority focuses on supportiveness. For example, families include positive, neutral, and negative contact with other members. Although it may not be socially acceptable to discuss the difficult aspects of family life, it should not be surprising that conflict is a normal part of families, given the emotional context of these interactions. Over the last 20 years, there has been growing recognition that some families harbour conflict of such severity that it can be referred to as neglect and abuse. **Abuse** can be of different types: physical, emotional, and financial. The role of families in abuse is evident when looking at the statistics for elder abuse—almost three-quarters of elder abuse is perpetrated by either the spouse or adult children (Statistics Canada, 2002g). Sometimes, this abuse began much earlier in life; other times, perpetrators transfer the abuse that they suffered in their own lives. However, much of this type of behaviour is hidden. Wiehe (1998) estimates that only 1 in 14 cases comes to the attention of authorities. There is some suggestion from both small qualitative studies and large population-based studies that contrary to popular belief and to official statistics, abuse of men could be greater than that of women (Pillemer and Finkelhor, 1988; Pritchard, 2002). Cultural prescriptions of images of men and, relatedly, the way in which abuse becomes defined could account for this.

Friendships are different from family relationships, characterized more by voluntary involvement, affective bonds, and consensus, and less by obligation than are kin ties. Our friends are likely to be age peers, to be similar to us in such characteristics as gender and socio-economic status, to share common experiences, and to have lived through similar transitions in society. They are especially important for companionship, emotional support, affection, and quick integration (Chappell, 1983; Lee, 1985). Friendships tend to fade away and reactivate if circumstances permit rather than to end on a bad note. As we journey throughout our lives, we accumulate a large number of social relationships. The concept of **convoy of social support** depicts the dynamic aspect of social interaction over time (Antonucci, 1985).

Structured Interaction

Even when we are not ill, informal networks are structured by our social position and vary by the same social determinants we have been discussing as affecting self-care. For example, the social networks of women and men differ from one another. Married men typically rely more on their wives for emotional support, whereas women rely more on their children and their friends (Gurung,

Taylor, and Seeman, 2003). Similarly, Lynch (1998) reports that among their larger social network of spouses, children, and friends or other relatives, men perceive the most positive support as coming from their wives, while women perceive the most positive support as coming from their children. Interestingly, perceptions of positive support do not increase with age but remain largely stable. However, perceptions of how demanding all three types of relationships are decrease across age groups. Yet such perceptions do not differ by gender; men and women perceive others to be just as demanding. (See Chapter 5 for a discussion of social capital.)

Gender differences are especially dramatic in the area of child care; women are the ones who nurture, socialize, and raise society's children. This entrenched gendered division of labour in parenting is especially poignant for men who take on this role. Even though the social and economic contexts of our lives are changing as more Canadian women work in paid labour and have fewer children, and as more fathers adopt the primary child care role, it is still uncommon for men to be the main nurturers of children In a study of Canadian fathers who are primary caregivers of their children (primarily stay-at-home and single fathers), Doucet (2006) reveals the very feminine world of raising children. The fathers in this study, like those in others (e.g., Pruett, 2000; Parke, 1996), described their caregiving as characterized by physical play, much activity had a 'rough' edge. It included more physical risk-taking and outdoor adventures. They were aware of parenting differently than mothers and spoke about mothers' emotional connections with their children established through pregnancy, birth, and breast-feeding. Importantly, fathers were made aware that they are living in a woman's world; playgroups, playgrounds, schools, homes of other children, and girls' sleepovers are all primarily woman-centred. Within such contexts, men were often treated as outsiders, experiencing suspicion, lack of acceptance, and scrutiny. Concern when it comes to girls' sleepovers was so powerful that some fathers avoid them. Most men eventually became accepted—by 'proving' themselves, by having particular women (sometimes their wives) helping to bridge their relationships with mothers, and by meeting other mothers in public places where heterosexual meanings were less likely to imbue cross-gender interaction.

Most of the fathers in Doucet's study noted that it is becoming easier as more dads become primary caregivers to their children, revealing their awareness that gendered roles not only structure our experiences but also shape new meanings for those very roles. While social structure typically evolves slowly, it is nevertheless dynamic in nature. Fathers as primary parents illustrate the interaction between structure and agency, wherein our enactment of roles is neither inflexible nor unchangeable. We have agency in how we choose to live within societal structures, and our enactment in turn influences that structure in the future.

We have only touched upon a few of the many studies of self-care and informal support during healthy times. Although not receiving as much attention as during times of illness, it is nevertheless an important and popular area of research. The discussion above is intended to provide a sampling of the questions and issues that fall within the area and to suggest that sociology, as a discipline, has much to offer by way of helping us understand the complex world within which we live. We turn now to self- and informal care in times of ill health, an area in which researchers have been busy for several decades.

SELF-CARE WHEN ILL

The Lived Experience of Self-Care when Ill

A **self-care model** of illness views lay persons as being at the centre of health care and therefore as the primary providers of health care. Self-care in the face of illness involves self-assessment, self-monitoring, and self-treatment. It includes consultation with family members, friends, and formal care providers; decisions regarding such things as what health-care professionals to see (if any), what medications to take (if any), and what other treatment options to use for symptom management (especially pain and discomfort); and management of our emotions, including fear, anxiety, and frustration. Our daily routines must often be adapted either to maintain activities or to postpone or cancel them. Self-care that is a response to symptoms is referred to as **illness behaviour**. When we experience symptomatology, we seek to understand the meaning and choice of a course of action. Self-care that is oriented toward becoming well or adjusting to chronic illness or disability and encompasses the management of activities when ill is referred to as **restorative self-care** or **sick-role behaviour**.

How we respond to symptomatology varies depending in part on the seriousness with which the symptom is perceived. For example, most people say that they would consult a physician immediately if they suddenly and inexplicably lost weight, encountered shortness of breath, or had frequent headaches. These symptoms are perceived as a potential threat to health. However, an upset stomach, bowel irregularity, and difficulty sleeping tend to call for self-treatment rather than the help of a professional. Over-the-counter medication is a popular form of self-treatment, especially for pain, coughs, bowel irregularity, tranquilizing, and sleeping (Segall and Goldstein, 1989; Segall, 1990). Reactive self-care becomes even more important in older age because so many of the health conditions experienced by seniors are chronic rather than acute in nature. Seniors often live day in and day out with persistent symptomatology (such as pain from arthritis), which they must manage and for which medicine is often unable to offer sufficient help (Baker and Stern, 1993).

Health professionals often view self-management of chronic illness in terms of techniques and strategies to be learned through structured education. In contrast, those living with conditions such as arthritis tend to identify it as a process invoked to bring order into their lives. Kralik and colleagues (2004) reported that persons with arthritis create a sense of order by recognizing and monitoring the limitations imposed on their lives; mobilizing resources; managing a shift in their self-identity; and balancing, pacing, planning, and prioritizing. Through trial and error within their daily life experiences, they reconstruct their identities and their daily lives.

Our causal attributions for illnesses are important in terms of the treatment options we choose. French, Maissi, and Marteau (2004) concluded that several reviews of the research in this area demonstrate a weak to moderate relationship between causal attribution and the emotional impact of the illness and the coping strategies employed. Interestingly, given the prominence of the biomedical model in Western health care, the large *United States General Social Survey* indicates that, overall, non-biologically based treatment options are more popular than those that are biologically focused. Talking to family and friends about symptoms of mental health problems (including major depression, schizophrenia, alcohol dependence, cocaine dependence, and 'troubled' behaviour) is recommended by 96 per cent of the sample; in contrast, prescription medication is recommended by 60 per cent. Depression and schizophrenia elicit the most professional, biologically based treatment options. Alcohol and drug dependence tend to elicit therapy and self-help groups as the most favoured treatment options. Beliefs in biological causes of disorder (such as chemical imbalances and genetics) are more likely to be associated with treatment options that are biologically based (such as psychiatrist, prescription medication, mental hospitals, general doctor). Put another way, beliefs in the causes of a problem are related to beliefs about appropriate treatment options. Many favour a combination of both biologically and non-biologically based treatment options.

There is much research on our beliefs about the causes of coronary heart disease (CHD) and related events such as myocardial infarction or heart attacks. Several studies suggest that the major causes include chronic stress and lifestyle factors such as smoking and diet. In addition, most people list more than one cause (French, Maissi, and Marteau, 2004). French and colleagues (2004) studied first-time heart attack patients, with an interest in exploring the reasoning involved in causal beliefs. They found that many people actively search for causes and, like other studies, confirm that attributions are often made to stress, heredity, and behaviours such as smoking, diet, and exercise. While people list several causes for their conditions, they tend to choose one triggering factor, usually smoking or stress. These authors argue that heart attack patients are motivated to seek causal attributions to help control their emotions; this involves avoiding blaming themselves or others while also searching for personal control over future heart attacks. Within this process, they view stress as an uncontrollable demand but the response to it as controllable.

Beliefs and behaviours can change over time and over the course of an illness or condition. Studying whiplash victims, Linnel and Easton (2006) report that it is only over time, when an injury does not heal quickly, that a person becomes more likely to expect the condition to last longer and with more severe consequences. A protracted timeline is not part of our cultural beliefs about whiplash. Even those with a prolonged recovery do not report extreme levels of pain and believe that they have much control over their symptoms.

Beliefs about mental illness by those who are mentally ill seem to differ substantially from the physical illness model so commonly adopted in research and by health-care practitioners. As Kinderman and colleagues (2006) note, most researchers study mental illness from a physical illness perspective, focusing on beliefs such as causation, trajectory, nature, consequences, and treatability. As these authors argue, there are a number of reasons to suggest that a physical health model is inappropriate for mental illness. For example, those with psychiatric problems may not have a set of internally consistent, coherent, and relatively stable beliefs about their illness. As well, those suffering from certain illnesses such as schizophrenia may have severe conceptual disorganization resulting in beliefs that are confused, inconsistent, and/or contradictory. Finally, those with mental health problems are afflicted at the level of the self, so that distinguishing between the illness and the self may not be possible. That is, they may not distinguish a disease entity that is separate from the self, and some whom others believe are mentally ill may not believe they have an illness.

Kinderman and colleagues studied individuals with a diagnosis of schizophrenia. They found that while in-patients and outpatients differed from one another in their beliefs about their conditions, both groups held beliefs that were dramatically different from the assumptions of physical health models. In-patients with schizophrenia did not separate their psychotic problems from their selves. Instead, their problems were considered part of who they are. They also revealed a lack of coherence and consistency in their beliefs about this part of themselves. They were confused and were trying to understand what was happening while simultaneously holding contradictory beliefs. When they did use professional language (such as the term schizophrenia) to try to understand their experience, it had a meaning that differed from that of the professional. Among outpatients, however, a clear delineation between their illness and their selves did occur, although it included time. They distinguished between their past ill selves and their current selves who were in remission. They were distant from and able to appraise their past selves. Outpatients were also characterized by an absence of personal agency. Unlike in-patients, outpatients were fatalistic, lacking hope, struggle, or puzzlement.

Structural Influences on Self-Care when Ill

When we are sick, social location continues to matter. The same factors with which you are now familiar (socio-economic status, gender, race/ethnicity, age) intersect in a multitude of ways to contextualize and impact self-care in times of illness.

Chronic illness receives much attention in this area because its long-term nature means that those afflicted must learn to manage their daily routines while living with illness. With many chronic illnesses, the person's quality of life depends on how they self-manage their illness. They must minimize the disease progression and its impact, typically drawing primarily on self-care but also on professional care. Self-care strategies vary, often by disease, because different diseases have different effects on our functioning.

Gender differences in self-care during times of illnesses are well established. As noted in Chapter 2 and earlier in this chapter, women tend to have more symptoms, have greater morbidity, and are more likely than men to seek informal assistance as well as professional help. They also are likely to have greater knowledge of and experience with concerns related to health. Among those with heart disease, Sharpe, Clark, and Janz (1991) found that women experienced lowered physical functioning and less adherence to prescribed exercise regimens than men. Women and men were equally likely to comply with medication advice. Burnette, Mui, and Zodikoff (2004) report that women with coronary heart disease change their behaviours, adapt to their environments, and use equipment more than men. Women are also much more likely to use prayer, meditation, or other helpers. Men, however, are more likely to engage in physical activities.

Because knowledge is often a prerequisite for action, it is perhaps not surprising that education is related to self-care when ill. Katz (1998) reports that, among those with rheumatoid arthritis, 13 or more years of education seems to be the important cut-off. People with this education level are more likely to use a heated pool, tub, or shower, relaxation methods, and stress control and to avoid certain foods. Interestingly, those with 12 years of education emerge as distinctive, sometimes using less of a particular self-care strategy than those with less education. Knowledge has been described as a necessary but not sufficient condition for effective self-care, something that has important implications for programming (Beeney and Dunn, 1990). That is, information and 'education' programs that transfer information may be necessary, but they cannot guarantee compliance. Because we know something does not mean we will act upon it.

Especially with changes in communication technology, health information has burgeoned. The availability of this technology, notably the computer and the Internet, means that access to self-care information is greater than it has ever been. This availability provides those with mobility difficulties ready access because they do not have to leave the home. Arguably, older adults can benefit more from this than those in younger age groups because their health is the most likely to deteriorate. On the other hand, preventive strategies are best begun when younger. Yet there is a common stereotype that seniors are unwilling to use the computer, stemming from a perceived resistance to change (McCann and Giles, 2002). Empirical support for this stereotype is lacking, although those older today have typically had less exposure to and use of computer technology than have college and university generations.

Wagner and Wagner (2003) report the results of a community-wide intervention that sent every resident a handbook described as a self-care reference guide, established a toll-free nurse-line for advice, created an on-line computerized health information database, held workshops for residents and health-care professionals on self-care, and set up a limited number of information kiosks in public places. These resources were advertised on billboards, radio, and print. Prior to the intervention, older adults were less likely to use books, computers, or a telephone helpline to obtain health information. This is due to a **cohort effect** rather than an **aging effect**. Previous generations of seniors were not exposed to computer technology; however, after the intervention, older adults increased their use of health information (specifically, the telephone helpline and the Internet) as much as younger or middle-aged adults. Their increased use of books for health information was greater than the increase for younger adults and similar to that for middle-aged adults. The study demonstrates older adults' interest in, willingness to, and ability to use new technologies.

Like other social structural factors, ethnicity also provides context and helps pattern our self-care responses when we are ill. Studying Chinese-Canadian and European-Canadian women with diabetes, Anderson and colleagues (1995) found that while culture-specific beliefs are evident (for example, Chinese-Canadian women believe ginseng is helpful when managing their diabetes), this does not preclude the use of Western medicine. Chappell and Lai's (1998) research later confirmed this finding among Chinese Canadians living in British Columbia. Western medicine is used just as often as among Canadians generally, with traditional Chinese medicine used simultaneously, especially among Chinese Canadians who practise traditional ancestor worship. One of the reasons for the use of Western services is their coverage under Medicare. We do not know what the use of these services would look like if both Western and traditional Chinese medicine were insured for the user.

Because so few Chinese-Canadian seniors speak English, they are largely unable to access information about their conditions, a major difference with the European-Canadian women in Anderson and colleagues' study. However, Chinese-Canadian women managed their diet regimes better than European-Canadian women, a finding the authors attribute to the lack of English among Chinese Canadians that meant they tended to stay at home and not work in the labour force, giving them more time and flexibility to manage their own diets. Contrary to the findings noted earlier in this section regarding education, the authors found lower levels of education related to better dietary management and medication routines—again explained in terms of language barriers and unemployment. The intersection of ethnicity and socio-economic status is evident here.

Importantly, while we all engage in self-care, we do not necessarily do so to the exclusion of other forms of care. We can engage in self-care while also receiving informal care and formal care services (see Chapter 4).

CAREGIVING

Although we all interact with others in varying contexts and to varying degrees, including different forms of helping one another, it is when health fails and we cannot continue our daily lives without assistance that everyday social interaction and social support is referred to as **caregiving**. The defining characteristics of **informal care** receipt are that the recipient cannot carry out the activity for themselves—assistance is required, and it is primarily unpaid. Perhaps the most obvious form of caregiving that comes to mind is care of children, especially when they are young. During adulthood, care is usually provided due to illness or disability. Caregiving becomes especially important for older adults because, as we saw in the last chapter, physical health declines as we age. This will become an even more important issue in the future; today's baby boom generation may spend more years caring for a parent than for dependent children (Atchley and Barusch, 2004).

Terms such as the **sandwich generation, hidden victims**, and the **generation-in-the-middle** have become popular for describing the notion that caregivers to older adults are often their middle-aged children, who have multiple demands. They can be caring for their parents, still raising their children, and working in paid labour. However, Canadian research has demonstrated the infrequency with which this actually occurs—children who are caring for a parent tend to have completed their own child-rearing (Penning, 1998; Rosenthal, 1986). Williams (2005) has shown that no more than a quarter of middle-aged caregivers are caring for parents while also raising their children. The term **serial caregiving** is a more apt descriptor of the fact that women are more likely to experience raising children, followed by caring for parents, and then caring for their husbands.

The concept of caregiving is complex. Social interaction might include several components of which only some constitute informal caregiving. For example, a daughter taking her elderly mother shopping might include elements of emotional support, negative emotional interaction, assistance, and companionship. Furthermore, the participants may not interpret the encounter in a similar manner. The daughter might define it as care whereas the mother might see it as a visit. Similarly, we think of informal care as more affective and less instrumental than formal services, although formal care workers can become 'like family', and family often provides technical assistance.

Some countries have programs that pay family caregivers, blurring the lines between informal and formal care. For example, Veterans' Affairs Canada has a program that will modestly pay family members. In Norway, family caregivers can receive training and be paid. In both of these instances, the caregiver is provided some monetary compensation, but his or her role remains essentially unchanged. In Britain, 'community care helpers' are paid 'symbolically' to care for single persons in their neighbourhood; the intent is to inject the affective side of family relations into the interaction (Ungerson, 2000). In this instance,

Table 3.2   Informal and Formal Care: Some Figures

Most common activities in home care:	Housework
	Shopping
	Meal preparation
	Person care
Hours provided by formal services	< 30%
Hours provided by family and friends	> 70%
Number of seniors receiving all care from informal sources	40%

Sources: S.A. Lafrenière et al. 2003. 'Dependent Seniors at Home: Formal and Informal Help', *Health Reports*. Statistics Canada Catalogue no. 82-003-XIE. 14, 4: 31–9; K. Cranswick. 2003. 'Caring for an Aging Society', *General Social Survey, Cycle 16*. Statistics Canada Catalogue no. 89-582-XWE.

an informal caring relationship is at least partially recreated through minimum compensation to willing individuals. There is, in other words, much fuzziness around the term 'informal care'; nevertheless, the distinction between informal and formal (paid care; see Chapter 4) is useful. There is much research on both informal and formal care, especially within gerontological literature.

As noted earlier, although not recognized as such until the 1970s, informal care is the dominant form of care in any society, far more prevalent than care we receive from the formal health-care system. Despite media attention on the latter, it is family and friends we first turn to when we become ill. Summarizing research on caregiving to seniors (those requiring the most informal care), Kane, Evans, and MacFayden (1990) report that the informal network provides 75 to 85 per cent of the total personal care received in industrialized countries. This is regardless of whether the country provides universal comprehensive health insurance. As Table 3.2 shows, over 70 per cent of home care to older adults is provided by family and friends.

The changing demographics including the aging of the baby boom generation and decreased fertility rates are therefore of concern. Such changes translate into an increasing proportion of elderly women without any surviving children. In fact, Keefe, Legare, and Carriere (2004) estimate that the proportion of older parents without any surviving children will increase as much as 50 per cent from 2001 to 2031. While they project that the proportion of older adults (those aged 65 and older) will remain relatively stable over this same period, the number will increase as the overall size of the elderly population grows. However, if the trend for men's life expectancy to catch up to that of women continues, there may be more caregivers available in future. While recent studies suggest that men are becoming more involved in childcare and unpaid housework (e.g., Keefe and Side, 2003), they do not appear to be more involved in caregiving to older adults. However, the younger generation of men might, as they age, engage in care for seniors when they themselves are older. In addition, siblings to date tend not to be very involved in providing care, but with fewer children available, they might become more important. As the baby boom generation becomes elderly, they will have few children but many siblings. Friends and neighbours are another potential source of assistance currently not utilized extensively. Box 3.2 provides an example of a very giving caregiver.

Box 3.2
A Caregiving Career

Maggie started caregiving when she was 47 years old, caring for her 79-year-old, widowed mother, who had pancreatic cancer. Maggie drove her mother to various health-care appointments, advocated within the health-care system for her needs, and provided both physical and emotional care. Following her mother's death (just eight weeks after diagnosis), Maggie inherited the care of a 90-year-old-aunt and an 81-year-old uncle. Her aunt was in a nursing home and so she visited, shopped for things not provided by the home, and took her on outings, including stays at her own home. Her uncle lived in his log cabin several hours from the city where Maggie lived. She called him weekly and visited monthly, bringing him groceries and other necessities. After he entered nursing-home care, she provided the same care as for her aunt. Her uncle died 18 months after her mother; her aunt lived another year and a half.

After their deaths, Maggie did not caregive for a year, until two of her sisters-in-law, both in their 70s, took ill. One, who had been deaf throughout her life, lived with Maggie and her husband for several months until suitable housing could be found. For both, she made health-care appointments, bought clothing, did their finances, and visited at least weekly, depending on their needs. This routine continued for 11 years for one sister-in-law and 27 years for the other. For some time before she died, one of her sisters-in-law did not recognize Maggie; nevertheless, Maggie continued her weekly visits and acted as an advocate on her behalf, especially after she entered nursing-home care.

At the time she began to provide care to her sisters-in-law, Maggie's husband, who had been diabetic and asthmatic for some time, also began to require full-time care. She cared for him for 23 years, again with little outside assistance, including home care. He had macular degeneration and, during his last five years, went into a deep depression that made things especially difficult for Maggie. Three years into caring for her sisters-in-law and her husband, her foster sister's health also declined. She cared for her for 26 years.

While caring for her husband, sisters-in-law, and foster sister, Maggie always took two weeks off each year, when she would not visit, or in the case of her husband provide care (he would enter respite). A friend would sometimes care for her husband one night a week so she could play bridge. She says gardening and other interests in which she immersed herself provided much needed relief. After her husband's death, she continued caring for one sister-in-law for four more years and her foster sister for two more years after that. Shortly after her husband's death, she also began assisting a long-term neighbour and friend who had become widowed. They married, but he died five months later. She had 'wonderful' home support when caring for him. After he died, a year passed with no caregiving demands. Then another neighbour and friend developed cancer. Maggie provided care for a year before this woman passed away.

As a result of her experiences, Maggie was instrumental in helping to establish local support groups for caregivers. When asked why she did so much, her humble response was, 'It's part of life, you do what life hands you.' According to Maggie, the worst thing about caregiving was 'accepting responsibilities that you think are beyond your strengths'. Were there satisfactions in the experiences? Maggie mentions personal growth, knowing you've made a contribution, and knowing you're doing something valuable.

Source: From a conversation with an inspiring caregiver.

The Experience of Caregiving

The social psychological study of caregiving is broad. It can include a phenomenological study of the meaning of caregiving experiences, a constructionist perspective on the social evolution of that meaning, a narrative study of the unfolding of the experience from its beginning to its ending, a social interactionist study of the changing relationship between the caregiver and the ill person, or the interaction between a caregiver and the formal health system. The areas of study and specific research questions are endless.

For example, Gage-Rancoeur and Purden (2003) used participant observation to study the development and evolution of caregiving during and after hospital stays among daughters of hospitalized cardiac patients. Daughters' caregiving was characterized by a non-linear process that included seeking knowledge of the situation, consolidation of their understanding, and acting on the knowledge. In managing the experience, they moved back and forth between these three dimensions and did so within different caregiving styles. When asked their reasons for becoming involved as caregivers to their parents, the most frequent reasons given were close family ties and helping each other. Other reasons were that other family members assist in other ways, they were chosen to do so through family dynamics, and that they were an only child and there was no one else. Sinding (2003) reports additional reasons for becoming involved in caregiving. She spoke to carers involved with persons dying of cancer, reporting that the perception that health professionals were doing their best but were 'run off their feet' in a work situation of constraint led carers to become more involved than they might otherwise have been.

Caring for someone differs depending on the illness and its consequent demands for care. An important dimension is whether the illness is short or long term. Another common distinction is that between physical and mental disorders. While physical illness can bring with it many caregiving tasks required to help the sick person, mental illness is quite different in character because the person providing care has to relate to different cognitive abilities. Among shared consequences for caregivers to those with either physical or cognitive disorders are anxiety and depression, economic difficulties, and work problems (Magliano et al., 2005).

Magliano and colleagues (2005) studied caregiving to those with schizophrenia and long-term heart, brain, diabetes, renal, or bronco-pulmonary diseases in a large sample in Italy. They found that objective demands were highest for the neurological diseases, with subjective burden highest for both neurological diseases and schizophrenia. As these authors point out, brain disorders and schizophrenia can both have many cognitive and behavioural symptoms, resulting in reduced autonomy and relational skills. It is often difficult for family members to understand the meaning of some of the symptoms. As well, family members often overestimate the patient's control over their symptoms. The fewer burdens experienced by those caring for persons with diabetes or heart, renal, or bronco-pulmonary disease could result from a slower progression of the disease and extended maintenance of quality of life, a better understanding of the condition, the later age of onset, and the availability of information about the illness.

Schizophrenia, though, emerged as distinctive when compared with these other diseases. In particular, these caregivers had significantly weaker social networks, a circumstance related to increased levels of burden. The authors speculate that this is related to the social stigma around schizophrenia, which was not present for the physical illnesses studied, and the less professional support available. The similarities and differences between the brain disease and schizophrenic groups highlight the fact that caregivers can experience considerable burden from this role, which may or may not adversely affect their quality of life. Caring for those with brain disease resulted in high levels of burden but not inadequate quality of life or overall well-being for these caregivers. Caregiving to those with schizophrenia resulted in high burden and inadequate well-being.

Parents of children with severe mental illness have unique experiences with atypical demands. The meaning of parental care in this situation incorporates themes of living with sorrow, anguish, constant worry, guilt, and shame; coming to terms with difficulties; and hoping for a better life for the child. Here, parental caregiving is often life long, characterized by grief, stigma, and worries about the future (when they may no longer be present to care for their child) (Pejlert, 2001). They, like others and their caregivers, must navigate competing messages from the media and health-care system (Meadows, Thurston, and Berenson, 2001).

Autism is an example of such an illness; it is a developmental disorder, often accompanied by mental retardation and characterized by behaviours such as perseverations, aggressions, tantrums, headbanging, and self-injury, together with a lack of communication and social skills (Gray, 1994). Caregiving for an autistic child is more stressful than parenting a child with other disabilities, such as mental retardation, Down's syndrome, cystic fibrosis, and chronic and fatal physical illness (Weiss, 2002). Caregivers, usually mothers, experience depression, anxiety, anger, and the need to cope with sometimes difficult behaviours (Gray, 2002) as described above (Dunn et al., 2001; Weiss, 2002).

Thus, autism not only impacts the child who has the disability but it also has the potential to act as a major stressor on the family, affecting the relationships between parents and those between the autistic child and his or her non-autistic siblings (Schopler and Mesibov, 1994). Relationships with siblings are often characterized by less interaction between a sibling with autism and one without (Stoneman, 2001); siblings of children with autism can have more peer problems, adjustment problems, and decreased level of intimacy, nurturance, and prosocial behaviour when compared to children without a sibling with autism (Kaminsky and Dewey, 2001).

The issue of caregiver burden has received much attention in the research literature, especially regarding caring for the aged. Much of the interest in caregiver burden has focused on the demands of caring for someone who is ill and/or disabled and the negative effects on the person providing care. Typically **burden** is considered the physical, psychological, emotional, social, and financial problems resulting from caring for a person who is impaired (George and Gwyther, 1986). It can refer to objective or subjective aspects. The former refers to the demands associated with the needs of the person receiving the care, the time it takes and the actual tasks that must be performed (e.g., changing diapers, transferring the person to and from bed, cooking, and feeding). The latter refers to the emotional reactions of the care provider, including such feelings as anxiety, lowered morale, and depression.

Much of the research in this area confirms that caregiving is burdensome. It can result in any number of emotional and psychological outcomes such as those listed above (as well as stress and strain), physical health declines on the part of the caregiver, social isolation, and loneliness (Hughes et al., 1999). Such findings has led to much discussion about what should be done to assist and support caregivers. However, for quite some time, the focus remained on the burden of caregiving without much attention paid to any possible satisfactions or positive aspects of the experience. The assumption was that caregiving was difficult and that there was nothing good about it. This is somewhat akin to studying marriage and asking spouses about only the annoying habits of their partner, without ever asking what they enjoy about the relationship or whether they want to stay married and why.

Researchers have recently begun asking caregivers not only about the burdens of caregiving but also about the satisfactions they derive from caregiving, whether they want to continue in the role, and how well they think they are coping. They have discovered that almost all caregivers can point to things they enjoy (such as something involving the personal relationship with the care recipient—watching him or her improve, seeing him or her happy, being close to him or her, or being able to help or give back what life has given them). The overwhelming majority of caregivers believe they are coping well, that the burdens they experience are not overwhelming and occur intermittently rather than continuously. Almost all want to continue providing care (Chappell and Litkenhaus, 1995; Keating et al., 1999).

Furthermore, while burden affects their overall well-being, caregivers can experience this burden while also maintaining a good quality of life. In other words, the stress of a particular role does not necessarily undermine overall quality of life. Our multiple roles comprise our quality of life, albeit some weigh more heavily than others depending on which ones are most salient to us. When examining and focusing on one role such as caregiving (or parenting, work, or friendship), it is important that we not assume that it either comprises the totality of a person's life or that there are not also other influences on his or her overall well-being. In terms of caregiving, it means that not all caregivers are overwhelmed. As a result, governments can focus on those who do require assistance.

Pearlin and colleagues' (1990) **stress-process model** of caregiving is a particularly popular theoretical model for examining the stress of caregiving (see Figure 3.1). This model argues that background characteristics including caregiving history and socio-economic characteristics affect caregiver burden, viewed as a subjective primary stressor. Such burden in turn affects outcomes such as depression and physical health. It also acts indirectly, through intrapsychic strains such as self-esteem and competence as well as through role strain such as family conflict and economic problems, to further affect these outcomes. Social support and coping strategies mediate this process. While still frequently used by researchers today, this model is often modified. Yates, Tennstedt, and Chang (1999), for example, incorporate the concept of appraisal by viewing burden as a secondary appraisal variable because it reflects a subjective assessment made by the caregiver.

Macro Societal Forces

Structural influences are especially relevant to informal care. Caring and intergenerational relations epitomize social relationality and the public good. Social structures, such as those represented by government, employers, and health insurers, place limitations on the availability of formal help; these limitations necessitate informal care. Current economic and political changes are characterized by a globalization of investment, finance, advertising and consumption markets; information and communication technologies; and neo-liberalism. This political agenda seeks to promote privatization, deregulation, and significant structural change in national bureaucracies; decreases in welfare programs and public services; and liberalization of trade and monetary policies (Navarro,

Figure 3.1   A Stress-Process Model

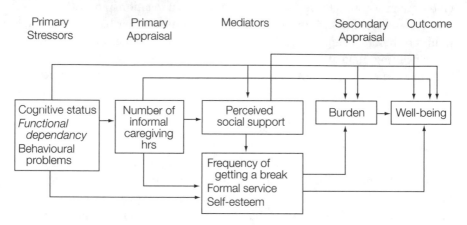

Source: N.L. Chappell and R.C. Reid. 2002. 'Burden and Well-Being among Caregivers: Examining the Distinction', *The Gerontologist* 42, 6: 772–80.

2002a). Within this perspective, the state's role is complementary to and facilitative of the private sector rather than setting limits to it as typified by the welfare state (Meyer, 2000).

The new rhetoric acknowledges the contributions of families and other informal networks, a clear break with the past wherein informal caregivers were silent partners in care, invisibly adapting to the formal health-care system. However, the primacy given to economic markets within neo-liberalism means that it does not recognize unpaid work. Yet as Bakker (1998) and Gough (2000) have noted, the unpaid work of reproduction, nurturing, and caring allows the realization of market relations. Altruistic collective behaviour in the private sphere of the household enables individualistically oriented market behaviour. Caring for the young, the old, the sick, the disabled, and those who cannot work results in more productive workers and consumers for capitalist economies. Because caring work is largely women's work, women contribute in critical ways to the neo-liberal agenda, without recognition or support. Indeed, McDaniel (2002) describes globalization's influence on caregiving as eclipsing, noting that the gendered nature of citizenship extends beyond labour force participation to social reproduction, unpaid work, and identities shaped by class and race. With increasing acceptance of privatization, increased burdens are placed on families, primarily women, to undertake even more caregiving. Increased demands are occurring as access to resources (both private and public) is being reduced (Chappell and Penning, 2005). (The marketization of caring within neo-liberalism is discussed in Chapter 5.)

Class inequalities have increased within the current climate of neo-liberalism (Navarro, 2002a), with research now showing increases in the gap between rich and poor, increased unemployment, decreased social expenditures, transfers of income from labour to capital, undermined working-class rights and unions, and increased part-time, home-based work, self-employment, contracting out, and temporary work (Coburn, 2001). The influence of these factors on access to and the provision of informal care means that those with lower incomes are more likely to have their parent(s) live with them in old age (Tennstedt and Chang, 1998). The middle classes have more options open to them, allowing for care at a distance. They are more likely to assume care management, to purchase services (such as suitable housing, formal services, and assistive devices), and to provide less direct physical care than members of lower classes (Bengtson, Lawton, and Silverstein, 1994). Those with more resources also tend to work in occupations that allow greater flexibility to accommodate caregiving. For example, professionals and managers can often arrive to work late, leave early, and take work home, while clerical and blue-collar workers are more likely to have to reduce their hours of work to accommodate care (Neal et al., 1993; Ursula, 2004).

Women predominate as caregivers due to both social structure and ideology. The majority of women can expect to provide care—to their children, to their spouses, and to their parents. In old age, wives tend to care for their spouses when the latter's health fails, while daughters tend to provide care to their mothers (who tend to be widowed by the time they need substantial assistance). Ideological factors portray paid work as primary for men and caregiving as primary and natural for women (Walker et al., 1998). A son is less likely than a daughter to offer care to an aging parent but is more likely to provide services when asked. He is also more likely to rely on his spouse or sister as the primary caregiver and to support the primary caregiver as a peripheral helper or to be involved in particular tasks as a secondary caregiver.

Among older adults receiving assistance for long-term health problems, women, those who are unmarried, those who are elderly, and those in poor health are more likely to be receiving informal care than men, those who are married, those who are younger, and those in better health. Ninety-three per cent of those who are receiving care have assistance with household tasks (such as help with shopping, heavy housework, or yard work) and not with the basic activities of daily living that are required for survival (such as eating or going to the bathroom) (Keating et al., 1999). The caregivers to these seniors tend to be middle-aged women, usually wives and daughters (Chappell and Litkenhaus, 1995).

The fact that women tend to be nurturers and carers in society is true at all ages. They are more likely than men to accept major responsibility for the organization and provision of care, to provide more total hours of caregiving, and to provide specific types of care and support, such as homemaking assistance, personal care, and emotional support. Men are more likely to perform instrumental activities, such as home maintenance and repair. Driving and help with finances are just as likely to be undertaken by men as by women (Frederick and Fast, 1999; Wilson, 2000). Sons do, however, become primary caregivers when they are only children, have only brothers, or live closer to the parents than their siblings. It is also worth noting that, as Harris and Bichler (1997) suggest, children may feel more comfortable providing care (especially personal care) to a parent of the same sex. Because women generally live longer than men, there are more of them to be cared for, perhaps also contributing to the smaller number of caregiving sons.

How and why gender differences continue to emerge is open to debate (see Chapter 2), but differential cultural scripts are powerful influences on beliefs and actions. In a novel piece of research, Benrud and Reddy (1998) read descriptions of gender differences in acute and chronic conditions that put either women or men at a health disadvantage to 333 diverse people. Both men and women attributed the condition to relatively uncontrollable, constitutional factors such as biology when the gender difference disadvantaged women. In contrast, both women and men believed the condition was due primarily to relatively controllable, nonconstitutional factors (such as their behaviour) when the gender difference disadvantaged men.

Ethnic Minority Culture

Cultural beliefs during illness are not well understood, partly because subcultural groups vary from one another. It is recognized, though, that this can be an especially salient area. North-American women of Vietnamese descent, for example, often report not ever having mammograms. Among some Asian-American/Pacific-Islander women, fatalism, cultural beliefs regarding karma and causes of illness (such as the belief that cancer is punishment for not living 'right'), modesty, and a preference for Eastern medicine can prevent breast cancer screening (Sadler et al., 2001). While there is variation among different Aboriginal peoples, some American-Indian and Alaskan-Native groups believe cancer is punishment for wrong doing, the result of a curse, or a way of preventing other women from experiencing it. In addition, some believe it can be caused by searching for it. This is related to the belief that language itself can influence what happens; discussing cancer thereby produces it (Rajaram and Rashisidi, 1998).

Unfortunately, racial, ethnic and minority groups often share structural disadvantages (Chappell, 2007a, 2007b). Especially in the United States, racial differences have long been documented as greater than age variations, and they tend to remain even among those of similar socio-economic status (Blau, Oser, and Stephens, 1979; Sutton and Peraud, 1989). The continuing inequities in income and assets, educational background, and societal factors for minorities is documented in the United States (Takamura, 2002) and other Western countries such as Great Britain (Bajekal et al., 2004). These disparities are often most evident among the elderly population due to a historic lack of education and employment opportunities, cumulative disadvantages throughout their lives (Nazroo et al., 2004). In Canada, Aboriginal groups stand as an obvious example (McDonald et al., 2001). The impacts on informal care are therefore evident in terms of class differences, as noted above. Because cultural minorities tend to have lower social-class standing, they have fewer resources, and all of the implications that lower-class life brings. In addition, those who emigrate from other countries may face formal service systems that are designed for the host society and not congruent with their culture.

When it comes to informal care receipt (though not provision), structural inequalities do not necessarily translate into disadvantage. While poorer health can result in greater caregiving demands, family and social support is high (Moriarty and Butt, 2004). This is a good example of the fact that while larger structural forces impose constraints and facilitate certain actions, we also live our lives very much at the local level. Although social structure can constrain our actions, we nevertheless engage in interpretive practice and reflexive formulation of possibilities and take action drawing on our skills, capabilities, and socially learned roles (Hendricks, 2003; see Chapter 1). Being closer to home inevitably encompasses our relationships with those close to us, particularly our families. Family values and behaviours derive from the cultural context of our lives. For cultural minorities, that culture often includes a hybridizing of the donor culture and the receiving culture, sometimes referred to as **bi-culturalism**. New **transnational identities** consist of a blending of the two cultures (Chen, 1997; Van Ziegert, 2002).

Much research suggests that ethnic sub-cultures value familism more highly, providing greater social support and more care when health declines (Chappell, McDonald, and Stones, 2007). In the 1980s, this translated into an assumption that members of these groups did not need formal care services, an assumption that was subsequently questioned on both methodological and empirical grounds. Methodologically, the term 'friend' varies across cultural groups—for example, Aboriginal and black peoples often consider what whites call 'acquaintances' as friends. Culturally insensitive measures may contribute to the belief that ethnic minorities have larger and stronger networks.

Another methodological issue arises from the virtual impossibility to empirically disentangle ethnic group effects from economic and class disadvantage—said another way, ethnic minorities might indeed have more and better caregiving when ill, but this may not be a subcultural influence. Rather, it may be a situation created by economic necessity because they cannot afford other options such as formal care services or supportive housing. Among those who can afford it, available services may be culturally insensitive and/or discriminatory, making them undesirable. Ethnic minorities often face barriers to accessing health-care services, including a lack of health-care workers who speak their language or understand their culture (Koehn, 2005). Many subcultural groups also experience excellent social support and care (Bajekall et al., 2004; Moriarty and Butt, 2004). Minority groups could of course experience better informal support both out of necessity and as a result of cultural norms and values; the two are not mutually exclusive.

Finally, while subcultural groups care for their members when they become ill, it is not clear that this differs substantially from whites. In fact, almost all people, whether part of the majority or a minority, have network ties and are close to at least some of them. Almost all of us have regular contact with our family and friends and, as already noted, we provide care when a family member becomes ill. In fact, Chappell and Kusch (2007) have shown how, among Chinese Canadians for whom filial piety is still embraced (respect and care for older adults is an obligation explicitly taught from a very young age), the provision of care does not differ as much as expected from that of other Canadians. They are much more likely to live with their elderly parents even when both parents are still living and there is a greater involvement of sons, but otherwise their patterns are very similar to non-Chinese-Canadian behaviours. Westerners, like those of other cultures and despite rhetoric of capitalistic individualism and a cult of youth, nevertheless care for family and friends (Chappell, 2003).

So, are all groups similar in caring for members but different in how that care is enacted (with sons performing some tasks that in other cultures daughters may perform) or do cultural minorities provide more and better care? If they do, which groups do and to what extent is it due to economic necessity and to what extent is it due to cultural norms and values? There is some evidence, albeit limited, that as immigrant ethnic groups gain in socio-economic status, they become more similar to non-immigrants in their interaction patterns. For example, in Canada, older generation Chinese people live in ethnic enclaves (Chinatowns), but current immigrants who are younger, well-educated, have well paying jobs, and face less discrimination, are settling among members of the host society (Li, 1998). Similarly, Moriarty and Butt (2004) report that new immigrant black, South Asian, and Chinese people in Great Britain with higher levels of education and professional employment are living less geographically proximate to others from their ethnic groups than did earlier migrants.

CONCLUSIONS

Self-care is the pre-eminent form of care, both in health and in illness. It includes our health beliefs and personal health behaviours regarding being healthy, staying healthy, being sick, and recovering from illness. In illness, self-care turns to self-assessment, monitoring, and questions of whom to consult, as well as whether and what treatment options to embrace. A self-care model places the lay person, not the health-care professional or the health-care system, at the centre of health care. Sociological interest from a social psychological perspective has added much to our understanding of what we mean by positive health, how we experience it, what beliefs we hold, how we decide what behaviours to engage in, and how complex the concept of lifestyle is. And it has contributed much to our understanding of how we interpret symptoms, how we experience and manage our lives when we have chronic illnesses, what we believe causes certain illnesses, and how those beliefs influence our subsequent actions.

The research cited in this chapter demonstrates the range of such a perspective, as well as its importance and recognition of human agency. Each life is experienced personally, within a unique biography that we draw on in our ongoing interpretations of our lives as meaningful and in our decisions within the context of our everyday lives. Social psychological perspectives are especially good at portraying and understanding life at that experiential level.

Human agency, though, is constrained and enacted within a social structural environment. Our discussion of structural determinants of self-care when healthy included reference to socio-economic, gender, race, and ethnic differences in health beliefs and health behaviours. We learned about these factors as major influences shaping our lives, with those from lower socio-economic status, women, and members of ethnic minority groups often experiencing disadvantage. This, however, is not to deny that people from other groups do not live in disadvantage, but that the probability of someone from a lower class, who is female, or who belongs to an ethnic minority living in disadvantage is greater than it is for those from higher classes, men, or whites. In addition, health beliefs and health behaviours are complicated; for example, research has not confirmed that women or ethnic minority people are always more likely to hold the 'wrong' beliefs or engage in risky health behaviours. Similarly, structural influences are evident when we are ill. In this chapter we learned that lower socio-economic circumstance, ethnic minority group status, old age, and being female are aligned with certain health-care beliefs and practices, but not always in expected ways. This is a complex area of study, one in which we must not hasten to generalize too quickly, lest we err.

Social interaction and social support represent other structural influences. We are all embedded within social environments; we live our lives interacting with others in multiple and often overlapping contexts. The social is constantly evolving, sometimes slower and sometimes faster. Although the composition of family is fluid, we are still embedded within family. Families are usually supportive, but there are negative elements and in more extreme cases there may be abuse. The influence of families and other social networks should not be underestimated. And while we speak about all of these structural factors as if they are separate from individuals, it is individuals who populate, construct, reconstruct, and participate in these social structures. They are not inherently separate from us. For example, there are no families without the individuals who comprise them. While a sociological perspective argues that those structures are greater than the sum of their parts, the individuals who comprise them in turn influence that structure.

Although most of the media and political attention targets the formal health-care system discussed in the next chapter, in fact, the vast majority of care when we are ill or disabled comes from the informal network of family and friends. Referred to as caregiving, or caring, it encompasses a popular area of research, especially in gerontology, a stage of life when physical health declines and assistance is often needed. Social psychological research targets the meaning of the caregiving experience, decisions regarding notions of caring for one's parents including the types of care to provide, and the relationship between care provider and care receiver. Structural determinants of caregiving include current restructuring of governments and of the welfare state to place more demands on families, especially women, to provide the informal care. While there are many beliefs about differences between majority and ethnic minority groups in terms of the greater care provided among the latter, evidence to date is not conclusive. Even if they do provide more care, it is not clear that this emanates from cultural norms or whether it is more from economic necessity or from both. It is clear that whatever the structural forces at work, the consequences are experienced at the individual level; it is the individual who must adapt, embrace, or otherwise cope with her or his environment.

Questions for Critical Thought

1. We often talk about 'healthy lifestyles', yet research to date suggests that we do not act in such a rational manner. What is the evidence? What can we conclude from it?
2. Devise a question that you believe is important to study in relation to self-care when we are healthy. What is your question, why do you believe it is important, and how would you study it (generally)?
3. Why is the study of the social determinants of self-care and informal care (whether in health or in illness) so complex?
4. If women continue to be the primary caregivers within society, how can lives be organized to ensure equity and fairness between men and women?
5. What is the relevance for informal caregivers of current trends involving economic globalization?

Suggestions for Further Reading

Bajekal, M., D. Bland, I. Grewal, S. Karlsen, and J. Nazroo. 2004. 'Ethnic Differences in Influences on Quality of Life at Older Ages: A Quantitative Analysis', *Ageing and Society* 24, 5: 709–28.

Chappell, N.L. 2007. 'Ethnicity and Quality of Life', in Walker and Mellenkopf, eds, *Quality of Life in Old Age*. Berlin: Springer, 179–94.

Eyles, J., M. Brimacombe, P. Chaulk, G. Stoddart, T. Pranger, and O. Moase. 2001. 'What Determines Health? To Where Should We Shift Resources? Attitudes towards Determinants of Health among Multiple Stakeholder Groups in Prince Edward Island, Canada', *Social Science & Medicine* 53, 12: 11611–19.

Kinderman, P., E. Setzu, F. Lobban, and P. Salmon. 2006. 'Illness Beliefs in Schizophrenia', *Social Science & Medicine* 63, 7: 1900–11.

McDaniel, S.A. 2002. 'Women's Changing Relations to the State and Citizenship: Caring and Intergenerational Relations in Globalizing Western Democracies', *Canadian Review of Sociology and Anthropology* 39, 2: 125–49.

Formal Care

Learning Objectives

In this chapter, you will learn that:

- The Canadian health-care system has developed with a primary focus on acute medical and hospital care.
- Medical and physician dominance over our health and health care are considered by some to be declining due to increasing corporate ownership and state interests in cost-cutting, as well as increasing interest in alternative health-care practices and other social movements.
- Complementary and alternative health services such as midwifery and chiropractic and naturopathic care are seeing increased public legitimacy and use.
- Canadians currently have more equitable access to general practitioners and hospital services than to other medical or non-medical services.
- In the past, patients' experiences with medical and hospital care tended to reflect a medical model of care and physician dominance. More recently, patients are seen as medical consumers with greater decision-making responsibility.
- Complementary and alternative medicine can be viewed as offering users opportunities for personal autonomy and control over care. They are increasing in popularity as medical dominance is threatened and the commercialization of health care increases.

INTRODUCTION

This chapter examines the various professions, therapeutic practices, and settings that form the Canadian health-care system. The following questions will be addressed: What changes have occurred over time in the way we treat health and illness care? How did some of the major health professions develop? What types of care are available to Canadians and what kinds do they use? To what extent do people rely on physician, hospital, and other forms of medical care, and to what extent do they use alternative services? What are the social and structural factors that influence access to care and the types, levels, and quality of care received? Finally, how do people experience the care that they receive and how are individual and social factors influential in defining these experiences? The chapter begins with a discussion of health professions (who does the work), then turns attention to health-care settings (where the work is done), followed by a section on experiencing health care, a social psychological perspective.

HEALTH PROFESSIONS

The Medical Profession and Provision of Medical Care

Historically, Canada's Aboriginal peoples viewed illness from within systems of religious beliefs. Illness was often seen as the result of individual actions such as breaking taboos. Since illness was the result of some foreign object or spirit having entered the space surrounding an individual, the job of the medicine man or woman (the shaman), was to remove the foreign object or spirit (Frideres, 2002). Different groups used different types of natural and supernatural interventions.

Over time and following contact with European settlers, Native populations were decimated and their health-care systems suppressed (Torrance, 1998). When the settlers arrived, they not only brought with them previously unknown communicable diseases (such as smallpox, cholera, typhus, influenza, and tuberculosis) but also the health-care beliefs and practices of their countries of origin. When they needed care, many relied on family members or others in the community on an informal basis. If and when they required more complicated treatment, they would often seek out one of a diverse range of health-care practitioners depending on what was available within their local communities.

Health care at this time was a pluralistic system in which no one type of health-care practitioner was dominant. Lay-trained midwives delivered babies in the home while other lay-trained persons performed surgery and set bones. Homeopathic doctors worked alongside allopathic practitioners in the open market. Most of the first allopathic medical practitioners (often referred to as the predecessors to modern or Western medicine) were either barber–surgeons from France who had received primitive training as apprentices or apothecaries who acted as general practitioners (GPs) dispensing available medicines. Allopaths treated illnesses with surgical interventions, drugs (such as castor oil, mercury, and quinine) and other therapies (such as immersion in cold water to cure a fever) designed to produce an effect opposite to that caused by the disease. Bloodletting was also used for a wide variety of ailments; other common treatments were the use of poultices, purging, and inducing vomiting. In contrast, homeopaths treated illnesses with drugs that would produce an effect similar to that caused by the illness (e.g., fever with a fever-producing drug). Eclectics (practitioners who used a variety of treatments) and other practitioners were also available.

Medical Education

It was largely during the late nineteenth and early twentieth centuries that medicine made the transition from 'a fragmented, largely poorly paid, and unheralded set of occupations' (Coburn, Torrance, and Kaufert, 1983: 418; see also Coburn, 2006: 434) to the dominant form of health care in Canada's medical division of labour. Changes to medical education were central to this transition. Early medicine was often based on little formal education—practitioners who did have training tended to bring it with them, primarily from Europe (Torrance, 1998). The first medical school in Canada was established in 1824 in St. Thomas, Ontario. By the turn of the century there were approximately 11 medical schools in the country. Because the state did not interfere in the medical marketplace during this period (Coburn, 1993), medicine was viewed as a trade by many physicians, and teaching in or operating a medical school was seen by these entrepreneur–physicians as a legitimate source of revenue. These medical schools taught several different types of medicine: allopathic, osteopathic, homeopathic, chiropractic, eclectic, botanical, and others. Often there were no entrance requirements other than the ability to pay tuition.

The ascendancy of modern scientific medicine gained added momentum from the publication of *Medical Education in the United States and Canada* (the Flexner Report), based on Abraham Flexner's 1904–05 review of Canadian and American medical schools and supported by the American Medical Association. This report was critical of the systems of medical education being offered in both countries, particularly of proprietary schools and those that did not have the facilities to teach laboratory-based scientific medicine (Flexner, 1910). Flexner called for some to be reorganized and others to be closed, arguing for the need to locate medical education within universities (such as McGill University; see photo below) and away from the strict control of practitioners.

Flexner's report had a major impact on medical education in Canada and the United States. It also helped establish the dominance of allopathic practitioners and laboratory-based scientific medicine as the norm for medical education and practice (Bolaria, 2002). However, Flexner was highly critical of all forms of medical sectarianism, including allopathy, homeopathy, osteopathy, and others. He noted that '[m]odern medicine has as little sympathy for allopathy as for homeopathy. It simply denies outright the relevancy or value of either doctrine' (1910: 156). According to Flexner, modern medicine did not belong to a sect but was a discipline in which knowledge was rationally applied to cure disease, in contrast to preconceived generalizations regarding diseases and their

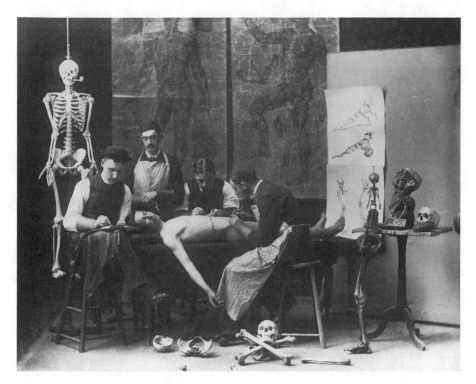

Anatomy study, McGill medical students, Montreal, QC, 1884. Wm. Notman & Son 1884, 19th century. Purchased from Associated Screen News Ltd. McCord Museum II-73328.

cures, like allopathy or homeopathy. Despite this criticism, Flexner showed a preference for allopathic medicine because it embraced modern scientific and laboratory techniques and thereby became part of modern medicine:

> Prior to the placing of medicine on a scientific basis, sectarianism was, of course, inevitable. Everyone started with some sort of preconceived notion; and from a logical point of view, one preconception is as good as another. Allopathy was just as sectarian as homeopathy. Indeed homeopathy was the inevitable retort to allopathy. . . . But now that allopathy has surrendered to modern medicine, is not homeopathy borne on the same current into the same harbor? (156)

The report asserted that the quality of education provided by most of the schools that Flexner reviewed was unacceptable. Based on the report, a number of sectarian medical schools were closed and medical schools that offered 'sectarian' courses (such as naturopathy, herbalism, homeopathy, and Eastern medicine) were informed that they would have to drop these courses from their curriculum or lose their accreditation. Only 8 of the 168 schools that Flexner reviewed were located in Canada; none were sectarian and none were closed. However, during this period, Canadians often went to the United States to get their medical training and consequently the changes that occurred there had an effect on Canadian medical education as well (Bonner, 1995).

Interestingly, the small proprietary and sectarian schools that Flexner was particularly critical of in the United States were more likely to admit women, racial minorities, and students with limited financial resources. As a consequence, the report also inhibited the economically underprivileged and women from pursuing careers in medicine (Beck, 2004). In general, the standardization of medical education advocated in the report led to North American medicine being dominated by well-off white males. By reducing the number of physicians serving disadvantaged communities, it also made it more difficult for people of colour, residents of rural areas, and those of limited means to obtain medical care (Beck, 2004), a pattern that continues today. Although the proportion of women graduating from Canadian medical schools has increased to the point where they currently outnumber male students (CIHI, 2006d), the majority of students continue to be from middle- or upper-middle-class families, with more limited enrolments from diverse racial/ethnic groups and rural areas.

Medical Dominance
By the mid-1900s, medicine had become the defining example of a profession in Canada, as well as the United States and other Western nations. While numerous definitions of the term have been proposed, Eliot Freidson, whose work had a major impact on sociological thinking in this area, defined a profession as 'an occupation which has assumed a dominant position in the division of labour, so that it gains control over the determination of the substance of its own work' (1970a: xvii). He also suggested that medicine enjoyed a high degree of **professional dominance**, including **autonomy** (the ability to control one's own work) as well as **dominance** (the ability to assert control over others, including other occupations in the health-care field).

The medical profession's ability to acquire and maintain professional dominance is frequently attributed to its expert knowledge. In the nineteenth century, this expertise included the germ theory of disease (defined by the view that disease is generally caused by germs, bacteria, or other micro-organisms) and associated medical and scientific discoveries (due to well-publicized advances in antiseptic surgery, vaccination, and public sanitation) that increased public confidence in the superiority of modern scientific medical practices. However, others argue that, in reality, medicine's success in gaining professional autonomy and dominance had little to do with the validity of medical theories or the utility of their approach (Starr, 1982). Instead, for Freidson (1970a, 1970b) and others, such success was attained and then preserved primarily through gaining support from the public, elites, and powerful professional associations. This included convincing the state elite to issue a state-sanctioned monopoly over the definition and treatment of illness as well as over decisions regarding access to specialists and medical tests, admission to hospitals, and acquisition of medications. It also included being granted the right to self-regulation and the power to establish standards of practice and training and to discipline its members (Welsh et al., 2004). Along similar lines, Navarro notes: '[I]t would be wrong to assume that mechanistic medicine was the result of the piling up of scientific discoveries . . . Science and technology are not the motors of history. Nor is the medical profession the shaper of the history of medicine' (1988: 62). In his view, the socio-political context within which scientific discoveries take place and professionals operate is one that is characterized by continuous struggle and competition between different views and positions. '[S]uccess depends on the articulation of these positions within the dominant power relationships in that society, of which class relationships are the determinants' (63).

Some argue that medicine's high degree of autonomy and control over the nature and conditions of its work as well as over other health-care workers (core features of medical dominance) have declined in recent years, and are now relics of the past (Freund and McGuire, 1999). Several different versions of this argument are evident within the sociological literature. The **deprofessionalization** argument (see Haug, 1973, 1988; Haug and Lavin, 1983) asserts that physician autonomy is being challenged as people become increasingly educated and knowledgeable about health and illness. According to Haug, deprofessionalization represents a 'loss . . . of [physicians'] unique qualities, particularly their monopoly over knowledge, public belief in their service ethos, and expectations or work autonomy and authority over clients' (1973: 197). The social forces responsible for this loss include: (1) increased reliance on computerized information systems (which effectively reduce physicians' monopoly over medical knowledge); (2) increases in the educational levels, interest, and assertiveness of the lay public together with increases in the likelihood that people will challenge medical authority; (3) increasing specialization within medicine (thereby increasing physicians' dependence upon one another as well as experts outside the profession, which diffuses the power of individual physicians); (4) the emergence and growth of the consumer self-care movement together with the proliferation of paraprofessionals (e.g., physicians' assistants); and (5) increasing public dissatisfaction with the costs of medical care and a questioning of its unselfish commitment toward the provision of care.

In contrast, the **proletarianization** argument, advanced by some political economists, suggests that capitalism will eventually cause all workers, including medical and other professionals, to gradually lose control over the terms and conditions of their work. According to McKinlay and Stoeckle, who are among the main proponents of this argument, proletarianization refers to 'the process by which an occupational category is divested of control over certain prerogatives relating to the location, content, and accessibility of its task activities, thereby subordinating it to the broader requirements of production under advanced capitalism' (1998: 200). Along similar lines, Coburn and colleagues (1983: 430) attribute the proletarianization of medicine to forces operating at two levels: (1) more proximate causes such as increasing state involvement in health and health care through national health insurance, increasing elite dissatisfaction with medical claims regarding efficacy, increasing competition from other health occupations, and more active self-help and consumer groups; and (2) more distant causes such as changing class structure associated with adjustments in the form of capitalism (e.g., the transition from entrepreneurial to advanced or monopoly capitalism). They note:

> The health-care system is undergoing the same processes of commodification and change to a more bureaucratized and rationalized mode of production as occurred earlier regarding factory and office work. Just as these earlier developments produced the proletarianization of segments of lower-level white-collar work, so recent changes are leading to medicine's new 'contradictory class location' (Wright, 1979). Physicians are now part of a group having some of the characteristics of the petite bourgeoisie and some of the characteristics of the traditional working class. (1983: 428)

In 1999, Coburn focused on the impact of transformations in class structure associated with the subsequent transition toward global capitalism, noting that globalization further helped to decrease the power of the medical profession. More recently, Coburn (2006) writes that while different capitalist economies accommodate medicine in somewhat different ways (as salaried employees of the state, as fee-for-service practitioners within national health insurance plans, as private entrepreneurs in the marketplace, or as some combination of these), in all of these situations medicine currently has less control than it did in its heyday from the 1950s through 1970s. He partly attributes this decline to changes within the nature of capitalism, which reduced congruence between state bureaucrats' and corporate managers' interests on the one hand and medical interests on the other.

Little consensus has been reached regarding the validity of the deprofessionalization and proletarianization arguments. According to Navarro (1988: 61), for example, the medical profession did not lose professional dominance because it never had it in the first place. Instead, dominance was always in the hands of the ruling elite. He also argues that despite the changes that are occurring and reducing medical professionals' autonomy, these do not represent a process of proletarianization. There is little similarity between physicians and real proletarian workers (with regard to such things as the need for state credentials, supervision of others, and control over the means of production), and professionals align more closely with capital than with labour. For his part, Freidson (1984, 1985) has continued to argue that medical dominance has not declined in recent years but that physicians remain the major sources of health-care expertise in our society, and that this will continue into the twenty-first century. In response to the deprofessionalization argument, he notes:

> The professions . . . continue to possess a monopoly over at least some important segment of formal knowledge that does not shrink over time, even though both competitors and rising levels of lay knowledge may nibble away at its edges. New knowledge is constantly acquired that takes the place of what has been lost and thereby maintains the knowledge gap. Similarly, while the power of computer technology in storing codified knowledge cannot be ignored, it is the members of each profession who determine what is to be stored and how it is to be done, and who are equipped to interpret and employ what is retrieved effectively. (1984, cited in Wolinsky, 1988: 40)

In response to arguments regarding medical proletarianization, Freidson asserts that while the autonomy of individual physicians might be reduced, this does not mean that the autonomy of the profession itself has declined (Wolinsky, 1988). Although the profession has encountered some challenges and an increasing internal stratification (increasing division between elite and other practitioners differentiated on the basis of education, discipline/expertise, or administrative positions), he maintains that medicine as a profession will have little difficulty maintaining its power. Freidson believes that medicine will retain control over the major factors responsible for professional autonomy: credentialism (control over training and the right to practise) and monitoring adherence to practice standards.

Consumerism and Corporatization

In more recent years, debates over the challenges to medical dominance posed by deprofessionalization or proletarianization have been recast into discussions regarding the implications of modern trends toward increasing **consumerism** and **managerialism** (Willis, 2006). According to Freidson (2001), professionalism, consumerism, and managerialism represent three different types of control over work. In professionalism, those within an occupation assume control; in the free market, consumers take the lead; and in bureaucracies, managers have the authority to define and coordinate people's work.

To some, consumerism is linked to individual empowerment and the emergence of a culture of social rights of citizens. Its consequences include changes in patients' attitudes and behaviours with respect to the medical profession (including demands for greater information and participation in health-care decision-making, reduced adherence to medical regimens, recourse to self-care and to alternative therapies, and increased official and legal complaints); the rise of consumer groups and a consumer-based rights movement; and greater institutional involvement (e.g., lay membership on committees; see Tousijn, 2006).

Yet, as Tousijn notes, evidence to support the notion of a 'savvy patient striv-ing for control over his or her illness is far from supported by evidence' (2006: 472). Not all patients are interested in or attempt to enact such control. Factors such as the age and education level of the patient and the nature and seriousness of the illness are also relevant to whether individuals wish to be actively involved in their care. As well, while doctors are aware of changes in patient attitudes and behaviours in the direction of greater involvement and self-care, they do not appear to regard these changes as threatening their autonomy. Freidson also sug-gests that consumerism reflects a utopian image:

> The ideology of the free market permeates our thought today, providing our assumptions about what is reasonable and what is not. In the ideal-typical form of the free market . . . there exists only individuals in interaction, making their own decisions to buy or to sell without any constraints imposed by organ-izations or socially organized entities of any kind. . . . This utopian image dom-inates the way we think about health care . . . even though little resembling the free market is to be found in reality. . . . [T]oday, the market in which health care takes place is organized by massive public and private insuring and health-care organizations, and consumer choice is heavily constrained by government regulation, insurance contracts, and the complex, esoteric character of the information bearing on those choices . . . It is simply grotesque to think of health care today as even potentially a truly free market . . . Insofar as there is competition, it is between organizations rather than individuals, and those organizations are highly bureaucratic in character, formally structured by hier-archy rather than by free interaction of individuals . . . (2003: 169–70)

In Friedson's view, the consumer health movement has had little impact on physicians, and public confidence in physicians has not declined any more than it has for other professional groups. Finally, Annandale (1998: 230) contends that consumerism does not live up to its promise as a vehicle for individual empowerment and that even as consumers, patients often have limited choice. Rather, consumerism is a political strategy whereby the state is able to introduce cuts to health care, implement a market-based system, and thereby move past the power of the medical profession. All are done in the name of the consumer.

The **corporatization** thesis suggests that, rather than consumerism, it is increasing corporate ownership and bureaucratic control (managerialism) over many aspects of medical work that increasingly threaten medical dominance and autonomy (Light and Levine, 1988). In fact, doctors themselves reportedly express greater concern about the impact of increasing managerialism—a model of work based on jobs and tasks designed to fit organization and economic needs under the control of managers. Managerial control emphasizes such things as performance appraisal, management by objectives, benchmarking, and quality assurance. This focus includes increased monitoring (e.g., through electronic health records) and standardizing of medical procedures and practices across jurisdictions in order to increase efficiency and to lower costs, as well as attempts to influence medical practice patterns (e.g., through emphasis on evidence-based medicine). As a result, medical practitioners can no longer draw only on their own diagnostic and treatment preferences, but must be able to defend their actions as compared with accepted medical practice (Willis, 2006: 423).

Research suggests that as hospitals and health-care delivery sites become part of large, integrated health-care systems that are often owned by for-profit corporations, increasing numbers of physicians become employees of hospitals or larger health care systems. Administrators become more involved in regulating the work of physicians, a shift that may compromise the ability of physicians, as a group, to maintain control over their own and other occupations (Hartley, 2002). In the United States, the majority of licensed physicians are now salaried employees working within corporately owned practices and clinics (Freund and McGuire, 1999). In Canada, however, this is not the case—73 per cent of physicians work in privately owned individual or group practices as private entrepreneurs and are paid on a fee-for-service basis by a third party (usually government) for the services they provide (Health Canada, 2005a). Yet, in Canada, governmental authorities have assumed an increasingly central role in monitoring and regulating doctors' work. In addition, the ability of the medical profession to direct and control the work of other health-care workers is declining as health-care managers increasingly assume this role and as other health professionals increasingly assume responsibility for work previously considered within the sole domain of physicians.

Yet, as Tousijn (2006) points out, such changes to the workplace are not imposed on medicine but are negotiated. Moreover, physicians remain in control of a specialized body of knowledge that managerial staff cannot access. They also remain in control of the main determinants of physician autonomy: credentialing (i.e., over training standards and rights to practise) and over the monitoring of practice standards (Annandale, 1998; Freidson, 2003).

Access to and Utilization of Physician Services
It is widely believed that Canadians have equitable access to health care as a result of Medicare (see Chapter 5). Universal health-care coverage has been implemented to ensure delivery of services on the basis of need rather than ability to pay. As such, it recognizes individuals' needs for health care based on differences in their health status. **Equity of care access** has been defined as 'the effectiveness of the health system in distributing services to populations on the basis of their relative need for health care' (Watson et al., 2005).

To what extent do Canadians currently have access to and make use of physician services? About 80 per cent visit a GP at least once in a given year. In 2005, 77 per cent of Canadians aged 18 to 64 and 88 per cent of those aged 65 and older consulted a GP in the previous year (Nabalamba and Millar, 2007).

People are less likely to see medical specialists such as dermatologists, geriatricians, pediatricians, psychiatrists, and surgeons, which typically require referrals from a GP. In 2005, approximately one in every four Canadians aged 18 to 64 and one in three Canadians aged 65 and older saw a medical specialist one or more times in the previous year (Nabalamba and Millar, 2007).

As noted earlier, people have equitable access to care when they receive services in accordance with health-related needs rather than social factors such as income or race/ethnicity or gender. The argument that Canadians at various income levels have equitable access to GP and hospital care is supported by evidence indicating that health-related need is one of the major factors associated with the receipt of care and that, in recent years, people have been able to access GPs regardless of their income levels (Dunlop, Coyte, and McIsaac, 2000; Nabalamba and Millar, 2007). However, equitable access to GPs does not mean that other structural factors have no impact on care access or that the level and quality of care received is equitable.

In 2004, only 20 per cent of Canadian family physicians accepted new patients without restrictions (CIHI, 2006), suggesting that factors other than health needs are being considered when it comes to accessing physician services. Recent research also suggests a pro-wealthy bias with regard to the use of specialist services: given similar health needs, those with higher incomes and socio-economic status (SES) are more likely to visit medical specialists and to do so more often than those with lower incomes (Dunlop, Coyte, and McIsaac, 2000; Nabalamba and Millar, 2007; van Doorslaer, Masseria, and Koolman, 2006). Findings such as these suggest a referral bias on the part of primary care physicians as well as wealthier patients' abilities to better negotiate the system. Furthermore, the service received might not be equitable among those accessing physician care. A growing body of research indicates that physicians' treatment decisions often vary depending on patients' levels of income and SES (McKinlay, Potter, and Feldman, 1996; O'Malley et al., 2001).

Finally, what impact will other social factors such as provincial and regional differences, rural or urban residence, race, ethnicity, age, gender, and sexual orientation have? Provincial and territorial variations in access and barriers to medical care services have been reported. For example, Wilson and Rosenberg (2002: 232) note that people living in the Atlantic provinces experience geographic barriers to care, including transportation and availability problems, more frequently than the rest of the Canadian population. Access to physician services also varies across provinces. In 1999, the number of physicians per 1000 people ranged from a low of 9.2 in Nunavut to a high of 21.2 in Quebec (Chan and Barer, 2000).

Geographic differences have also been reported *within* provinces. For the most part, rural communities are more poorly served than urban areas (Eales, Keating, and Prior, 2002). A review of studies conducted in various locales points to reduced access to GPs and particularly to specialists per capita as well as less availability of other health-care professionals and services (such as therapists, counsellors, palliative care, and mental health services) in rural than in urban areas (Casey, Call, and Klingner, 2001; Chan and Barer, 2000; Nagarajan, 2004; Thommasen, 2000). In 2004, over 20 per cent of Canada's population lived in rural areas with less than 10,000 residents; only about 16 per cent of GPs and 2 per cent of medical specialists worked in these areas. The distribution of specialists is more geographically varied than that of GPs (van Doorslaer, Masseria, and Koolman, 2006). Similarly, Nabalamba and Millar (2007) report lower use of specialist services among people living in rural areas. With regard to specific medical services, a recent Canadian study found that over 90 per cent of rural residents had access to routine medical services (e.g., ambulatory, basic laboratory, and X-ray services). However, less than two-thirds had access to more specialized services (e.g., ultrasound, fluoroscopy, blood banks, and chemotherapy), and only 9 per cent had access to sophisticated medical technologies (e.g., CT scans and nuclear medicine) (Buske, 2000).

With regard to ethnic and racial factors, several US studies have shown that racialized minority patients are less likely to visit physicians or to be referred to specialists, less likely to receive preventive care, and are frequently treated less aggressively than whites. For example, a study by the Institute of Medicine in the United States reviewed over 100 studies focusing on the quality of health care among various racial and ethnic groups while taking into account differences in disease severity, other illnesses, location of care, age, and gender. The findings were fairly consistent—most studies showed that minorities were less likely to receive needed services (Smedley, Stith, and Nelson, 2005). This result was not related to ethnic and racial differences in preferences for treatment (although such differences also exist). Instead, it suggests the importance of two factors: (1) how the health-care system operates, including cultural and linguistic barriers to equitable care, differences in health insurance (a major influence in the United States), and differences in where care is received; and (2) the care offered by the health-care providers themselves, including biases, stereotypes, and clinical uncertainty, that operate to the disadvantage of minorities. For example, evidence suggests that physicians' treatment decisions vary in part depending on patients' race/ethnicity (van Ryn and Burke, 2000).

In contrast, evidence from the United Kingdom, which has universal access to medical care, suggests equivalent use of physician and preventive care services by both racialized minorities and whites (Smaje, 2000). In Canada, relationships remain somewhat unclear and contradictory results are evident. Some studies report ethnic minority groups use fewer health services; for example, Nabalamba and Millar (2007) found that visible minorities and Aboriginal people are less likely to report specialist consultations than whites. On the other hand, others report that ethnic groups use similar or more health-care services. For example, Blais and Maïga (1999) found no differences in the number of medical services used in a year by non-Canadian born versus native Quebecers. However, in their study, ethnic groups used specialists more.

Recent studies also focus on immigrant health and health care. Kliewer and Kazanjian (2000) report that physician visits in Manitoba and British Columbia were about 40 per cent lower among first-year immigrants than the general population. Similarly, McDonald and Kennedy (2004) found that immigrants were less likely to have and to have visited a family physician in the past year. Utilization became similar within six to eight years of arrival. A study conducted in Ontario by Wen, Goel, and Williams (1996) found that immigrants and other ethnic/cultural groups usually had equal access to GPs but often showed lower use of hospital emergency rooms. Another study comparing immigrant and Canadian-born women's postpartum experiences in accessing and using health services in the first four weeks following hospital discharge (Sword, Watt, and Krueger, 2006) found that immigrant women were as able as Canadian-born women to access health-care services (e.g., obstetrician, public health-care nursing). However, they were more likely to have learning needs that were unmet during their hospital stays, financial needs, less ability to access household help, and less access to social support (e.g., from family members and friends) and financial assistance, often because they did not know where to go.

Finally, age and gender differences in access to medical care are also evident. The vast majority of older adults report having seen a physician in the past year (89 per cent), and their use of medical specialists has increased over the past two decades. However, lack of interest and expertise on the part of the medical community in dealing with the largely chronic health problems of an aging population has also been reported (Forbes, Jackson, and Kraus, 1987). Physicians appear to spend less time with older patients even though they generally have more health problems. This trend could occur because older adults with generally uncurable chronic conditions may be considered inappropriate candidates for curative treatments and may therefore be treated less aggressively. For example, a study conducted by Ganz (1992) reports that older women with breast cancer are less likely to be offered breast conserving surgery as a treatment option during the early stages of cancer than are younger women. These and other findings suggest that older adults may occupy a marginal position in the modern health-care system. The fact that chronic rather than acute illness tends to prevail in later life suggests a mismatch between the health-care needs of an aging population and the health-care system available to meet those needs.

A somewhat similar situation is evident among women. Sociologists have long noted the tendency to **medicalize** (the process whereby an activity or condition becomes defined as an illness to be treated under medical authority) women's lives such that many aspects of their lives and bodies are seen as unhealthy or pathological (thus as diseases) and therefore in need of medical intervention (Findlay and Miller, 2002). These include premenstrual and menstrual cramps and irregularities; contraception, abortion, pregnancy, childbirth, and menopause; and physical appearance (weight, beauty), all of which tend to be defined in medical terms with medicines, hormones, and surgical interventions commonly employed as treatments. Medical authorities have also laid claim to other elements of women's lives such as child-rearing, where doctors (e.g., Dr Spock) have become acknowledged experts in the raising of 'healthy' children. Finally, not only women's physical health but also their mental health has become heavily medicalized. Given this situation, it is not surprising that women use more medical services than men. Women are more likely than men to report visiting a GP in a given year and also tend to be over-medicated. This finding is especially true with regard to psychotropic drugs and sedatives; women and older adults are the most likely to be prescribed tranquilizers and sleeping pills (Graham and Vidal-Zeballos, 1998).

Yet there is a paradox with regard to relationships between gender and the receipt of medical care. While on the one hand women tend to be targeted for increased attention by medical-care providers, on the other, less interest in and attention to women is evident when in contact with health authorities. For example, a US experimental study conducted to examine the impact of gender and other patient characteristics (age, class, race) on doctors' practices (diagnostic and management) with regard to coronary heart disease (CHD) found that while class and race had no impact, patient gender had a significant impact on the doctors' behaviour: women were asked fewer questions, received fewer examinations, and had fewer CHD diagnostic tests ordered (Arber et al., 2006). The discrepancies were greatest in the case of middle-aged women, leading the authors to conclude that there is **gendered ageism** in doctors' behaviours.

Nursing Care
Despite the visibility of physicians within our medical care system, modern health care also involves a wide variety of other health personnel—laboratory technicians, rehabilitation therapists (physiotherapists, occupational therapists), and nurses. Collectively, health occupations comprise a considerable part of the Canadian work force (895,000 people in 2003). The vast majority of these health-care workers are nurses (see Figure 4.1). Currently, registered, licensed practical, and registered psychiatric nurses (RNs, LPNs, and RPNs, respectively) represent almost one-half of all health-care workers in Canada (CIHI, 2006c). In 2001, the number of registered nurses working in hospitals or other health-care settings totalled over 231,000—approximately 750 nurses per 100,000 people (CIHI, 2004b).

Nursing Care in a Historical Perspective
Historically and today, the story of nursing is closely linked to that of medicine, as well as to family care and to the work carried out by nuns in religious and charitable institutions. In Canada, as elsewhere, family members have long been providing care for the ill at home as part of the informal (unpaid) domestic economy. The providers of such care are generally women, with nursing care regarded as consistent with women's roles and natural abilities (Benoit, 1998).

Figure 4.1   Number of Health-Care Professionals per 100,000 Population, Canada, 2003

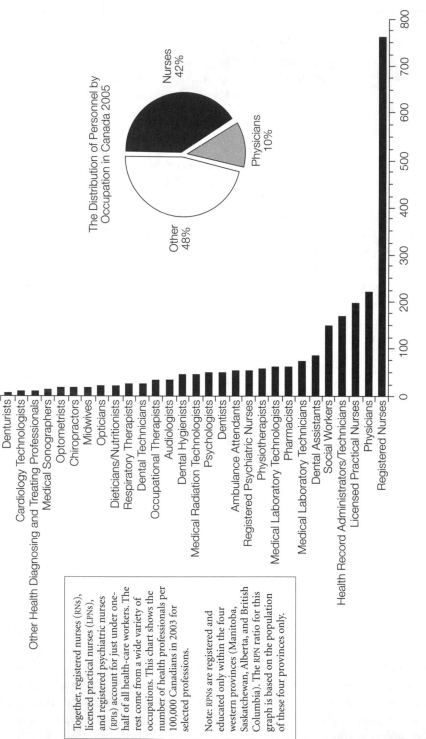

Together, registered nurses (RNs), licenced practical nurses (LPNs), and registered psychiatric nurses (RPIs) account for just under one-half of all health-care workers. The rest come from a wide variety of occupations. This chart shows the number of health professionals per 100,000 Canadians in 2003 for selected professions.

Note: RPNs are registered and educated only within the four western provinces (Manitoba, Saskatchewan, Alberta, and British Columbia). The RPN ratio for this graph is based on the population of these four provinces only.

The Distribution of Personnel by Occupation in Canada 2005

Nurses 42%

Physicians 10%

Other 48%

Source: CIHI, 2005a. *Canada's Health Care Providers—2005 Chartbook*. Ottawa: Canadian Institute for Health Information.

Nursing care was taught by mothers to daughters as part of a female apprentice-ship or learned by domestic servants as a duty, not as a job (Reverby, 1996). Thus, in this context, caring (nursing) was unpaid labour of love.

The practice of nursing as a formal occupation was also influenced by the work of untrained nurses and nuns who cared for those in need (i.e., those with-out families to care for them or without the necessary financial resources). Some of the earliest hospitals were public institutions that catered to the ailing poor. They were often dirty and overcrowded and as a result mortality rates were extremely high. Many of those who worked in these settings were lay nurses—those who had nowhere else to go, sometimes recovering patients themselves. Often they were poverty stricken, unmarried, or widowed women. In the eigh-teenth and nineteenth centuries, hospitals were also established by religious orders to care for those who were ill as a result of the various epidemics (small-pox, influenza, scarlet fever, typhoid, and tuberculosis) that threatened the pop-ulation of the time. Those who worked in these settings were often nuns engaged in charitable work on behalf of the church (Goulet, 2003).

Therefore, like medicine, nursing began as an activity that was not necessar-ily based on specialized knowledge and training. However, unlike medicine, nursing had its origins in work that was done by women, was often unpaid or paid very little, and was grounded in familial caring or other selfless or charita-ble acts of kindness. As described by Wotherspoon (2002), the medical division of labour therefore reproduced the patriarchal structure of the day.

Nursing Education
Florence Nightingale (1820–1910) is widely credited with helping to establish nursing as a profession; her ideas formed the basis for subsequent nursing edu-cation and training programs in Canada, Great Britain, and the United States. She felt that nurses had to be women since only women had the necessary char-acter attributes—they should be responsible, clean, hard-working, obedient, and caring. Because these attributes could not be taught, she sought women who had good reputations and character. Her goal was to see hospitals managed by well-educated and competent (female, middle- and upper-middle class) nurses who, at the same time, were completely supportive of and subservient to (male, upper-class) doctors. Consistent with this perspective, Nightingale's training program emphasized discipline, order, and practical skills. Emphasis was placed on recruiting those who had the necessary personal attributes and then fine-tuning these through training. The primary focus of students' training consist-ed of supervised practical nursing (clinical) work on hospital wards.

The first formal training programs for nurses were established in hospitals rather than universities or other formal educational settings. In Canada, the first program for nurses opened in St Catherine's, Ontario, in 1874. Established by two nurses from Florence Nightingale's school in the United Kingdom and a doctor, it offered a two-year program based on practical nursing experience in

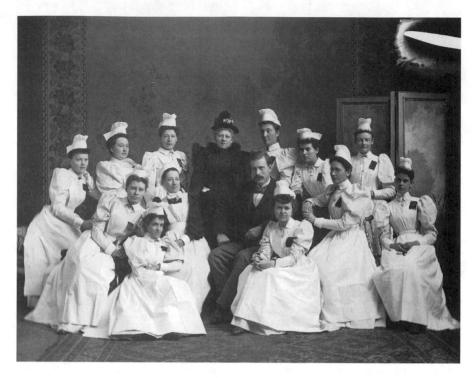

Nurses of the General Hospital, Montreal, QC, 1894 Wm. Notman & Son 1894, 19th century. Purchased from Associated Screen News Ltd. McCord Museum II-105877.

the hospital setting. By 1900 there were 20 hospital-based nursing schools; by 1909 there were 170; and by 1930 there were approximately 220 (Wotherspoon, 2002: 88).

According to Torrance (1998), establishing nursing programs within the hospital system ensured the availability of a constant and inexpensive supply of nurses to work within these settings. Thus, it appealed to the administrative, governmental, and other authorities responsible for running the hospitals. However, it was a system that exploited nursing students to carry out most of the hospitals' work. Because nursing students represented the vast majority of staff, their formal educational training was inadequate; student nurses often put in extremely long hours (60 or 70 hours per week) for several years in exchange for room and board and access to educational supplies (Freund and McGuire, 1999). Yet the hospitals usually offered little or no work to them following graduation, relying instead on a subsequent cohort of nursing students.

It was not until 1919 that the first Canadian university-based degree program in nursing was established at the University of British Columbia. Early university-based programs continued to reflect established thinking about nursing practice, emphasizing technical skills, following orders, and adhering to established practise rather than developing nursing knowledge (research). This approach limited the ability to enhance nursing status relative to other university-educated occupational groups (Wotherspoon, 2002). Moreover, a division developed between those trained in and committed to the hospital service system and those who saw the need to develop the profession through university-based education and research. Although the *Survey of Nursing Education*, written in 1932 by G. Weir and co-sponsored by the Canadian Nursing and Medical Associations (CNA, CMA), recommended that nursing schools be removed from hospital control and placed within the provincial government education system, it was not until the 1960s (following a further Royal Commission report) that non-hospital-based nursing education programs developed on a larger scale.

Nursing as a Profession and Medical Dominance
While medicine is almost always considered a professional occupation, nursing (as well as other medical occupations) is often classified as paraprofessional. According to Freidson (1970b), this is because nurses occupy subordinate positions relative to medical practitioners. This position can be attributed to four characteristics of nurses and their roles: (1) their technical knowledge derives from medicine and needs to be approved by physicians; (2) they usually assist physicians in their work rather than replace them in terms of diagnosis and treatment; (3) their work tends to take place at the request of physicians (that is, under 'doctors' orders'); and (4) they lack the prestige associated with medicine.

What accounts for nurses' subordination to medicine? Some argue that it is an outcome of the political process whereby medicine managed to achieve professional dominance. For example, Torrance contends that

[b]ecause of the social origins of physicians, their association with medical institutions, and their favourable connections with socially and politically dominant groups, physicians with the aid of the state achieved dominance over the healing enterprise. The profession either absorbed competing occupations, drove them into a quasi-illegal status outside the official division of labour, or most common, lent them some legitimacy in exchange for a subordinate status as auxiliaries to medicine. (1998: 4)

He notes that unlike some other occupations, nursing represents an occupation that was restricted primarily through subordination to medicine.

Others argue that the power held by a predominantly male medical profession and the subordination of nursing may have had more to do with gender than with hierarchical position (Zelek and Phillips, 2003). Nursing was relatively unique as an occupation that was open to and eventually respectable for women. Yet from the outset, nursing was also characterized by low pay, subordination to physician authority, and a primary focus on caring rather than curing during a time that considered the latter to be much more important. According to Reverby (1996: 668), nursing was historically organized with the expectation that its purpose was to care as a duty. Thus, nurses were expected to act out of an altruistic obligation to care without thought of professional autonomy.

Nurses have long been working towards attaining professional status and have adopted various strategies in order to do so, including increasing educational requirements, developing their own specialized body of nursing knowledge, and establishing a nursing association to deal with standards of nursing practice and the disciplining of members. Nurses have also taken over some of the work routinely performed by physicians (e.g., taking blood pressure, administering medications) while handing over some of their less desirable tasks to nursing assistants. Various nursing specialties have been developed and in some jurisdictions, nurse practitioners with advanced training can now perform procedures that were once exclusively performed by physicians.

Yet debate is ongoing regarding the advisability and capability of nursing to acquire professional status as well as the strategies to be adopted for doing so. There are also different perspectives within nursing over whether it should attempt to achieve professionalization through an emphasis on higher education and a scientifically based nursing education or to embrace the caring/nurturing aspects of the nursing role. This debate is linked to differences of opinion regarding the appropriate level and type of educational preparation (scientific knowledge and research versus technique-focused curriculum and practical application). While the move away from hospital-based nursing training may have led to improved professional status for nursing in Canada, it also increased inequalities within nursing. Despite the emphasis on degree qualifications, most nursing graduates continue to receive their initial training in diploma programs, which has maintained the fragmentation of nursing into two streams—one more highly skilled and educated and the other service-oriented and less educated. As a consequence of advancing their credentialing and research policies, nurses are also contributing to a bifurcation of their occupation into an educated elite and a majority of low-paid support workers.

The ability of nursing to achieve professional status also remains questionable. Concerns include the fact that many nurses remain employed within structures (e.g., hospitals) that accord them limited autonomy and, despite internal stratification, nurses tend to have limited influence over the work of other professions in the health-care field. Yet arguments that medicine may be undergoing deprofessionalization also raise questions regarding the extent to which nursing will continue to be subordinate to medical authority. For example, over 40 years ago, Stein (1967) suggested that doctor–nurse interactions often reflect the rules of what he called 'the doctor–nurse game'. The rules of this game call for both parties to preserve the structure of the relationship—one in which physicians are superordinate and nurses subordinate—while at the same time allowing both to contribute to patient care. In the game, nurses learn how to give physicians advice while maintaining the appearance that they are deferring to physician authority:

Nurses use subtle non-verbal and cryptic verbal cues to communicate recommendations, which in retrospect appear to have been initiated by the doctor. The 'game' ensures that open disagreement is avoided and carries advantages for both parties: the doctor gains from the nurse's knowledge and experience, while the nurse gains increased self-esteem and professional satisfaction. . . .
(Hughes, 1988: 17)

In 1990, Stein re-examined the doctor–nurse game, finding that nurses were no longer willing to be subordinate and had unilaterally decided to stop playing the game. He attributed this finding to various changes that had taken place between the two time periods. These differences included declines in public esteem for and confidence in medicine, the increasing presence of women in medicine and men in nursing, nursing shortages, and the women's movement, as well as the changes in medical education that were increasing nurses' interests in professional status.

More recent trends may be somewhat less supportive of nurses' attempts to enhance their professional autonomy. As noted earlier in this chapter, increasing managerial control over health services represents another recent trend that may have major implications for health-care providers, including nurses. Among the strategies that managers have used to try to control costs and improve efficiency within hospital settings is implementing 'case mix groupings'—a system for defining the specific tasks and time required to provide care to a typical patient with a particular health problem. In a case mix system, patients are assigned a particular time/cost value and nurses are required to provide nursing care to them within specified time limits. Yet it has been argued that by reducing a nurse's decision-making power, such systems demean the autonomy/authority of the nurse. In the process, they also threaten the nurse's morale and challenge his or her commitment to providing the best care possible (Clarke, 2008).

Another strategy consists of developing less hierarchically structured **collaborative models of care** delivered by multidisciplinary and/or interdisciplinary teams of health-care providers that are interdependent and share power and responsibility for care. Those in favour of a team approach argue that it not only improves patient care but also the productivity of health-care providers. As well, researchers note that the boundaries between nurses' and physicians' work in hospital settings tend to become less clear as nurses increasingly take on some of the tasks (e.g., prescribing medications) previously performed by doctors (Allen, 2002).

However, others point out that despite the potential of collaborative models, nurses often remain reluctant to cross boundaries, their knowledge and roles tend to be devalued relative to that of medicine, and medical discourses tend to dominate within collaborative health-care teams (Coombs and Ersser, 2004; Hindmarsh and Pilnick, 2002). Researchers also point out that although collaborative health-care teams are often seen as limiting medical dominance, they actually reveal its structural embeddedness. For example, Bourgeault and Mulvale's (2006) qualitative study of such teams operating in Canada and the United States found that various institutional, regulatory, and economic factors both fostered and limited the success of collaborative health-care teams. They note that '[i]n Canada, this includes legislation and regulations created at a time when professional scopes of practice were more clearly demarcated and medical dominance more powerful'(491). As a result, medical dominance continues to be **structurally embedded** in public coverage of health-care services. And, insofar as public coverage preserves medical dominance, it also prevents models of care designed to reduce medical power from succeeding.

Complementary and Alternative Medicine (CAM)

Complementary and alternative medicine (CAM) is the label frequently used to refer to various forms of care generally considered outside the realm of conventional Western medicine or other health professions closely aligned with it (e.g., nursing, physical therapy, occupational therapy, psychiatry, psychology). Complementary medicine refers to those forms of care provided together with conventional medicine, while alternative medicine refers to care used instead of conventional medical care.

Major types of CAM change over time as existing therapies become part of conventional care and new approaches emerge. Current lists include alternative health-care systems such as naturopathic medicine, homeopathic medicine, traditional Chinese medicine (TCM), and Ayurveda; mind–body techniques such as meditation, prayer, mental healing, and art, music, or dance therapies; the use of natural and herbal substances and therapies, such as using shark cartilage to treat cancer; body manipulation techniques such as chiropractic medicine, osteopathy, massage therapy, as well as a host of others ; and therapies that rely on the use of energy fields (such as Therapeutic touch, Reiki, Johrei, Qi gong). See Box 4.1 for definitions of some of these practices.

CAM practitioners who were part of the health-service landscape prior to the early twentieth century included chiropractors, osteopaths, homeopaths, naturopaths, and TCM practitioners. Despite fairly widespread use at that time, by the turn of the century most were accorded little legitimacy and actively suppressed by orthodox medicine and licensing authorities. Historically, the medical profession's ability to attain professional dominance meant that it was also able to achieve legitimacy and power over other health-care occupations. While some competitors were subordinated to medical authority (such as pharmacists, nurses, anaesthetists), others saw their practices limited (such as osteopaths) or were excluded (such as chiropractors) from legitimate practice (Coburn, 1999). The ability of one group to exclude others from gaining access to the market is a process known as **social closure**. According to proponents of social closure theory, it is also the process that the medical profession uses in its efforts to create and maintain a monopoly within the health-care marketplace (Saks, 2001).

Box 4.1
Complementary and Alternative Care Definitions

Acupuncture ('AK-yoo-pungk-cher') is a method of healing developed in China at least 2,000 years ago. Today, acupuncture describes a family of procedures involving stimulation of anatomical points on the body by a variety of techniques. American practices of acupuncture incorporate medical traditions from China, Japan, Korea, and other countries. The acupuncture technique that has been most studied scientifically involves penetrating the skin with thin, solid, metallic needles that are manipulated by the hands or by electrical stimulation.

Aromatherapy ('ah-roam-uh-THER-ah-py') involves the use of essential oils (extracts or essences) from flowers, herbs, and trees to promote health and well-being.

Ayurveda ('ah-yur-VAY-dah') is a CAM whole medical system that has been practised primarily in the Indian subcontinent for 5,000 years. Ayurveda includes diet and herbal remedies and emphasizes the use of body, mind, and spirit in disease prevention and treatment.

Chiropractic ('kie-roh-PRAC-tic') is a CAM whole medical system. It focuses on the relationship between bodily structure (primarily that of the spine) and function, and how that relationship affects the preservation and restoration of health. Chiropractors use manipulative therapy as an integral treatment tool.

Dietary supplements are products (other than tobacco) taken by mouth that contain a 'dietary ingredient' intended to supplement the diet. Dietary ingredients may include vitamins, minerals, herbs or other botanicals, amino acids, and substances such as enzymes, organ tissues, and metabolites. Dietary supplements come in many forms, including extracts, concentrates, tablets, capsules, gel caps, liquids, and powders. They have special requirements for labelling. Under DSHEA, dietary supplements are considered foods, not drugs.

Electromagnetic fields (EMFs, also called electric and magnetic fields) are invisible lines of force that surround all electrical devices. The Earth also produces EMFs; electric fields are produced when there is thunderstorm activity, and magnetic fields are believed to be produced by electric currents flowing at the Earth's core.

Homeopathic ('home-ee-oh-PATH-ic') **medicine** is a CAM whole medical system. In homeopathic medicine, there is a belief that 'like cures like', meaning that small, highly diluted quantities of medicinal substances are given to cure symptoms, when the same substances given at higher or more concentrated doses would actually cause those symptoms.

Massage ('muh-SAHJ') **therapists** manipulate muscle and connective tissue to enhance function of those tissues and promote relaxation and well-being.

Naturopathic ('nay-chur-o-PATH-ic') **medicine**, or naturopathy, is a CAM whole medical system. Naturopathic medicine proposes that there is a healing power in the body that establishes, maintains, and restores health. Practitioners work with the patient with a goal of supporting this power, through treatments such as nutrition and lifestyle counselling, dietary supplements, medicinal plants, exercise, homeopathy, and treatments from traditional Chinese medicine.

Osteopathic ('ahs-tee-oh-PATH-ic') **medicine** is a form of conventional medicine that, in part, emphasizes diseases arising in the musculoskeletal system. There is an underlying belief that all of the body's systems work together, and disturbances in one system may affect function elsewhere in the body. Some osteopathic physicians practise osteopathic manipulation, a full-body system of hands-on techniques to alleviate pain, restore function, and promote health and well-being.

Qi gong ('chee-GUNG') is a component of traditional Chinese medicine that combines movement, meditation, and regulation of breathing to enhance the flow of qi (an ancient term given to what is believed to be vital energy) in the body, improve blood circulation, and enhance immune function.

Reiki ('RAY-kee') is a Japanese word representing Universal Life Energy. Reiki is based on the belief that when spiritual energy is channelled through a Reiki practitioner, the patient's spirit is healed, which in turn heals the physical body.

Therapeutic touch is derived from an ancient technique called laying-on of hands. It is based on the premise that it is the healing force of the therapist that affects the patient's recovery; healing is promoted when the body's energies are in balance; and, by passing their hands over the patient, healers can identify energy imbalances.

Traditional Chinese Medicine (TCM) is the current name for an ancient system of health care from China. TCM is based on a concept of balanced qi (pronounced 'chee'), or vital energy, that is believed to flow throughout the body. Qi is proposed to regulate a person's spiritual, emotional, mental, and physical balance and to be influenced by the opposing forces of yin (negative energy) and yang (positive energy). Disease is proposed to result from the flow of qi being disrupted and yin and yang becoming imbalanced. Among the components of TCM are herbal and nutritional therapy, restorative physical exercises, meditation, acupuncture, and remedial massage.

Source: National Institutes of Health National Centre for Complementary and Alternative Medicine. 2007. 'What is CAM?'. Available at http://nccam.nih.gov/health/whatiscam/#d6.

However, this dominance is constantly changing. In recent years, a number of other complementary and alternative medicine occupations have attempted and frequently succeeded in achieving professional recognition with enhanced legitimacy and higher incomes (Welsh et al., 2004). There is increasing consumer use and demand for CAM services, which has been attributed to a variety of factors: growing dissatisfaction with orthodox medicine, particularly in dealing with the increasingly common chronic health problems of the population; resurgent interest in natural methods of preventive health care; public desire for greater control over personal health care; and an increasingly ethnically and culturally diverse population whose citizens are accustomed to using a variety of treatment modalities.

In addition, there are signs that the medical profession, while still creating barriers at an institutional level, may be relaxing its resistance somewhat, at least on an informal level (Coburn, 1999). Some physicians are incorporating alternative approaches and techniques into their practices and medical schools are increasingly integrating CAM into their teaching curricula. The state is also relaxing its stance and is increasingly sympathetic to the ambitions of some of the more popular CAM occupations to professionalize (Kelner et al., 2006). For example, some provincial governments, such as Ontario and British Columbia, have recently made it possible for CAM occupations to gain official recognition within the existing health-care system (Kelner et al., 2006). Alternative health professions that have attained official recognition and are regulated (and therefore fall under provincial/territorial or federal legislation and are governed by a professional organization that sets standards of education and competence to practise) in one or more Canadian provinces include chiropractic (now legally recognized in 11 provinces and territories), midwifery, osteopathy, naturopathy, massage therapy, and acupuncture (see Figure 4.2). In the sections that follow, we examine a few of these professions.

Midwifery

Until the middle of the nineteenth century in Canada, female midwives were the principal attendants at childbirth (Bourgeault, 2000). Little is known about midwives who looked after Aboriginal women prior to European settlement. However, frontier families had access to several kinds of midwives, depending upon their economic situations and cultural backgrounds (Benoit, 1998). During this period, midwifery was not a formally organized profession but was primarily a locally organized system of women helping other women in time of need, with payment usually made in kind. Midwives were frequently women experienced in childbirth who lived in the area. They often functioned not only as midwives but also as nurses, housekeepers, and child-care workers after the birth. Their training was generally acquired through informal and sometimes formal apprenticeship to a more experienced midwife (Bourgeault, 2000).

Figure 4.2   Percentage of People Reporting Alternative Health-Care
Consultations in Past Year, by Sex

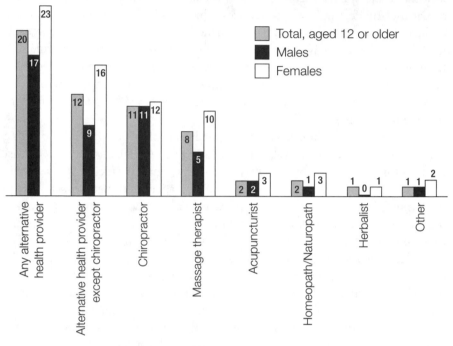

Type of alternative health care

Source: Adapted from J. Park. 2005. 'Use of Alternative Health Care'. *Health Reports* 16, 2: 39–42. Release
date: 15 March 2005. Available at: http://www.statcan.ca/bsolc/english/bsolc?catno=82-003-XIE.

The position of midwives changed during the latter 1800s and early 1900s
when childbirth was relocated from home to hospital and physicians gained control over it and the care of birthing women. In Upper Canada, for example, practising midwifery without a licence was declared illegal in 1866. Subsequently, the
Medical Practitioners Acts of most provincial governments restricted the performance of maternity services to licensed members of the College of Physicians
and Surgeons (Benoit et al., 2005) and maternity care came to be provided almost
entirely by medical and nursing personnel in hospital settings. While traditional
lay midwifery did not disappear, access was generally restricted to remote areas
where medical services were frequently unavailable (Benoit, 1998). There were
relatively few formally recognized midwives in Canada. According to Bourgeault
(2000: 172), Canada gained the distinction of being the only Western industrialized country without any formal provisions for midwifery care.

It was not until the latter half of the twentieth century that Canadian mid-wifery enjoyed a rebirth (Bourgeault, 2000). During the 1970s and 1980s there was increasing demand for the services provided by labour coaches (dulas) and lay midwives who worked unregulated in the private health sector, largely from middle-class women who were dissatisfied with mainstream medicalized health-care practices. This was also a time when many hospitals reorganized their maternity wards to promote family-centred care, revised outdated policies to allow fathers to witness the births of their children, and permitted newborns to stay in the room with their mothers (Benoit, Carroll, and Millar, 2002).

Researchers have suggested various reasons for this rebirth. According to Bourgeault (2000), consumer backlash to medicalized childbirth practices was promoted by the Home Birth Movement, which viewed birth as a normal life process that should be under the control of those giving birth and located with-in the home environment rather than a medical procedure carried out under physician control in hospital settings. As a result, the new midwifery came to be viewed as a symbol of women's regaining control over the reproductive process. Bourgeault also notes the importance of federal government cutbacks to provin-cial health-care funding for increasing interest in less costly alternatives to hospital-based birthing practices.

Whatever the reasons, it was not until the 1990s that midwifery finally attained legal status in several Canadian provinces. In 1993, Ontario became the first to legalize midwifery and integrate it into its publicly funded health-care system. Midwives can now practise legally in five provinces, with four of these (British Columbia, Manitoba, Ontario, and Quebec) including their services within Medicare (Benoit et al., 2005). From 1996 to 2001, the number of active registered midwives in Canada increased by 124.2 per cent (perhaps due to changes in the reg-ulatory environment rather than to actual increases in the number of midwives). The Canadian Institute for Health Information (CIHI, 2005a) reports a total of 413 active registered midwives in Canada in 2002, with over half located in Ontario. This figure likely reflects the fact that registration is not required as a condition of employment in most Canadian provinces (i.e., those in which midwifery is not reg-ulated). In contrast, the 2001 Canadian Census reports 4,705 midwives in Canada, an increase from the 2,895 reported in the 1996 Canadian Census (CIHI, 2004b).

There is debate regarding the benefits and drawbacks of recent changes in midwifery. Bourgeault (2000) suggests that midwifery in Ontario changed somewhat as a result of integration into the mainstream health-care system, moving from an amorphous social movement to something more bureaucrati-cally organized. For example, there was a shift from client regulation to profes-sional self-regulation. The educational model changed from an eclectic apprentice-based approach toward a university-based degree program. Along similar lines, Benoit (1998) notes that the eagerness to professionalize and the rush to embrace scientific knowledge can exclude lay and nursing members as well as practical knowledge.

Chiropractic Care

Although spinal manipulation is one of the oldest and most widely practised healing methods, chiropractic was not defined as a profession until 1895, when Daniel David Palmer, a Canadian who moved to the United States in 1865 at the age of 20, reportedly gave his first spinal adjustment. Palmer believed that vertebral subluxation (misalignment) was the cause of all disease and that chiropractic was a complete system of care—thus an alternative to allopathic or scientific medicine. Its focus was on relationships between bodily structure and function and their impact on overall health. Other chiropractic practitioners, known as 'Mixers', believed in combining spinal adjustment methods with other methods such as nutritional or physical therapy.

Although chiropractic has steadily gained acceptance and increased use, the Flexner Report was extremely critical of chiropractic care:

> The chiropractics . . . are not medical sectarians, though exceedingly desirous of masquerading as such; they are unconscionable quacks, whose printed advertisements are tissues of exaggeration, pretense, and misrepresentation of the most unqualifiedly mercenary character. The public prosecutor and the grand jury are the proper agencies for dealing with them. (158)

In part, Flexner's criticism reflected concern with the entrepreneurial nature of chiropractic enterprise at the time. When Palmer founded the first chiropractic college in the United States, the Palmer School of Chiropractic, the only admission requirement was reportedly a $450 entrance fee (Smith, 1969). While entrance requirements have changed, resistance to chiropractic care has continued, particularly in the United States with ongoing opposition from the American Medical Association. In Canada, resistance has also been noted (Coburn and Biggs, 1986). For example, as recently as 1972, the Canadian Medical Association reaffirmed its policy restricting physicians from making referrals to chiropractors.

Today chiropractic appears to have attained a measure of legitimacy in Canada and other countries (Meeker and Haldeman, 2002). It is now one of the few CAM groups to have been granted official self-regulatory status by provincial governments across the country and has had its own provincial and national associations for much longer than any other CAM group. In 1923, Alberta became the first jurisdiction outside of the United States to license chiropractic. Chiropractors' inclusion within provincial health insurance varies, with some jurisdictions offering partial coverage with restrictions (such as number of visits per year). Currently, chiropractors are the largest group of CAM practitioners in Canada and one of the largest groups of primary medical practitioners. In 2002 there were 6,418 registered (active licensed) chiropractors in Canada, 20.4 for every 100,000 people in the population (almost half were located in Ontario [CIHI, 2005a]). This figure represents an increase from 3,917 in 1993.

On the one hand, these developments suggest that the profession has been successful in ensuring its survival despite medicine's attempts to exclude and destroy it. On the other, such success may have come at a cost. Coburn (1993) argues that chiropractic's increased legitimation has led to a narrowed scope of practice. That is, chiropractic no longer represents a complete alternative or competitor to orthodox medicine but rather a specialist member of the team. He notes that chiropractic has been medicalized in the process—its focus is only on misalignments of the musculoskeletal system, its education consists of a great deal of basic medical science, and its early ties with naturopathy have been diminished.

To the extent that medicalization has taken place, it is incomplete. For example, chiropractic has for the most part been precluded from university affiliation. In the United States, only one university provides a program in chiropractic. Instead, training is located within specialized chiropractic colleges located outside the university system. In Canada, the profession has faced ongoing difficulties in its attempts to affiliate with a university, despite the fact that other health occupations such as nursing and midwifery are currently taught in universities (Grayson, 2002). There are two main chiropractic educational institutions in this country: the Canadian Memorial Chiropractic College was established in Toronto in 1945 and is where the vast majority of practising Canadian chiropractors received their training (Kelner et al., 2006); and the recently established program at the Université du Québec à Trois-Rivières (UQTR) is one of only a few university-based chiropractic programs in North America.

Naturopathy
Naturopathy is a form of holistic health care based on the assumptions that both health and illness are natural processes and that natural healing processes also exist in the body. The role of the naturopath is to work with the patient to activate and support these natural healing processes through the use of various therapies including nutrition, botanicals, homeopathy, physical therapies, hydrotherapy, acupuncture, and TCM.

Naturopathy originated in North America in the late 1800s—the first American School of Naturopathy was established in New York in 1905. The profession was licensed to practise in several states and provinces over the course of the 1920s and 1930s. However, like other sectarian medical practices, it went into decline as scientific medicine gained ascendancy. And like several other sectarian professions, naturopathy is now in the process of re-establishing its legitimacy (Verhoef, Boon, and Mutasingwa, 2006). In 2000–01, almost 500 naturopathic practitioners were licensed in Canada. Naturopathic medicine is currently regulated in four out of 10 Canadian provinces (British Columbia, Saskatchewan, Manitoba, and Ontario), with regulation pending in Alberta.

However, contrasts between sectarian medical practices are evident as well. For example, unlike midwifery and chiropractic care, naturopathic care is not insured under any provincial or territorial government health plan, although some private health insurance companies will reimburse patients (Verhoef, Boon, and Mutasingwa, 2006). While chiropractic care has restricted its scope of practice in order to achieve legitimacy, naturopathic medicine has broadened its scope. Naturopathic practitioners are trained in and draw upon a wide range of therapeutic and diagnostic procedures—most commonly nutritional counselling and supplementation, botanical medicine, and homeopathy. Verhoef, Boon, and Mutasingwa (2006) suggest that naturopathic medicine's draw on other therapeutic systems presents a challenge to the profession's attempts to achieve professional status. Because naturopathic medicine does not possess a unique body of knowledge, conflicts are likely to arise due to the overlap with other professions also vying for regulation.

Medical influence is evident within this profession as well. For example, the Canadian Association of Naturopathic Doctors (CAND) describes naturopathic medicine as a primary health-care system that blends modern scientific knowledge with natural forms of medicine. With regard to training, the naturopathic doctor, like conventional doctors, must complete pre-medical studies at university and then take a four-year, full-time accredited program. 'Training includes basic, medical, and clinical science; diagnostics; naturopathic principles and therapeutics; and extensive clinical experience' (CAND, 2007). In regulated provinces, they must also pass provincial and national licensing examinations. Canada currently has two training institutions accredited by the Council on Naturopathic Medical Education—the Canadian College of Naturopathic Medicine (established in 1978 in Toronto) and the Boucher Institute of Naturopathic Medicine (established in British Columbia in 2000).

Homeopathy

Homeopathy was developed by German physician Christian Samuel Hahnemann (1755–1843). Like early chiropractic and naturopathic forms of medical care, homeopathic medicine is considered a complete medical care system. It rests on the philosophy that illness can be cured through medical care that produces effects similar to the illness symptoms—that 'like cures like'. This theory is opposite to that on which allopathic medicine is based—that illness is best treated by drugs or other therapeutic procedures designed to bring about an effect opposite to that created by the disease. In homeopathy, very small amounts of highly diluted medicine (primarily herbal) are prescribed that, if given in larger doses, would produce the same or similar symptoms of illness in healthy people. It is also believed that therapeutic potency can be increased and side-effects reduced through serial dilution of the medicine (that is, repeatedly diluting the medicine with water or alcohol) accompanied by vigorous shaking between dilutions.

Internationally, homeopathy was one of the more prominent forms of therapy in the nineteenth century. In Canada, homeopaths began to operate in

Quebec and Ontario in the 1840s and were regulated in various locales (Upper Canada, Montreal, British Columbia) between 1859 and 1889 (Clarke, 2008). In North America, however, homeopathy's popularity waned following the release of the Flexner Report. Today, it is widely used in many parts of the world, but has not flourished in North America. Instead, homeopathy has been widely criticized with regard to its lack of scientific validity and the safety of its treatments.

During the last decade, however, there has been somewhat of a revival regarding homeopathy. Because homeopathy is not yet widely regulated—anyone can 'hang out a shingle' and call himself or herself a homeopath (Kelner et al., 2006)—and there is no central registry, determining an exact number of practitioners is difficult. Homeopathy is not only practised solely by homeopaths but also by other health-care practitioners, including naturopaths, chiropractors, and orthodox physicians (Northcott, 2002). Moreover, this small group is divided, with several colleges and associations. Statutory regulation is currently under way in several jurisdictions (e.g., Ontario) although hotly contested by those within the homeopathic community. Some wish to continue to practise their occupations free from external control; others seek professional recognition and designation.

Use of Complementary and Alternative Medicine
It is difficult to know exactly how many people use various forms of CAM. Much depends on what therapies are included. Canadian midwifery services, although legal and publicly funded in several provinces, remain an alternative for a relatively small although increasing number of women; midwives currently attend only two per cent of births nationally (Benoit et al., 2005). Women who use these services tend to be professional women with fairly high levels of education and income. As well, registered midwives tend to work in large urban centres rather than in rural areas. According to Benoit, Carroll, and Millar (2002), women of child-bearing age who live in rural and remote communities lack access to midwifery as well as to physician care.

Overall, it seems that about three-quarters of Canadians have used at least one type of alternative therapy at some point in their lives (Esmail, 2007). A 2003 Statistics Canada survey indicates that approximately 20 per cent of Canadians aged 12 and older reported using some type of complementary or alternative care during the preceding year (Park, 2005), marking an increase from 1994–95 when approximately 15 per cent of those aged 18 and older reported using such care. The most common forms of alternative care were chiropractic services (11 per cent), massage therapists (8 per cent), acupuncturists (2 per cent), and homeopaths or naturopaths (2 per cent) (Park, 2005). Other types of alternative care (including herbalists, reflexology, relaxation therapy, and spiritual healers) were seldom used. McFarland and colleagues (2002) report that in both Canada and the United States chiropractic was the most frequently used CAM treatment, with Canadian use three times that of the United

States. In both countries, there was little use of acupuncture, homeopathy/naturopathy, or massage therapy. In addition, people in both countries were very unlikely to have seen *only* a CAM provider but tended to access such care in conjunction with mainstream medical care.

In both Canada and the United States, CAM use is higher in western regions than in other regions. In Canada, CAM use varies from lows of 3.9 per cent in Nunavut to a high of 27.5 per cent in Alberta. This range is likely the result of provincial differences in health benefits and other policies—for example, chiropractic is not listed among insured health services in Newfoundland and Labrador, while Manitoba covers up to 12 visits per year within its provincial health-care plan. CAM use is also greater among women than men, although this difference is minor when it comes to chiropractic services. Higher CAM use among those with higher education and income (Park, 2005) likely reflects ability to pay because the costs of many such services are, at most, only partially covered by provincial health-care plans. In terms of age, those aged 35 to 44 are the most likely users, followed by those aged 25 to 34 (Health Canada, 1999a). Finally, CAM users are slightly less likely to report excellent health, more likely to report chronic conditions and problems with instrumental activities of daily living, and more likely to have seen a conventional physician in the previous year (even after adjustment for all other factors) than non-users (McFarland et al., 2002; Millar, 2001; Park, 2005).

Ethnic differences are also evident in the type of therapy used. Chiu and colleagues (2006) explored ethnic variations in CAM use by Chinese cancer patients living in British Columbia. They found that all of those interviewed used a combination of TCM and Western medicine. Their reasons included beliefs in the need to care for the body, mind, and spirit together with the view that herbal remedies were important in maintaining such balance; the failure of conventional medicine to deal with the side effects of cancer or to prevent recurrence; and the support of family and friends for CAM use. Both types of therapies were often used simultaneously to complement one another—Western medicine to alleviate acute health problems and TCM to treat chronic conditions in a more holistic way.

HEALTH-CARE SETTINGS

Hospitals
Historically the earliest Canadian hospitals, such as the Hôtel-Dieu Hospitals established in Quebec City (in 1639) and Montreal (in 1642; rebuilt in 1861), were created primarily for the ailing poor and generally provided domestic and custodial rather than medical care. They provided food, shelter, and support to the chronically ill who were poor and dying as well as those who had no family or were unable to access private sources of care. Those with contagious diseases as well as those with mental illnesses were turned away. Some of these hospitals

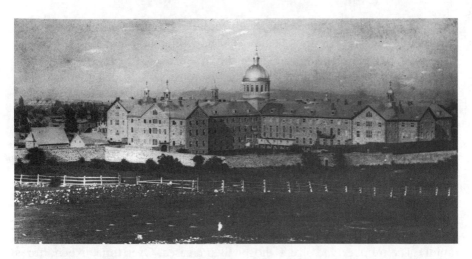

Hotel Dieu Hospital, Montreal, QC, about 1865. Anonymous. Gift of Mr David Ross McCord. McCord Museum MP-0000.1764.2.

were established by municipal governments; however, government funding was limited and, because the settings primarily serviced the poor, little income was generated. Other hospitals were established by charitable organizations or religious orders, the latter as settings wherein nuns could minister to the bodies as well as to the souls of the ill (Goulet, 2003).

Over the course of the nineteenth century, general hospitals became increasingly dedicated to the provision of medical rather than simply custodial care for the ailing poor and, by the 1870s, all major Canadian cities had general hospitals (often one for Protestants and one for Catholics). Specialized hospitals were created for those with contagious diseases. The poor and unsanitary conditions that often prevailed within these settings, the fact that they catered to the destitute and the dying, and the stigma associated with accepting services from such charitable organizations meant that few would access them if they had a choice (Goulet, 2003; Weitz, 1996a). For example, until the 1870s, doctors did not generally wear gloves or masks while performing surgery. Nor did they wash their hands or disinfect their instruments prior to moving from one patient to another (Goulet, 2003).

During the latter part of the nineteenth and early twentieth centuries, medical dominance and the increasing emphasis on scientific medicine created a need to locate care in settings where not only patients but also medical laboratories and technologies (such as X-rays) could be housed and surgeries performed. Florence Nightingale and other nursing reformers were also instrumental in establishing more sanitary and professionally operated institutions. Thus, hospitals became places where scientific medicine was practised, complex medical technology was located and could be accessed, and highly skilled medical training was provided. In the 1870s, doctors began to adopt various techniques for preventing post-surgical infection. Death became a less likely outcome of hospitalization. Over time not only the homeless and ailing poor but also the middle and upper classes began to draw upon the care provided within these settings (Torrance, 1998). Private and semi-private rooms were added to the public wards typical of such settings in order to accommodate their needs.

Yet according to Torrance (1998), it was not until the Depression and World War II that Canadian hospitals gradually transformed from relatively simple quasi-charitable organizations to large-scale modern bureaucratic organizations funded by public sources. After the war, in times of prosperity, the federal government began funding hospital construction and later universal hospital care so that care could be obtained at no direct charge to the patient and hospitals would become firmly established as the location for medical care.

Demand for hospital care and for new facilities and technology increased rapidly. The number and size of hospitals increased. Over time, expenditures also increased and staffing patterns changed toward a greater diversity of increasingly specialized health-care occupations. The share of health-care funding consumed by hospitals also increased, leading to federal/provincial government attempts to control hospital costs in the 1980s and 1990s (see Chapter 5).

Currently, hospital costs represent the single largest category (about one-third) of health expenditures in Canada (CIHI, 2001). Unlike countries such as the United States, which is witnessing increased proprietary and corporate ownership of hospital settings, Canadian hospital costs continue to be paid for by primarily public funds (federal, provincial, and municipal) as decreed in the Canada Health Act. Nevertheless, increasing concern about rising health-care costs has led to hospital closures and downsizing, especially in some rural areas where beds were rarely filled. For example, the number of hospitals and hospital beds declined during the 1980s and 1990s. From 1995–96 to 1999–2000, 275 acute-care hospitals closed, merged, or changed to provide other types of care. Health-care practices and procedures also changed considerably, including reduced in-patient hospital admissions, shorter hospital stays, and greater out-patient care (Health Canada, 2005). Whether these changes will eventually move acute-care hospital settings away from the centre to the periphery of our health-care system remains to be seen.

Access to and Utilization of Hospital Services
As noted earlier, Canada prides itself on having established a universal health-care system, ensuring that people have equitable access to care and receive services in accordance with health-related needs rather than social factors such as income, ethnicity, or gender. Thus, Canadians at various income levels are often said to have equitable access to both physician and hospital care. In general, Canadians are relatively unlikely to experience hospital care: in 2005, about 9 per cent of Canadians spent at least one night in hospital (Asada and Kephart, 2007). Yet a recently published report concludes that equity regarding the

allocation of primary health-care services in British Columbia varies depending on the type of service involved—whereas access to GP services is equitably distributed, this is less evident with regard to other health services such as hospital emergency services (Watson et al., 2005). There are indications that quality of care received may also vary. For example, a study of patients suffering heart attacks who went to various hospital emergency departments in Alberta from 1998 to 2002 found that those who lived in lower-income neighbourhoods were often treated less aggressively than those living in wealthier neighbourhoods, despite the fact that they were more likely to visit emergency departments. This finding may also reflect differences in the health services available within different neighbourhoods. On the other hand, others report little evidence that people living in lower-income neighbourhoods in Ontario face longer waits for elective surgery (which includes 22 common elective procedures such as cataract removal, hysterectomy, tonsillectomy, prostatectomy, and tubal ligation) than those in higher-income neighbourhoods (Shortt and Shaw, 2003).

Waiting times for hospital surgical care appear to vary from province to province, with longer waits in Prince Edward Island, Nova Scotia, Quebec, Manitoba, Saskatchewan, and Alberta. A review of studies conducted in various locales points to fewer and smaller hospitals in rural than urban areas (Casey, Call, and Klingner, 2001; Chan and Barer, 2000; Nagarajan, 2004; Thommassen, 2000). As well, differences in access and utilization emerge with regard to ethnic and racial factors. For example, several US studies have shown that racialized minority patients are more likely to be hospitalized in acute-care settings than whites—and the quality and treatment outcomes of hospital care are also found to be poorer (Smaje, 2000). In contrast, evidence from the United Kingdom suggests less use of hospital services by racialized minorities than by whites (Smaje, 2000). Along similar lines, an Ontario study found that immigrants and other ethnic/cultural groups often showed lower use of hospital emergency rooms when compared with non-immigrants (Wen, Goel, and Williams, 1996).

Finally, gender and age differences in access to and utilization of hospital care are also evident. Women are more likely to receive hospital care, due largely to the fact that the majority of births continue to take place in hospital settings. Yet they appear less likely than men to be recipients of aggressive medical and surgical care (e.g., cardiac surgery). With regard to age, although those aged 65 and older account for approximately 13 per cent of the Canadian population, they account for over 33 per cent of all acute-care hospital discharges and because they tend to be in hospital longer than younger individuals, they account for about 50 per cent of all days spent in hospitals (CIHI, 2001). However, despite this group's greater utilization of hospital services, a recent study of the effects of age on the care of people hospitalized with congestive heart failure found that older patients, especially older women with cardiac disease, tend to be treated less aggressively than those in younger age groups (Alter et al., 2002; Cujec et al., 2004).

Since the introduction of national hospital insurance, hospitalization rates have decreased for younger age groups but have continued to increase among older adults, leading to concern that older adults are using such services inappropriately as well as to discussions regarding the need to ration services to those most likely to benefit (i.e., younger age groups). Yet decisions about hospitalization are not made by older adults but by their physicians. The rates also reflect lack of access to services (such as home care) required for coping with long-term chronic illnesses and disabilities as well as with dying. A study recently conducted in Manitoba found that 40 per cent of all acute-care hospital days were used by about 5 per cent of patients. About two-thirds of these patients were aged 75 and older, many of whom were awaiting transfer to another type of care (i.e., nursing home care, home care, chronic care) (DeCoster, Bruce, and Kozyrskyi, 2005). In other words, they were in hospitals because other, possibly more appropriate types of care were not accessible.

Long-Term Residential Care

As hospitals became increasingly focused on providing high-tech medical and surgical care, their emphasis shifted to acute rather than chronic illnesses and conditions. This change left a gap for those with chronic illnesses requiring long-term care. At the same time, increases in life expectancy and declines in mortality brought about by improvements in public health (nutrition and public sanitation) meant that more and more people were living longer and that the prevalence of chronic illness and disability were increasing. As a result, long-term residential care settings, or nursing homes, were established to provide health care to those unable to function independently due to physical or cognitive disabilities. Individuals who reside in such facilities require high levels of personal care together with some nursing care or supervision.

In contrast to hospitals, residential care facilities are owned and operated by a mix of public and private sources. Nursing homes in Canada historically consisted of small independent owner-operated homes. Since 1971, many have been taken over by larger chains. Currently, just over one-half of all residential care facilities in Canada are owned and operated by governments, not-for-profit, or charitable or religious organizations. The remainder are owned by proprietary sources and operated on a for-profit basis (Berta et al., 2006; CIHI, 2005b).

The extent of public versus private ownership varies from province to province—95 per cent of residential care facilities in Saskatchewan are publicly owned and operated compared to 43 per cent in Ontario (CIHI, 2005b). The costs of care also vary. Unlike hospital care, where the costs are publicly insured under the Canada Health Act, residential care costs are set by each province. In general, costs are shared between residents and provincial/territorial governments, with governments covering the costs of the care up to a specified limit (i.e., personal care and nursing costs) and residents paying for the costs of their accommodation. However, daily charges vary from lows of $10 to $30 per day in

British Columbia, Saskatchewan, Manitoba, Quebec, Yukon, and the Northwest Territories to highs of over $90 per day in Newfoundland, Nova Scotia, and New Brunswick (CIHI, 2005b).

Provincial governments also assume responsibility for policies and regulations governing the care provided within long-term care settings. Consequently, provincial standards and the quality of care also vary from province to province. Differences in quality of care across organizations can be accounted for by structural factors such as size, type of ownership (for-profit v. not-for-profit), staffing levels, and type of care provided. Having more direct-care personnel (registered nurses, nurses' aides) is often associated with better care. In the United States, not-for-profit facilities have been found to provide more services and better quality of care and to have higher direct-care staffing levels and lower staff turnover than for-profit facilities. In Canada, where both not-for-profit and for-profit facilities are funded by government, research findings are similar. For example, a recent Ontario study found that staffing levels are significantly higher in government-owned and not-for-profit facilities (Berta, Laporte, and Valdmanis, 2005; Berta et al., 2006). Similarly, a British Columbia study reports that the average number of care hours provided by staff per resident was higher in not-for-profit facilities (McGregor et al., 2005: 645). Thus, since both are supported by public funds, the authors conclude that 'public money used to provide care to frail elderly people purchases significantly fewer direct care and support staff hours per resident-day in for-profit long-term care facilities than in not-for-profit facilities'.

In recent years, the involvement of proprietary interests in the provision of long-term care is increasing in several provinces (Berta, Laporte, and Valdmanis, 2005). In British Columbia, for example, observers report recent reductions in not-for-profit residential care facilities and a 'sixfold increase in corporate investment in residential care and assisted living facilities' (Cohen et al., 2005). This finding has generated concern regarding the implications for accessibility and quality of care within such settings.

Who Uses Long-Term Residential Care
At one time Canada was known for having very high levels of long-term care institutionalization. Currently, however, a relatively small proportion of Canadians are residents of such facilities. The vast majority (81 per cent; see McGregor et al., 2005) are aged 65 and older. In 2001, 9.2 per cent of women and 4.9 per cent of men aged 65 and older were residents in such facilities (CIHI, 2005b). Nevertheless, the likelihood of residential care placement also increases with age. In 1996 very few persons (2.1 per cent) aged 65 to 74 were in long-term residential care settings. However, this increased to 8.9 per cent of those aged 75 to 84 and 33.8 per cent of those aged 85 and older (Lindsay, 1999). Residents enter into care relatively late in life and therefore do not generally remain in such facilities very long; the median length of stay is approximately two years (CIHI, 2000).

As a result, the proportion of older adults who will spend some time in a facility of this type at some point in their lives is considerably higher than the proportion that is in care at any one time.

The likelihood of residence also varies by gender and socio-economic status as well as across provinces. Two-thirds of long-term care residents are women, reflecting the combined realities of differences in longevity, age- and gender-based poverty, and higher levels of chronic illness and disability among women, as well as their decreased access to informal community-based supports (CIHI, 2001). In addition to the influence of health problems (especially cognitive impairment), age, gender, and socio-economic status, social factors such as living alone and being without a spouse or other informal caregiver also influence the likelihood of being in long-term residential care (St John et al., 2002). Overall, it is the very old, women, and those with less access to social and economic resources who are the most likely recipients of this more privately focused and market-driven form of long-term care.

Home Care

The provision of health care within large institutions such as hospitals is a relatively recent phenomenon. Well into the nineteenth century, those who were sick were generally cared for at home, including those with limited financial resources but with family members available to provide care and middle-class and wealthier people able to secure privately paid care (Torrance, 1998). Although the formal health-care system moved toward doctors' offices, medical clinics, hospitals, and other medical-care settings, recent years have seen attempts to bring care 'closer to home'. Today, most care (self and informal) still occurs in the home.

Public (formal) home care programs were first introduced in Canada during the 1950s. At that time they tended to offer medical services only and were seen primarily as a means to shorten acute-care hospital stays. In the 1970s, however, home care was also seen as a means of limiting the number of people requiring long-term residential care (Chappell, 1994). In addition, there were those who argued that home care should not only be a substitute for institutional care but also a broader form of health care providing 'an array of services enabling Canadians, incapacitated in whole or in part, to live at home, often with the effect of preventing, delaying, or substituting for long-term care or acute-care alternatives' (Health Canada, 1990). The services should not only encompass biomedical services—those typically provided in medical or hospital-care settings—but should also include services that substitute for those provided by long-term care institutions or that prevent or delay institutionalization. This argument was based in part on research indicating that many of those who were being institutionalized did not require medical or nursing care but help with everyday activities such as housekeeping, meals, and transportation. Accordingly, despite opposition from those who considered such services social rather than health related, home care programs began to provide supportive services such as housekeeping and laundry, personal care services (e.g., help with bathing, getting dressed, and eating), home maintenance (e.g., home repairs, gardening), and help with transportation and respite services for those with long-term illnesses and disabilities.

By the late 1980s, home care programs were available in all provinces and territories. Like other health services, responsibility for home care rests with the provinces and territories. Consequently, home care policies, services, and delivery vary considerably (Coyte, 2000; Coyte and McKeever, 2001). Currently all provincial and territorial plans cover home support services (such as homemaking, personal care, meal services) and home nursing care (Ballinger, Zhang, and Hicks, 2001). Some plans also offer therapeutic services (physiotherapy and occupational, speech, and respiratory therapy), medical equipment and supplies, minor home repair and home maintenance, social services (such as friendly visiting services) as well as respite and palliative care. While respite care is designed to give family members a break from the demands of caregiving, palliative care is end-of-life care aimed at pain and symptom control for those who are in the advanced stages of life-threatening illness. Some provinces (e.g., Ontario, Newfoundland, and Prince Edward Island) require physician referral in order to access services, thereby preserving the gate-keeping function of physicians and the dominance of the biomedical approach. Some limit access to those in particular age (e.g., aged 65 and older) and income groups.

As with long-term residential care, the private health-care sector is more heavily involved. Across the country, home care services are delivered by both public and private sources and on both a for-profit and not-for-profit basis (Aronson, Denton, and Zeytinoglu, 2004). In some provinces home care workers are hired directly by publicly funded organizations. Most provinces offer a mix of publicly and privately funded services. Medical, nursing, and therapeutic services (such as occupational or physical therapy) are often delivered by publicly funded program staff, while support services such as personal care, homemaking assistance, meal preparation, and transportation services are often outsourced to for-profit or not-for-profit agencies external to government (Hollander and Pallan, 1995). Most programs also charge care recipients (often on a sliding scale depending upon income).

Since its introduction, home care has become an increasingly important component of the Canadian health-care system, substituting for care in hospitals and long-term care facilities. In recent years, home care has been one of the fastest-growing programs in the system (Williams, 1996). Canadian public expenditures on home care almost doubled over the course of the 1990s (from 2.3 per cent of the national health care budget in 1990–91 to 4.0 per cent in 1997–98; see also Figure 4.3). It has also attained prominence in government policy documents and rhetoric where it is often presented as an inexpensive and therefore attractive alternative to increasingly costly physician, hospital, and long-term residential care. The 1990s saw extensive review and restructuring of

Figure 4.3   Provincial–Territorial Hospital and Home Care Expenditures ($ Millions), 1980–81 to 2000–01

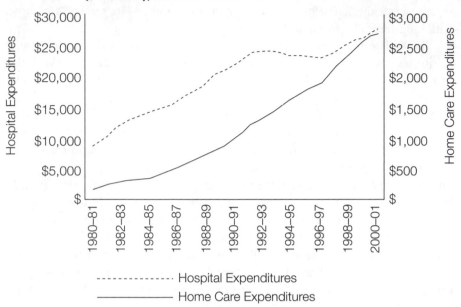

- - - - - - - - - - - - - Hospital Expenditures
———————— Home Care Expenditures

Source: R.J. Romanow, Commissioner. 2002. *Building on Values. The Future of Health Care in Canada.* Ottawa: Health Canada. Reproduced with the permission of the Minister of Public Works and Government Services Canada, 2008.

the Canadian health-care system, a process initiated in response to growing governmental concern over the current and future costs of health care as well as the system's effectiveness and efficiency (see Chapter 5). Home care, along with other community-based services, assumed a central role in the new health-care system that was being envisioned during this period—one that saw a redistribution of dollars from medical and institutional care to a broader base of community health services and a shift of decision-making power from professionals to individuals whose health was affected (Chappell, 1995). This new vision led to recommendations that home care become part of Canada's publicly insured and universally accessible health-care system (National Forum on Health, 1997).

To date, however, formal community-based home care has not emerged as a major component of Canada's universal health-care system. Instead, it remains politically and economically secondary and subordinate to the more medical components of the system. Therefore, despite being one of the fastest growing components within Canada's health-care system, home care continues to account for only a small proportion of Canada's total health-care budget. Also, despite increases in spending on home care, in some jurisdictions fewer people are receiving home care services than a decade ago and the services are more likely to be nursing care and other medically oriented services (such as mobile dialysis, chemotherapy, and palliative care) rather than home support services such as housekeeping, help with meals, shopping, or transportation (CIHI, 2007).

Who Uses Home Care

Figures for community care are difficult to access, particularly for privately paid services. However, it has been estimated that about 10 per cent of adults aged 65 and older and 2.5 per cent of those aged 18 and older received publicly funded or subsidized formal home care services in the preceding year (Wilkins and Park, 1998). Most received homemaker or home help services. Somewhat fewer received home nursing care or help with personal care activities, such as bathing, dressing, or getting in and out of bed, and meal preparation or meal delivery services.

People who receive home care services tend to be female, older (aged 65 and older), and not married or childless (Mitchell, Roos, and Shapiro, 2005). They also tend to be in relatively poor health. According to the *National Population Health Survey*, the likelihood of receiving these services is also higher for those with lower family incomes and for those who live alone. Access to home care services also varies across the country (see Figure 4.4).

There are also differences in access across rural and urban areas. Yet the importance of health-related differences in accounting for these variations remains unclear. For example, Penning and colleagues (forthcoming) found significant geographic differences in home care utilization over the course of the 1990s. Their study, conducted in British Columbia, found that people living in some health regions received more home support and home nursing care than those in other regions. Similarly, those living in rural areas generally received more home support hours and home nursing care visits than those living in other, predominantly more urban, areas. These differences were not due to such factors as age, gender, or income levels. While these findings provide little support for assertions that individuals living in rural areas receive less home support and home nursing care than those living in more urban areas, neither do they necessarily support conclusions that those living in rural areas tend to be relatively advantaged or, alternatively, that equitable care is received. As noted, assessing equitable access to care should take needs for health care into account. To the extent that those living in rural areas can be assumed to have greater needs for care than those living in more urban areas, their more extensive care seems appropriate. Whether the care provided is in proportion to need and whether the relationship between need and utilization is the same in different areas remain questions in need of further study.

As already noted, home care accounts for only a small proportion (4 per cent in 1997–98) of total national public health-care spending (Health Canada, 1998). Furthermore, recent increases in funding have not necessarily been accompanied by increases in the number of people receiving such care. Instead,

Figure 4.4   Number of Government-Sponsored Home Care Users per 1,000 Population, Actual versus Standardized, by Province/Territory and Canada, 2003

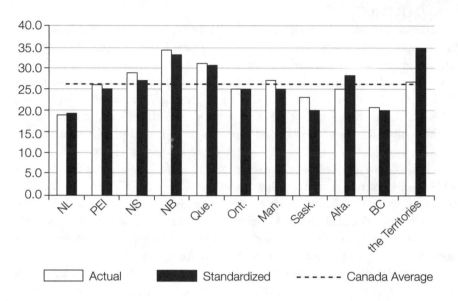

Source: CIHI. 2007. *Public-Sector Expenditures and Utilization of Home Care Services in Canada: Exploring the Data.* Ottawa: Canadian Institute of Health Information.

research recently conducted in British Columbia points to declines in the number of older adults receiving publicly funded home care services (including home support services as well as home nursing care) and the extent of care received in recent years (number of hours or visits; see Cohen et al., 2005; Penning, Brackley, and Allan, 2006). There are indications that services are being redirected towards those with more acute medical care needs, including people dying from cancer, AIDS, and other illnesses. Those most likely to rely on these services in the past were those with high levels of chronic illness and disability, older elderly women, those without access to informal sources of support, and those with lower levels of income (Coyte and McKeever, 2001; Penning, 2001). Evidence of service reductions together with decisions to shift from publicly to privately funded care will therefore have a disproportionate impact on these groups (Williams et al., 2001).

Other Forms of Community-Based Care

Typically, when we discuss health-care settings, we focus attention on hospitals, nursing homes, and other institutions. If we think about community-based settings, we may think about doctors' offices, walk-in clinics, other medical care settings (such as medical laboratories, blood donor clinics, or cancer screening centres), or home-based nursing or hospice care. It is less likely that our attention turns to other non-medically oriented settings. In fact, these may not be seen as health-care settings at all. Such settings include places where we practise self-care (sports and recreational facilities, health and education sites, and wellness centres), where we participate in mutual aid (support groups for those with a specific disease or addiction), and where we engage in more formally provided health as well as illness care services (weight-loss settings).

In many ways the importance of these settings to our health remains hidden, given the predominantly medical focus of our system. The vast majority of health-care resources are devoted to physician and hospital care—few are allocated to other forms, including those that focus on health promotion and disease prevention. Yet Canada has a long history of involvement, both nationally and internationally, in the development of health promotion programs and policies (see Chapters 5 and 6, on health policy and looking to the future).

EXPERIENCING FORMAL CARE

Medical and Hospital Care

Care-related experiences vary depending, in part, on the type of care involved. Sociologists have long been interested in doctor–patient relationships within and outside of hospital-care settings. As with illness experiences generally (see Chapter 2), they began by examining these relationships from the outside as defined by sources other than those receiving care. Initially their focus was on consensual aspects of the relationship that were regarded as objectively (normatively) defined. According to Parsons (1951), for example, the relationship was assumed to be voluntary in which both parties shared a common goal—restoring the patient's health. Doctors provided the best care they could and patients did everything they could to get well. The relationship was considered symbiotic and consensual: '[i]n the post-World War II era, physicians' control over medical care was based to a large degree on trust, and stemmed from knowledge of the personhood of the doctor and from the results of medical treatments . . .' (Jennings, 2006: 356–7). From Parsons's perspective, medical authorities (physicians) were the active agents in the illness encounter. Those who were ill were viewed largely as passive recipients of medical authority—their primary duty was to seek out and then comply with medical dictates for the purpose of getting better. Thus, a considerable amount of research during this period focused on how well patients complied with medical directives.

By the 1960s, however, the public had become increasingly critical of the medical profession and the type of care it often provided. Within sociology, attention was increasingly drawn to the medical model of care and the potentially adverse implications of medical authority and asymmetric doctor–patient interactions for patients' care-related experiences and outcomes. Rather than passive, willing recipients of physician benevolence, patients came to be seen as powerless victims of **professional dominance** (Freidson, 1970a, 1970b) and of a model of care that created and sustained **social distance** (a sense of separation or difference between social groups resulting in an inability to identify with each other) between doctors and their patients and accorded little importance to patients' perspectives or concerns. According to Mishler (1989), for example, physicians and patients tend to have different and conflicting agendas in the medical visit. The doctor's medical agenda focuses on biomedical evaluation and treatment, particularly in relation to acute or life-threatening conditions. In contrast, the patient's lifeworld agenda deals with personal fears, anxieties, and other everyday circumstances (including preventive care of those who are well, treatment of minor health conditions, and treatment of chronic health problems). In Mishler's view these two agendas often conflict with one another and make communication difficult. The result is a patient experience frequently characterized by poor communication, lack of access to information, limited involvement in decision-making, and inadequate concern for personal identities and psychosocial needs.

Research tended to support these concerns. For example, Korsch and Negrete (1972) observed 800 pediatric acute-care visits within a medical clinic and found that about one-fifth of the parents left the clinic without being informed about what was wrong with their child and almost one-half had no idea what had caused their child's illness. A quarter of the parents reported that they had not discussed their major concerns with the doctor because of lack of opportunity or encouragement. For their part, physicians tended to view the parents who felt that physicians had not met their expectations as 'grossly non-compliant'. Similarly, Waitzkin (1985) found that although the average patient–physician visit lasted 16.5 minutes, patients spent an average of only eight seconds asking questions. In addition, physicians believed that they spent an average of nine minutes providing information to their patients but actually spent an average of 40 seconds doing so. Even if physicians provided explanations for the illness to their patients, they rarely showed any interest in the patients' perspectives (Frank, 2002). Findings also revealed that about one-half of all physician visits were initiated for psychosocial rather than strictly biomedical reasons (Ashworth, Williamson, and Montano, 1984).

Some patients' experiences were worse than others. For example, physicians often preferred treating younger patients and held negative images of elderly patients; they often treated patients of different ethnic and social class backgrounds differently. More negative experiences were also reported in association with social characteristics such as being homosexual, homeless, unemployed, employed in the sex trade, or being on welfare. According to one study, hospital staff admitted treating patients they considered to be 'undesirable' less thoroughly than others (Mizrahi, 1986). Occasionally, this can lead to mistakes in diagnosis and treatment such as when a homeless person is brought unconscious to the emergency room and treated as if the condition was alcohol induced rather than the result of some other problem, such as a serious neurological problem (Freund and McGuire, 1999).

Patient empowerment and therefore patients' opportunities for involvement in decision-making regarding their care increased substantially from the 1960s onward. According to Potter and McKinlay (2005), as criticism of the power of the medical establishment increased, medical consumerism also grew, gradually transforming the doctor–patient relationship into a market transaction in which economic concerns played a central role. As consumers, patients had increased power and agency. The emergence of medical consumerism was associated with enabling patients to challenge their physicians and to gain the knowledge necessary to make educated decisions regarding treatment options: consumer-organized movements took their concerns to the courts and the doctor–patient relationship began to be viewed as a partnership, recognizing patients' rights and emphasizing the physician's duty to present all relevant information (Potter and McKinlay, 2005). Thus, laws around informed consent increasingly required that physicians provide patients with information concerning the potential benefits and risks of medical treatments and alternatives to allow patients to participate in decisions concerning their own medical care and treatment. The notion of patient as decision maker is not limited to legal doctrine but, within the last two decades, has become part of the culture of medicine itself. As a result, moral principles, such as the patient's right to self-determination and informed consent, have come to guide the way physicians approach medical decisions and treat their patients (Jennings, 2006; Zussman, 1993). By the 1990s, physicians not only acknowledged patients' basic right to make decisions relevant to their medical care but also often encouraged them to do so (Zussman, 1993). According to one study, while 88 per cent of the physicians studied in 1961 reported that they generally did not inform patients of a cancer diagnosis, by 1979 about 98 per cent reported that their policy was to inform patients (Novack et al., 1979).

There is ongoing debate regarding the extent to which patients actually want an active role in decision-making and exactly what this means. Some researchers report that only a small minority of patients are interested in assuming this role; many of those who do are those with long-term chronic illnesses and disabilities. However, Rier's (2000) first-hand sociological account of his own experiences as an intensive care unit (ICU) patient suggests that full disclosure of information to patients as well as patient negotiation and collaboration with physicians may be of little relevance to some of those who are critically ill. In addition, many patients express interest in receiving information so they can better comply with physicians' directives rather than to direct their own treatment. For example, from a study conducted in 11 European countries, Bastiaens and colleagues (2007: 33) report that older adults' desire for involvement in their care focused more on the caring relationship and a person-centred approach than on active decision-making. That is, they want to have a trusting relationship, to be respected, to have sufficient time during consultations, and to receive information—these elements are central to involvement.

Furthermore, the ideals of patient-centred care and opportunities for patients to participate in their care are not universally accessible. Patient age, education, and social class are related to the likelihood that physicians will give them information. In particular, those who are younger, have a college education, and reflect upper- or upper-middle-class backgrounds receive more information and more extensive explanations (Street, 1991; Waitzkin, 2000). Ethnic, racial, and language differences also exist. For example, Cooper-Patrick and colleagues (1999) report finding that African-American patients rate their visits with physicians as less participatory than whites. However, patients whose physicians are the same race as them rate their physicians' decision-making styles as more participatory. Gender differences are sometimes opposite to what is expected, with physicians giving more information to women than to men. Waitzkin (2000) suggests that gender and ethnic barriers in communication may have begun to improve somewhat as patients and physicians gain greater awareness of barriers to information giving, along with changes in the gender and ethnic composition of the medical profession. He reports that female physicians tend to spend more time with patients (giving information as well as listening to them) and devote more attention to the psychosocial aspects of care.

Other social factors also come into play. A study on the health-care needs of crack-using female prostitutes in Toronto found that although these women were heavy users of the health-care system and generally reported positive experiences, they also encountered structural barriers. Some cited their drug use as a key factor affecting the care they received: 'Lots of times if you go to the hospital to emergency with a really serious problem and you get turned away because you have addiction on your file. It's assumed that you're there for drugs . . . You're sloughed off. It's pretty common' (Butters and Erickson, 2003: 11).

In addition, empowerment and patient-centred care differs in meaning and importance in different settings. In 1992, Zussman (1992) spent six months in the ICUs of two large teaching hospitals in the United States. He reports that while patient autonomy has penetrated medical practice within this setting, it tends to be evident only when it comes to 'rituals of closure' such as signing informed consent forms or negotiating 'do not resuscitate' orders. Similarly, in an ethnographic study in the surgical wards of two general hospitals, Fox (1993) found that when patients tried to ask questions (such as why they felt the way they did, when they could expect to feel better, and when they could go home) the surgeons often ignored them. Instead, they focused their discussions with patients and their families around surgical care itself (its goals, its specific outcome, etc.). This focus on surgeon-centred themes gives patients few opportunities to introduce their own perspectives or concerns into the discussion.

Parke's (2007) research on the fit between older adults and acute-care hospitals reveals how large social structures and systems influence those they are designed to help. Although the research began with the assumption that the characteristics of hospitals and their employees are a poor fit for all older adults, the results indicated that this is true only for some. The research shows that it is not chronological age per se that creates problems but the relationships between vulnerable individuals and their functional disabilities and the environmental demands. Older adults capable of self-determination are no different from younger adults; they are capable of seeking autonomy and of participating in decision-making. Those who can function independently and are cognitively alert can decide to cooperate with the environment or choose not to conform.

However, if the needs of the individual (typically those who are frail, cognitively impaired, and unable to make their own decisions or to function independently) do not fit, the patients are unpopular with staff members, who feel incompetent because they cannot properly meet their chronic-care needs in an environment established to meet acute-care needs. These patients demand more time than the system allows; they require special attention; they cannot cooperate or comply. The architectural features, bureaucratic conditions, chaotic atmosphere, and employee attitudes all contribute to difficulty meeting the needs of these patients. However, staff members interpret these patients, rather than patient *care*, as difficult.

Among those who are cognitively capable, greater involvement in decision-making has been found to be positive for patients' care experiences. Patients report being least satisfied with narrowly biomedical visits and most satisfied with visits in which the physician adopts a participatory decision-making style (Cooper-Patrick et al., 1999). Individuals who receive such care tend to have better preventive health outcomes (such as quitting smoking and engaging in long-term exercise and weight loss) as well as adherence to medical treatment and other aspects of physical and mental health. Finally, both quantitative and qualitative studies indicate that, when physicians listen well and show care and compassion, patients' psychological well-being, physiological symptoms, and functional health outcomes all tend to improve (Stewart, 2003).

Despite the increasing focus on patient empowerment and its positive implications for patient care-related experiences and health outcomes, there are also suggestions that medical consumerism can have negative implications. For example, Zussman (1993) suggests that rather than pointing to greater collaboration between patients and physicians, consumerism may signify physicians distancing themselves from their patients and abdicating their responsibility for some decisions. The focus on locating individual responsibility in the hands of the patient, according to Potter and McKinlay (2005), reflects the fact that the consumer model that served to empower patients subsequently gave way to a corporate model toward the end of the twentieth century. As a result, both patients and physicians faced a loss of status. Within this model, corporate ownership and management accompanied by profit-making and cost-reduction agendas gradually replaced patient care as the dominant objectives of health care. For example, Waitzkin (2000) suggests that within this model medical practitioners often function as double agents (serving as gatekeepers who are required to restrict access to specialists, emergency care, and other services in order to keep costs down while continuing as advocates for patients). Financial concerns limit open communication (in that patients have to make a strong case to gatekeepers justifying their need to access services). Under these conditions, patients' trust of physicians may be jeopardized and the doctor–patient relationship may become nonexistent in the twenty-first century: 'Today . . . the word "relationship" as applied to the doctor–patient experience may be a misnomer . . . One could ask, for example, if a person's most recent physician visit was more akin to their encounter with their last cab driver, or the person who sold them their last pair of shoes' (Potter and McKinlay, 2005: 465). In Potter and McKinlay's view, what happens between a doctor and a patient may be more accurately described as an encounter rather than a relationship.

Complementary and Alternative Medicine

There is debate regarding the reasons for the increased popularity and use of alternative therapies in recent years. One explanation is that it reflects patient dissatisfaction with their experiences with conventional medicine in Western societies, including dissatisfaction due to ineffective medical treatments, the adverse effects of conventional medical therapies, and poor doctor–patient communication and relationships (Boon et al., 1999). Thus, researchers have reported that users of CAM say they have less confidence in the efficacy of conventional medicine (Gray et al., 1997) as well as more satisfying, personal relationships with CAM practitioners compared to the rather brief and technical consultations they tend to experience in conventional medical care (Frank, 2002). Increased use of complementary and alternative medicines represents the increased importance of being treated as 'a whole person', especially for contemporary health consumers who reject being objectified by traditional doctors.

Others argue that patients are turning to CAM primarily for ideological reasons, including their beliefs in holistic health or an alternative lifestyle (Sharma, 1992). Goldner (2004) reports finding that most clients as well as practitioners define their participation in CAM as a form of activism and as being part of a larger social movement—although each acts individually, they are united in their challenge to Western medicine. Through a common ideology, a diffuse social movement is comprised of those who identify with others of like mind (Goldner, 2004).

Still others link patient participation in CAM to patients' acceptance of personal responsibility for health accompanied by their desires for personal control over treatment decisions. The need to exercise a measure of control over treatment decisions may reflect the illness experience itself. For example,

Foote-Ardah (2003) examined meanings of CAM use in the everyday lives of people with HIV; those who reported having used some form of CAM over the course of their illness saw it as one way they could increase control and thereby try to cope with the uncertainties of their illness. Along somewhat similar lines, Verhoef, Boon, and Mutasingwa's (2006) review of studies examining reasons behind CAM use among cancer patients suggests that one of the main reasons is that it represents a basis for hope.

Patients' use of CAM has also been attributed to the increasing commercialization of health care and emphasis on medical consumerism. Thompson (2003: 84) suggests that the growth and mainstreaming of CAM has led patients as consumers to see Western medicine simply as one system of healing among others. The natural-health marketplace is a pluralistic, decentralized marketplace offering many alternatives and founded on notions of consumer choice and allows individuals to 'engage in an interactive, self-producing consumption experience'. Thompson's analyses of the illness narratives of two women suffering from chronic illnesses (multiple sclerosis, chronic fatigue syndrome, and fibromyalgia) suggested that their use of various natural-health alternatives enabled them to cope with their bodies suddenly failing and their dissatisfaction with available medical options. While they viewed their medical care (including diagnoses, treatment options, and long-term prognoses) as disempowering, they regarded their explorations of the world of natural-health alternatives as journeys of self-discovery. These journeys were conducted in partnership with natural-health experts. Holistic practitioners were seen as supportive guides who helped individuals discover their personal paths to wellness. Thus, CAM enabled these women to resist the identities assigned by conventional medicine and to re-script them in more positive ways that emphasized self-discovery and personal transformation. They were able to construct their chronic illnesses as 'an opportunity for discovering their inner regenerative potential and expanding their spiritual horizons' (81).

It seems that many of us act pragmatically and choose whatever works from a pluralistic marketplace. Researchers have reported that rather than being pushed toward CAM use because of a deep philosophical commitment to a complementary/alternative paradigm, many simply 'hedge their bets' and use both. Boon and colleagues (1999) report finding that few of those they studied drew a clear line between CAM and conventional medical care. Instead, most saw their options as a smorgasbord from which they could choose a unique treatment protocol. Although some individuals expressed disappointment with the outcome of their conventional medical care and others described deep belief in the complementary/alternative philosophy, most used both systems simultaneously.

Does this mean that patients do so without reflecting on the risks involved? Based on her qualitative study of people with Parkinson's disease who use various forms of CAM, Low (2004) reports that the people she studied were prepared to try almost anything that might prove helpful but also thought about the risks involved (e.g., health risks from the therapies themselves, risks of being taken advantage of). They also used various strategies to try and manage those risks, such as checking credentials and rationalizing the risks. However, Low also reports that people are often constrained in their ability to exercise reflexivity in managing the risks associated with the use of CAM by various social factors (such as social class, race/ethnicity, age, health status, access to information). In other words, they exercise agency as health-care consumers, but they do so within socially structured situations.

Long-Term Care: Institutional and Home

Sociologists have long drawn attention to the negative implications of long-term residential and institutional care on patient experiences—including their ability to exercise personal autonomy and agency, their interactions with care providers, and sense of self, identity, and well-being. One of the earliest and best-known studies to focus on the experiences of those living in institutional settings was conducted by Erving Goffman (1961), who examined the mental hospital with a focus on the world of the patient–inmate. Goffman saw nursing homes and other institutions established to care for groups such as those who are blind and for prisoners as one type of **total institution**, defined as 'a place of residence and work where a large number of like-situated individuals, cut off from the wider society for an appreciable period of time, together lead an enclosed, formally administered round of life' (Goffman, 1961: xiii). His interest lay in the characteristics of these institutions and the impact of residence and of the medical model of care adopted within such settings for the structure of the residents' selves. Goffman envisioned the residents as engaged in a **moral career** in which their identities of themselves and others gradually change within a process of humiliation and degradation (**mortification**) of the self.

Subsequent studies drew on Goffman's work to examine the moral career of nursing home patients (Gustafson, 1972), the social conditions that led to patient abuse in nursing homes (Stannard, 1973), and the negative implications for patient care of the bureaucratic organization of nursing homes (Myles, 1978). Throughout this work, the patient experience was considered largely negative. Two decades of research documented problems with patient care, use of physical restraints, and misuse and inappropriate use of psychotropic drugs and chemical restraints (Harrington, 1996). Commenting on the situation in the United States, Harrington noted that although high-quality nursing home care is available, it has probably had more quality of care problems than any other type of health-care organization. Such problems were often linked to inadequate staffing (few registered nurses) and staff training and turnover due to low wages along with medicalization and lack of attention to residents' quality of life. According to Harrington, a major deterrent to improving quality of care within such facilities is the proprietary operation by investor-owned corporations.

Over time, however, sociologists also began to view patients as actively involved in assigning meaning to their experiences and in creating a social world through their interactions within such settings. Diamond (1992, 2000) reported that on one hand, the medical model of care dominated the organization of nursing homes. However, he also challenged the notion of patients as passive recipients of care and therefore as acted upon rather than acting. Based on his participant observation study conducted while he was employed as a nursing assistant in several US nursing homes, Diamond suggested that most patients are conscious of the world in which they live and participate actively in its daily construction. Often this activity is evident around actions of daily living such as eating and bathing. Along similar lines, Kane and colleagues (1997) reported that nursing home residents express satisfaction with choice and control over everyday issues. They found that nursing home residents tend to attach importance to choice and control over matters such as bedtime, rising time, food, roommates, care routines, use of money, use of the telephone, trips out of the nursing home, and contact with the physician.

Canadian research by Funk (2002) confirms variability in resident preferences for involvement in decision-making depending on the area examined. Residents of the nursing homes she studied said they preferred more say in less technical decisions and in more personally relevant decisions (such as deciding their own bedtime rather than deciding between two medications with differing effects on quality of life). Forty-three per cent preferred full, independent decision-making. Individual self-confidence and educational levels were important to whether or not people wanted a say in everyday decisions; however, education was especially important in their preference to be involved in 'big ticket' decisions affecting their lives. This researcher warns of the practical difficulties of enacting personal empowerment in a setting where routinization without individual involvement has been standardized.

As residents of long-term care institutions are actively involved to varying degrees (a choice to be disengaged can also be viewed as active decision-making), so too are the staff of these facilities. For example, caring for those with severe intellectual and developmental disabilities who live in an institution can be emotionally and physically demanding and sometimes dangerous work. Lundgren and Browner (1990) have shown how psychiatric technicians have a culture of support for one another that enables them to partially oppose institutional polices when they believe them to inhibit the delivery of proper care and to do so without jeopardizing their own interests as employees. Those studied were all women. They believed in providing empathic, nurturing care to the residents and they received great satisfaction from doing so. Informal socialization, some on-the-job autonomy, and opportunity for co-worker solidarity were all essential ingredients for this work culture to flourish. Covering for late arrivals to work and taking walks to de-stress were just two of the strategies developed for coping with a high-pressure work environment. Importantly, injecting personal meaning into their work in terms of providing individualized affection and respect to each resident enabled them to resist the institutional definition of their work as primarily custodial and clerical while simultaneously meeting their job requirements. Lundgren and Browner (1990) suggest that the non-confrontational and nurturing solution developed by these workers reflects the political struggles of women and demonstrates the humanizing potential of women in an increasingly efficient and instrumental work world.

With recent shifts away from institutional care toward community-based care, researchers have begun to direct greater attention to the experience of home-based care. Their research points to the importance of home for the personal identities of care recipients and the difficulties that introducing care within this setting can pose (Martin-Matthews, 2007). As noted by Rubinstein (1990), home is a key cultural symbol embedded with meanings associated with personal control, security, comfort, familiarity, autonomy, protection, and positive emotions. Being at home while sick suggests one is less sick than when one has to leave the home, thereby implying a more active personhood. Similarly, Kontos (2000) notes that home is a place where control over one's own life can be freely exercised. Care in the home therefore evokes images that are less depersonalized, more humane, and more individualized than care in an institution whether it be a hospital, group-home, or nursing home setting (Holstein, 1990).

When services enter the home, the setting is changed to become the site of service provision. This transformation challenges residents because service providers become a powerful influence within their private domains. Dill's (1990) account of this process finds that while nurses and social workers bring different perspectives into the home (nurses focus more on physical functioning and medical conditions, while social workers focus more on family relationships and socio-emotional functioning), both bring a clinical lens that emphasizes pathological factors, thus producing particular representations of the resident. These representations must be scripted into standardized descriptions to meet the documentary reality of the jobs.

Based on an ethnographic study of senior tenants living in supportive housing, Kontos (2000) notes that the tenants' understanding of their home as home was threatened by staff and management policies, procedures, guidelines, and constraints, all of which restricted the tenants' independence. Rather than simply accept these constraints, residents engaged in strategies to oppose what they perceived as staff interference, the negation of home, and the conversion of home space into institutional space.

Research also attests to the importance of the personal relationships established with home care staff. It has been suggested that the literature both romanticizes the affective ties between workers and clients as well as overstates the exploitative nature of the relationship; the reality lies somewhere between the two (Stacey, 2005). Clients sometimes form bonds with home care workers such that they become close friends or **fictive kin**, effectively part of the family. Thus, care work often blurs the lines between informal and formal care, possibly lead-ing to situations where workers go above and beyond the call of duty, devoting extra hours of care and taking on extra work. It can also lead to close emotion-al ties and friendships between workers and those they are caring for. As one of the home care workers in Stacey's study notes:

> Kelly, a white 60-year-old aide, often let her client sleep at her home, even though the terms of their contract forbad this. Kelly was paid for three hours of care a day, but often spent a week of uninterrupted time with her elderly client. She was aware of breaking the rules, but said that both she and the client liked the companionship and that the client was afraid to stay alone at night in her home. Kelly explained that 'It's not an issue, we're friends. We enjoy each other's company and we go out to eat together.' (2005: 839–40)

Along with other health-care services, home care is undergoing a transition toward a system characterized by increasing emphasis on consumerism and market-based care together with privatization, cuts, and rationing of services. For example, Aronson and Neysmith (2001) note that home care is being rapid-ly reorganized along market-modelled lines and that service users are increas-ingly required to translate their needs for care into market terms and therefore to redefine themselves as consumers (or customers). Aronson's longitudinal qualitative study of elderly women's accounts of home care rationing in Ontario contradicts those who see this transition as giving service users opportunities for greater empowerment and control. Because many service users were limited in their capacity to navigate the home care marketplace on their own, they ex-perienced insecurity and subordination within an unpredictable system offering a meagre supply of services. They did not feel free to exercise consumer choice nor to demand quality within a mixed economy of home care (Aronson, 2002a).

Nevertheless, within these constraints, Aronson (2002) and Neysmith (2006) report that these women attempted to assert personal agency and were actively involved in shaping their needs to cope within unstable and diminishing home care provision. For example, while some felt that they were being 'pushed over the edge' as a result of the insufficient and depersonalized care, others attempted to 'take charge' and actively impress their needs and identities on home care provi-sion or to 'restrain their expectations' and adjust silently and stoically to the shortcomings of the system. Thus, Aronson notes that '[h]ome care's front line emerged as a complex site of struggle for identity and agency—a struggle in which elderly people engage with inventiveness and determination but also with dwindling support, few witnesses, and mounting isolation' (Aronson, 2002: 399).

CONCLUSIONS

This chapter has highlighted the development and challenges facing various components of Canada's formal health-care system, including medical and allied health professions such as physicians and nurses; complementary and alternative care professions such as midwifery, chiropractic, and naturopathic care; medical-care settings such as acute-care hospitals and long-term care institutions; as well as home- and community-based care. It has also explored the provision and receipt of care from the points of view of various care providers and care recipients.

Throughout the twentieth century, Canada's system of care has focused primarily on the provision of medical care for acute conditions within hospital settings in a system that has been dominated by physicians and therefore reflected medical interests. To date, other health-care workers have largely been subservient to medical-care practitioners or have been forced to function outside of the primary, publicly funded health-care system. This system of care has come under increasing public and state criticism and is currently undergoing dramatic change, including reductions to medical exclusivity and hospital budgets, as well as increased recognition of alternative care providers, therapeutic techniques, and settings for care. These changes have been accompanied by public dissatisfaction with medical dominance and the perceived inadequacies of medical care, increasing interests in pursuing alternative forms of care (such as natural childbirth and more holistic care), governmental interest in cost control, and increasing corporate and market-based interests in health care.

What the future holds remains unclear. On the one hand, many see recent transitions as reflecting successful challenges to the medical profession and state control over population health. As medical care increasingly becomes one of many health professions, health care is being democratized. In the process, citizens are empowered to make choices and select among available alternatives to adopt the types of care they believe best suit their own needs. On the other, the choices being made increasingly involve replacing publicly funded care with options that lie outside of our publicly funded health-care system. Corporate- and market-based interests are increasingly involved and users are required to pay for care. These private-pay options have always been the major services available for long-term care of older adults and others with chronic-care needs in our population. Current trends may make this the option of choice for other segments of the population, thereby increasing the likelihood of inequities (by income, gender, race, etc.) in access to care. At the same time, the resilience of the existing medically focused care system suggests that aspects of medical care will remain publicly funded at least for some time to come. For example, recent trends toward enhancing community-based home care services have been accompanied by the medicalization of the services being offered. To address these issues is to venture into the realm of health policy, which is the focus of Chapter 5.

Questions for Critical Thought

1. It has been suggested that medical dominance is currently in decline and that medicine is gradually becoming just one health-care profession among others within a more pluralistic health-care system. Present arguments for and against this view.

2. Discuss the relevance of gender and social class for understanding relationships between who provides care, the types of care provided, and the status of those receiving care.

3. Various explanations have been given for why complementary and alternative care use is increasing. Assess the relative merits of each.

4. Compare and contrast people's experiences with (a) physicians and alternative care providers and (b) hospitals and other institutional care settings versus home and community-based care.

5. Canada's health-care system is often described as equitable. Yet we noted that evidence of equitable access to general practitioners and hospital care does not mean that access to other services is equitable, that structural factors other than income have no impact on access to care, or that the level and quality of care received is equitable. How equitable is Canada's health-care system?

Suggestions for Further Reading

Benoit, C., S. Wrede, I. Bourgeault, J. Sandall, R. de Vries, and E.R. van Teijlingen. 2005. 'Understanding the Social Organization of Maternity Care Systems: Midwifery as a Touchstone', *Sociology of Health and Illness* 27, 6: 722–37.

Coburn, D. 2006. 'Medical Dominance Then and Now: Critical Reflections', *Health Sociology Review* 15: 432–43.

Diamond, T. 1996. 'Social Policy and Everyday Life in Nursing Homes: A Critical Ethnography', in P. Brown, ed, *Perspectives in Medical Sociology*. Prospect Heights, IL: Waveland Press, 684–702.

Freidson, E. 1970. *Profession of Medicine*. New York: Dodd Mead.

Kelner, M., B. Wellman, S. Welsh, and H. Boon. 2006. 'How Far Can Complementary and Alternative Medicine Go? The Case of Chiropractic and Homeopathy', *Social Science and Medicine* 63: 2617–27.

Torrance, G.W. 1998. 'Hospitals as Health Factories', in D. Coburn, C. Coburn, C. D'Arcy, and G.M. Torrance, eds, *Health and Canadian Society: Sociological Perspectives*. Toronto: University of Toronto Press, 438–55.

Chapter 5

Health-Care Policy

Learning Objectives:
In this chapter, you will learn that:

- Canada's health-care system is under provincial jurisdiction; only physician and acute hospital care are covered by Canada's national health-insurance program (Medicare).
- Canadian health-care reform of the 1990s represents a retrenchment back to a medical model of care, contrary to the vision of health-care reform that promoted a broader vision of health and illness and argued for a shift from institutional to community-based care, health promotion, and disease prevention.
- A major reason for the direction of health-care reform is the globalization of American-style capitalism. Another major reason is entrenched vested interests.
- The consequences of the globalization of capitalism include a widening gap between rich and poor and greater health and health-care inequalities.
- Alternatives to the current system include health promotion and disease prevention within a comprehensive social determinants of health model that will facilitate individual agency and both individual and population health.

HEALTH CARE AS SOCIAL POLICY

In this brief look at the sociology of health and health care, we have examined theoretical approaches to the subfield, health as it varies across a number of statuses, the predominance of self and informal care, and our Canadian health-care system and services within it. That brings us to social policy. **Social policy** simply refers to a plan intended to influence and determine decisions and actions with respect to social affairs. Our interest here is in policy created by governments, or **public policy**, and particularly one type of public social policy, namely health policy. Health policy is especially important to a sociological perspective because it has consequences for people's health and health care and can result in differential resources and access to care within the population. In this chapter, we analyze health-care policy and its implications for health, self-care, informal care, and the formal services that are available to us. As such, the chapter illustrates the relationship between structural, macro arrangements (policy), and individual agency.

The chapter begins with a brief description of Canada's health-care system, followed by an examination of the contemporary Canadian health-care reform process that began in the 1990s, including the arguments made for change, the vision behind replacing the existing system, and some of the changes that are taking place. Whether these changes are leading us to the vision of a new and more appropriate system is also examined, to assist in our assessment of the consequences of structural reform for individuals and groups. Some of the reasons for the types of changes that are occurring are presented, followed by a discussion of the types of reform necessary to achieve the vision put forward in the 1990s and to facilitate individual agency for both our health and health care.

SOME BACKGROUND ON CANADA'S HEALTH-CARE SYSTEM

While the federal government plays an important role through funding, health care is a provincial responsibility. In this federal system, the government has less authority than in countries with more centralized governments. Furthermore, while Canada has a publicly funded system, only hospitals and physician services are universally insured through Medicare because, at the time it was established, these services were unquestioningly accepted as providing the most appropriate care for ensuring the nation's health. They were embraced within a system designed to be equitable so that any citizen in need would receive care irrespective of his or her ability to pay. This system did not and does not represent socialized medicine. Instead, physicians primarily operate as private entrepreneurs with guaranteed incomes and are primarily paid on a fee-for-service basis.

The Medical Care Act, which established Medicare, was passed in 1966. By 1972, all provinces and territories had joined the program so that Medicare was available throughout the country. At that time, the federal government paid one half of the costs of physician and hospital services provided by each province and territory, conditional on their meeting a number of criteria. These requirements included universal coverage, reasonable access to services, portability of benefits across provinces or territories, comprehensive services, and non-profit administration by a public agency. Although these criteria are still operative, the federal government no longer pays half of all costs; it now makes lump sum transfers to the provinces and territories untied to the amount spent by the latter. If any province or territory violates the conditions upon which access to federal funding is based, such as by allowing extra billing or user fees, the federal government can reduce its payments to the offending province or territory by an amount equal to the total of all extra billing and user charges. This practice removes incentives for extra billing and user charges, but only so long as the federal government transfers significant financial assistance to the provinces for health-care services. Funding from the federal government has varied over the years; however, 2001 saw a return to larger health-care transfers.

Prior to the establishment of Medicare, an individual's economic resources were a partial determinant of the receipt of care. Since Medicare was introduced, those who have worse health (lower-income groups, seniors, and women) tend to receive more services irrespective of their ability to pay (McDonald et al., 1973; Manga, 1978; Broyles et al., 1983). A similar shift took place in the United Kingdom after universal Medicare was introduced there (Rein, 1969; Stewart and Enterline, 1961). That is, research has shown that universal medicare allows those in need to receive care and that care is not dependent on the ability to pay.

All health-care services except acute-care hospitals and physician services are excluded from Medicare. Home care and home support services[1] and practitioners such as chiropractors, naturopaths, and physiotherapists as well as prescription medications (unless provided within an acute-care hospital) are outside of our publicly funded system. Each jurisdiction (province, territory, region) has its own mix of these services with variation in the services available, the referral mechanisms in place, and the user fees charged (if any). These non-Medicare services were expanded as part of all provincial programs during the 1970s and 1980s.

By the late 1980s, all levels of government had become increasingly concerned with continually escalating costs and were dissatisfied with their fiscal arrangements. The federal government especially disliked the high costs associated with funding an area of provincial responsibility; the provinces especially disliked what they perceived as federal interference in their jurisdictions. There was widespread questioning of the value of medicine, which was fuelled by concerns regarding the aging of the population (since older adults are prone to chronic conditions for which medicine has no cure). For the first time since Medicare was established, the 1990s saw governments refocus their attention away from concerns with health-care, issues of equity, and the extension of equal financial protection and access to all or most of those in the population, and toward issues of efficiency and cost-effectiveness. This shift was a major challenge because, when Medicare began, no mechanisms had been devised to evaluate medical interventions or to ensure cost accountability.

Nevertheless, a remarkably consistent **vision for health-care reform** emerged throughout the country and indeed throughout much of the industrialized world. According to this vision, a new health-care system would incorporate the following aspects: a broader definition of health (beyond medicine) inclusive of social and psychological aspects; collaboration between multiple sectors (including the informal, volunteer, and private for-profit sectors); a change of focus away from cure alone to also include health promotion and disease prevention and from institution-based to community-based care; greater opportunities for citizen participation in decision-making about health choices and health policies; decentralized regional health authorities instead of provincial systems; improved human-resources planning with an emphasis on alternatives to the fee-for-service method; council-like entities for enhancing the efficiency of managing services; and increased funds for health services research, especially on utilization, technology assessment, program or system evaluation, and information systems (Mhatre and Deber, 1992).

This vision, embraced by governments and the populace, provided a blueprint for a more appropriate system of care that would not exceed the cost of the existing system. It was consistent with the basic principles that underlie Medicare and are endorsed by most Canadians: equity, compassion, collective responsibility, individual responsibility, respect for others, efficiency, and effectiveness. It promised a more appropriate yet cost-effective system for an aging society (Chappell, 2007c). Although various aspects of the 1990s vision for health-care reform were not new, a political will to act was. The vision therefore provides an important benchmark against which we can assess the reform process taking place throughout the 1990s and later.

HEALTH-CARE REFORM

By the late 1990s, all of the provinces and territories were actively engaged in reforming their health-care systems. Representing the largest single expense in the pubic health-care system, hospitals (private, non-profit agencies with global budgets) were the first target of cuts. Long-term or chronic-care beds in hospitals, deemed as not the 'proper' business of acute-care hospitals, were cut, as were hospitals that had historically operated at substantially less than full capacity (such as many hospitals in rural Saskatchewan). Hospital budgets were often frozen or increased only modestly (Chappell, 1993a, 1993b). In-hospital medical interventions were performed more and more as day surgeries (Deber et al., 1998). That is, hospitals became streamlined to focus on their acute-care mandate (and not custodial or long-term care) and to perform many of their interventions on an outpatient rather than an in-patient basis. Given this refocus, it was argued that many post-surgery services that had been available at public expense only when people were in hospital should now also be available in the community. Roy Romanow (2002), in his final report as head of the Commission on the Future of Health Care in Canada, recommended that short-term home care (referring specifically to post-acute hospital care including medication management and rehabilitation services) be made available within Medicare. While not incorporated into Medicare, which would have made these services difficult to dismantle, the federal government subsequently transferred monies to the provinces for the enhancement of short-term post-acute care. (See Box 5.1 for the timeline of key health-care system landmarks.)

Box 5.1
Canada's Health-Care System: Selected Timeline

1867
British North American Act passed: federal government responsible for marine hospitals and quarantine; provincial/territorial governments responsible for hospitals, asylums, charities, and charitable institutions.

1897 to 1919
Federal Department of Agriculture handles federal health responsibilities until 1 September 1919, when first federal Department of Health created.

1920 to 1942
Municipal hospital plans established in Manitoba, Saskatchewan, and Alberta; Royal Commission on Health Insurance, British Columbia and Alberta pass health insurance legislation, but without an operating program; Federal Dominion Council of Health created in 1940; Federal Interdepartmental Advisory Committee on Health Insurance created in 1942.

1947
Saskatchewan initiates provincial universal public hospital insurance plan, 1 January.

1948
National Health Grants Program, federal; provides grants to provinces and territories to support health-related initiatives, including hospital construction, public health, professional training, provincial surveys, and public health research.

1949
British Columbia creates limited provincial hospital insurance plan; Newfoundland joins Canada, has a cottage hospital insurance plan.

1950
Alberta creates limited provincial hospital insurance plan, 1 July.

1957
Hospital Insurance and Diagnostic Services Act, federal, proclaimed (Royal Assent) 1 May; provides 50/50 cost sharing for provincial and territorial hospital insurance plans, in force 1 July 1958.

1958 to 1961
All 10 provinces and the Northwest Territories and the Yukon had hospital insurance plans with federal cost sharing by 1961. In this year, the federal government creates the Royal Commission on Health Services to study need for health insurance and health services; appoint Emmet M. Hall as Chair.

1962
Saskatchewan creates medical insurance plan for physicians' services, 1 July; doctors in province strike for 23 days.

1964
Royal Commission on Health Services, federal, reports; recommends national health-care program.

1965
British Columbia creates provincial medical plan.

1966
Canada Assistance Plan (CAP), federal, introduced; provides cost-sharing for social services, including health care not covered under hospital plans, for those in need, Royal Assent July, effective 1 April.

Medical Care Act, federal, proclaimed (Royal Assent), 19 December; provides 50/50 cost sharing for provincial/territorial medical insurance plans, in force 1 July 1968.

1968 to 1972
All 10 provinces and the Northwest Territories and the Yukon had medical insurance plans with federal cost sharing by 1972.

1977
Federal–Provincial Fiscal Arrangements and Established Programs Financing Act (EPF) federal cost-sharing shifts to block funding.

1979
Federal government creates Health Services Review; Emmet M. Hall appointed Special Commissioner to re-evaluate publicly funded health-care system.

1980 to 1983
Health Services Review report released in 1980, recommends ending user fees, extra billing, setting national standards; provincial/territorial reciprocal billing agreement for in-patient hospital services provided out-of-province/territory in 1981; federal EPF amended, removing revenue guarantee and amending funding formula in 1982; Royal Commission on Hospital and Nursing Home Costs, Newfoundland, begins in 1983 (reports in 1984); Comite d'étude sur la promotion de la santé, Quebec, begins 1983 (reports 1984); La Commission d'énquête sur les services de santé et les services sociaux, Quebec, begins 1983 (reports 1987); Federal Task Force on the Allocation of Health Care Resources begins 1983 (reports 1984).

1984

The Canada Health Act, federal, passes, combines hospital and medical acts; sets conditions and criteria on portability, accessibility, universality, comprehensiveness, public administration; bans user fees and extra billing. All provinces and territories must be in compliance by 1 April 1987.

Provincial/territorial reciprocal billing agreement for out-patient hospital services provided out-of-province/territory.

1985 to 2001

Virtually all provinces and territories establish health-care review committees, panels, councils, commissions, task forces, and/or discussions throughout this period, many establishing more than one.

1986

Federal transfer payments rate of growth reduced.

1988

Provincial/territorial governments (except Quebec) sign reciprocal billing agreement for physicians' services provided out-of-province/territory.

1989 to 1994

Further reductions in federal transfer payments.

1991

National Task Force on Health Information, federal, reports; leads to creation of Canadian Institute of Health Information.

1994

National Forum on Health, federal, created to discuss health care with Canadians, chaired by the prime minister, begins, recommends reforms in 1997.

1995

Federal EPF and CAP merged into block funding under the Canada Health and Social Transfer (CHST), to support health care, post-secondary education, and social services, begins 1 April 1996.

1999

Social Union Framework Agreement (SUFA) in force; federal, provincial, and territorial governments (except Quebec) agree to collective approach to social policy and program development, including health.

2000

First Ministers' Communiqué on Health, announced 11 September.

2001

Standing Senate Committee on Social Affairs, Science and Technology review (Kirby Committee), federal, begins 1 March, publishes recommendations 2002; Commission on the Future of Health Care in Canada (Romanow Commission), federal, begins, reports 2002.

2003

First Ministers' Accord on Health Care Renewal announced; Health Council of Canada established to monitor and report on progress of Accord reforms.

2004

Federal CHST split into two transfers: the Canada Health Transfer (CHT) and the Canada Social Transfer (CST); First Ministers' A 10-Year Plan to Strengthen Health Care.

Source: Health Canada. 2005a. *Canada's Health Care System*. Available at: http://www.hc-sc.gc.ca/hcs-sss/pubs/care-soins/2005-hcs-sss/time-chron_e.html. Accessed 4 May 2007. Reproduced with the permission of the Minister of Public Works and Government Services Canada, 2008.

Initially, attempts were also made to limit the number of practising physicians. Ten per cent reductions in new admissions and post-graduate training in medical schools were agreed to, as were tighter restrictions on foreign-trained physicians' practice, and differential fees for physicians who settled in under-serviced areas. By 2005, however, some provinces (such as British Columbia) were beginning to expand medical school enrolments, and Prime Minister Paul Martin was urging greater use of foreign-trained doctors. To date, incentives for physicians to work in under-serviced areas have been largely unsuccessful. Aggregate caps on physician billings have been negotiated with some provincial medical associations, but physician work stoppages and work-to-rule campaigns have tended to result in increases rather than decreases to physician remuneration (Alberta and British Columbia are but two examples). Currently, user fees are being charged in some areas where they did not exist before (such as for medical equipment in Manitoba); income testing is being imposed for higher room and board fees in long-term care facilities (such as in British Columbia); and private for-pay services are growing (especially in Alberta and British Columbia).

During the 1990s, the addition of new long-term nursing home beds to the system was halted and community care budgets increased somewhat. Yet the fact that these budgets were already small meant that percentage increases translated into relatively little additional funding. The Romanow Report made no mention of long-term home care, despite the fact that gerontologists have long recognized that seniors tend to require such care. Rather, attention focused on recommendations for enhancing short-term home care—post-acute care, short-term mental health problems (a curious recommendation given the chronic nature of such problems that require longer term solutions), and pallia- tive care services (appropriately short-term). Compared with long-term chron- ic care for seniors, post-acute care is intensive and expensive, requiring a large portion of the comparatively small overall home care budgets.

The focus on short-term home care has important consequences for long- term home care, services that had been slowly building in the 1970s and 1980s. A recent study conducted by Penning, Brackley, and Allen (2006) asked whether the restructuring of health services that occurred within 1990s health-care reform in British Columbia was facilitating access to community care as the vision suggested or whether it was contrary to this vision. They argued that if the evidence was more consistent with cost cutting, medicalization, or profitiza- tion, then such restructuring is not achieving the goals specified in the vision. They distinguish between home nursing care and home support services, both provided within community home care. The former is often considered med- ically necessary and therefore a medical service. The latter, on the other hand, is typically considered a social service, is contracted out by most provinces, and is delivered by a mix of for-profit and not-for-profit agencies. With data spanning the 1990s, the authors found that the number of people receiving home support decreased or remained stable over the years but the hours and visits per person (the intensity of care) increased. For home nursing, the number of people and visits either declined or remained the same; however, the intensity of care decreased somewhat.

Such results suggest the intent of health-care reform is not being imple- mented, but that service (and cost) reductions are targeting social care compo- nents within the overall home care service system. Given that fewer clients receive home support services but that those who do receive a greater intensity of service, there appears to be a redirection of services away from clients who have less medical need and more potential for prevention and toward more medically intensive post-acute care. Through this transition, home care is increasingly becoming a **medical support system**, less comprehensive than that envisioned in the 1990s, and one with little social care. For older adults, this sys- tem represents a major shift in service provision.

This transition is occurring at a time when other research in the same province points to the preventive function of home care/home support. Hollander (2001) compared four health units: two had implemented cuts to homemaking-only services as directed by the provincial government in the 1990s (that is, those who received homemaking service but no other service had this service cut) and two had not followed this directive. Those who were cut from the service later cost the government more in terms of increased use of hospital beds, increased use of home care services, and increased admission to nursing homes. These overall cost increases were not apparent until the second year after the cuts and were greater still in year three. Also, the costs were higher for the group that had been cut even though more of them died (and thus cost the system nothing in terms of services received). These findings suggest that social services such as homemaking have preventive and maintenance functions for health in addition to and beyond their cost effectiveness.

Other research demonstrates that home care allows clients to stay in their own homes, is preferred by them, and is also less costly than nursing home care. Hollander and Chappell (2001) compared the costs of home care and nursing home care for clients receiving the same level of care in British Columbia from 1987 to 1997. Home care costs were 40 per cent to 75 per cent of facility care costs, with differentials decreasing with greater levels of care. The costs for home care increased during times of transition (when a client is changing levels of care) but were still less than nursing home costs. The only time home care costs exceeded nursing home costs was when someone died. Importantly, these increased costs were due to hospitalization, not to home care services per se. While those living at home generally die in hospital, nursing home residents usually die within these institutions; they are often not transferred to hospitals, thus keeping costs down. Such findings suggest that the costs of receiving care at home can be reduced further if cost-effective alternatives to dying in expensive acute-care hospitals are found.

In another study, Chappell and colleagues (2004) compared the costs of long-term home care and nursing home care for clients with similar levels of health need, including the costs of informal care provided by family members. Data were collected on time spent providing care by members of the informal network and by formal workers. Costs to government and to families were computed. Again, home care costs were lower when controlling for level of need of the client and when costing the time for family care at minimum wage. While these studies suggest that home care services are a more cost-effective option, it is important to remember that they are dependent on the availability of an informal caregiver. If there is no one available, services in the home may not be an option.

Another arena of change was **regionalization**. Regionalization (including restructuring of health services from a provincial to a regional level) was highly touted following the creation of the National Forum on Health (established by the federal government to advise on the public's views regarding health-care system improvements) in the late 1990s. Most provinces regionalized based on the argument that it would allow for decision-making and service integration at the local level. Thus, local communities and service users would have greater say in what services were provided, thereby tailoring services to local needs. However, as enacted, regional restructuring was at best only partial, encompassing hospital services and community care, but excluding both physician services and drug coverage (Chappell, McDonald, and Stones, 2007). That is, the major decision-makers (such as physicians, who are estimated to control approximately 80 per cent of public health-care costs, including hospital admissions, prescription drugs, laboratory tests, and return visits) and major cost escalators (drugs) were omitted. Thus, regionalization integrates a historically well-established and powerful vested interest (acute-care hospitals) with a weak distant cousin (home care). Given this particular marriage, it is not surprising that only short-term, post-hospital home care was recognized in the Romanow report and in subsequent health accords between the federal and provincial governments.

Interestingly, despite the importance attributed to regionalization and the resources allocated to it, there is little research on whether it can provide more efficient and appropriate health care. Those in favour argue for its ability to bring services 'closer to home'. However, Allan and Penning's (2001) research before and one year after regionalization finds no differences in terms of visits to specialists, in-patient hospital separations, or home care use. Differences between regions decreased in terms of visits to general practitioners, outpatient hospital separations, and home nursing care, suggesting increased standardization between regions. Other research (Penning, Allan, and Brackley, 2001) compared three regions that differed in their socio-demographic composition and also found that the use of acute-care hospital services, physician services, and community-based home care prior to and for two years after regionalization was similar in each of the regions. These two studies suggest that regionalization is leading to more similarity rather than to increased dissimilarity in service delivery, as would be expected given differentiated needs between regions (a rationale for regionalizing).

A LACK OF PROGRESS

Although the vision of health-care reform included health promotion and illness prevention, reform to date (as we've discussed above), has focused on physician and hospital care. Little attention has been directed towards home care (especially long-term care) or the larger structural elements of the community such as the workplace and educational institutions. When health authorities include health promotion and illness prevention activities, they tend to focus on little more than the provision of information about healthy lifestyles such as proper nutrition or the harmful effects of smoking. Part of the difficulty lies in the all-encompassing nature of health promotion. Health authorities often do not know where to direct their efforts, given their lack of jurisdiction over such areas as education and the workplace. Nevertheless, there are examples of what they could be doing, some of which are elaborated on below.

A health promotion perspective recognizes upstream factors—psychosocial and environmental factors—as influencing health. This view is consistent with the broad World Health Organization (WHO) definition of health discussed earlier (see Chapters 1 and 2). It is also consistent with early reports released by our federal government on the importance of a health promotion perspective. In 1986 both the Lalonde report and the Epp report put Canada at the forefront of arguing for this approach (see below for an elaboration). Determinants of health within this perspective include peace, shelter, education, food, income, a stable ecosystem, sustainable resources, social justice, equity, and personal health beliefs and behaviours. This perspective recognizes individual choice (agency) and self-care as well as the effects of structural position within society. For example, Aboriginal people living on isolated Northern reserves have access to few fresh fruits and vegetables in winter; those exposed to harmful chemicals at work often have little choice in the effects they ultimately suffer. While we have agency, there are limits.

Individual risk behaviours, such as smoking and poor eating habits, were the focus of early health promotion endeavours, resulting in charges of **blaming the victim** for his or her own health problems. Broader approaches were evident by the 1990s (Goodman, 2000; Merzel and D'Afflitti, 2003). **Social ecology**, a prominent and popular approach today, posits a set of principles for examining interdependencies between individual and aggregate manifestations of health problems. Individual, group, organizational, community, and policy influences on health are all acknowledged (Stokols, 1996). The need for collaboration across sectors and levels is also emphasized. This perspective argues for enhancing social, environmental, and economic conditions as well as individual capacities (Chappell et al., 2006). Another approach, adopted by the Canadian government, is a **population health perspective** (sometimes also referred to as the **social determinants of health perspective**; see Eyles et al., 2001). For example, its Healthy Living website (http://www.hc-sc.gc.ca/hl-vs/index_e.html) refers to nutrition, social contacts, and physical activity, acknowledging that where we live, work, learn, and play all affect our healthy living choices (see Box 5.2). The Canadian public also largely accepts this perspective.

Building healthy environments that encourage physical activity is an example of a health promotion approach. Following research showing that developing public parks and trails encourages higher levels of physical activity, Napolitano and colleagues (2006) implemented and evaluated a communications-based campaign within an employment site to encourage awareness of local walking paths. Promotional material included flyers, e-mails, website postings, and biweekly information booths. After one month, 65 per cent of employees within that site correctly identified walking path signs (increased from 51 per cent a month earlier), 75.5 per cent were familiar with physical activity messages around the workplace (increased from 64.6 per cent) and walking activity increased three and a half times.

In another example, those opposed to condom availability argue that the health promotion approach increases adolescent sexual activity. To test the veracity of this concern, an HIV prevention program for Latino adolescents in a US city incorporated the promotion and distribution of condoms. Sexual activity among Latino adolescents was compared with that of adolescents living in another city where the HIV prevention program did not incorporate such a strategy. A comparison of the two cities showed that males in the intervention city

Box 5.2
The Integrated Pan-Canadian Healthy Living Strategy

The Healthy Living Strategy provides a conceptual framework for sustained action based on Healthy Living. It envisions a healthy nation in which all Canadians experience the conditions that support the attainment of good health. The goals of the Strategy are to improve overall health outcomes and to reduce health disparities. Grounded in a population health approach, the initial emphasis is on healthy eating, physical activity, and their relationship to healthy weights.

Included in the Strategy are pan-Canadian healthy living targets—which seek to obtain a 20 per cent increase in the proportion of Canadians who are physically active, eat healthy, and are at healthy body weights. While ambitious, these targets can be achieved through collaborative action and will serve to sustain momentum from the 10 percentage point, year 2010 physical activity target set by Ministers responsible for Physical Activity, Recreation, and Sport in 2003.

While the Healthy Living goals and targets provide a standard reference point for all sectors to measure the success of their own strategies and interventions, to be successful, coordinated effort is required. Proposed action has developed through intersectoral working groups, and will be considered in the implementation of the Strategy.

The Strategy offers a means to ensure greater alignment, coordination, and direction for all sectors, and provides a forum for multiple players to align efforts and to work collaboratively to address common risk factors. This integration ensures that stakeholders are better and more broadly informed, thereby facilitating greater synergy and improved identification of opportunities across sectors. The intersectoral nature of the Healthy Living Strategy also provides a national context and reference point for all sectors, governments, and Aboriginal organizations to measure success of their own strategies and interventions.

Source: Public Health Agency of Canada. 2005. 'Healthy Living'. Available at: http://www.phac-aspc.gc.ca/hl-vs-strat/index.html. Reproduced with the permission of the Minister of Public Works and Government Services Canada, 2008.

were less likely than those in the comparison city to initiate first sexual activity; females in the intervention city were less likely to have multiple partners; and there was no effect on the onset of sexual activity for females, the chances of multiple partners for males, or the frequency of sex for either males or females. Promoting and distributing condoms did not increase sexual activity among adolescents (Sellers, McGraw, and McKinlay, 1994).

In Mexico City, where 60 per cent of contraceptives are provided by pharmacy workers (rather than physicians), Pick, Poortinga, and Givaudan (2003) developed a training program and print materials for pharmacists on condom use and HIV prevention. They compared four groups—one received training only, one received materials only, one received both, and one received neither but did have a tour of a pharmaceutical company. Those who received training only or training and materials increased their knowledge, reduced their mistaken beliefs about HIV/AIDS and its prevention, and held more positive attitudes and norms about their role as educators. Those receiving both the training and materials had the greatest increase in condom sales and in providing information to clients. The results were still evident three months after the intervention.

Other examples abound. In terms of bicycle helmet use, Farley, Haddad, and Brown (1996) showed that a four-year program mainly involving communication strategies and community organization (so bicycle helmets were readily available) and targeted to elementary-school children in one region of Quebec was effective. Compared with municipalities not exposed to the campaign, helmet use increased from 1.3 per cent to 33 per cent among young cyclists in the community where the program was launched. Importantly, the benefits were not evenly distributed; it was only one third as effective in poorer areas.

Many of these health promotion programs receive one-shot funding and are vulnerable to the political whims of the day. When Prime Minister Harper's Conservatives won a minority government in 2006, they cut funding to many programs that fall within this arena. The following are only a few examples of programs for which funding was totally eliminated:

- Canada Policy Research Networks
- Canadian Heritage Support to Canadian Volunteerism Initiative
- Canadian Volunteerism Initiative
- Community Access Program, Internet access for communities at libraries, post offices, community centres
- Court Challenges Program
- Environment: Youth International Internship Program
- First Nations and Inuit Tobacco Control Program
- Foreign Affairs and Public Diplomacy Program
- Foreign Affairs Youth International Internship Program
- HRD Adult Learning and Literacy programs (funding eliminated for some programs, reduced for others)
- HRD Youth Employment Programs (funding eliminated for some programs, reduced for others)
- Royal Canadian Mounted Police Drug Impaired Driving Program Training

Another hindrance to health promotion is fragmentation between government ministries. The need for jurisdictions such as health, education, employment, and sport to work together has been widely recognized. However, there is little evidence that such co-operation is happening. To the contrary, there is some evidence that greater fragmentation may be occurring. (See Box 5.3.) For example, one consequence of the Romanow Report has been a refocusing of

Box 5.3
Treating Addictions

Several addiction support groups are available in most Canadian cities, all established around one specific addiction. For example, support groups for alcohol, smoking, and gambling addictions are all distinct and separate from one another. But what if there exists an addiction-prone personality whereby some people are more likely to become addicted and if 'cured' of one addiction develop another? Barnes and colleagues (2000) developed an Addiction Prone Personality Scale that is scientifically rigorous and predicts substance misuse behaviour such as alcoholism and smoking. Anderson and colleagues (1999) demonstrated the predictability of this measure for both men and women and across age groups (Barnes et al., 2005). It is important to note that personality is not the whole story; these same researchers also found that youth raised in families with parental alcoholism, high stress, and low family cohesion, as well as those whose peers smoked marijuana, were also more likely to partake in heavy marijuana smoking. Similarly, Tucker et al. (2002) reported that adolescents embedded in pro-smoking environments and who had parents who approved of smoking were much more likely to smoke.

Why is this important? If addiction is a generalized tendency, like the host response (see Chapter 3), treating addictions separately will solve little. The person who quits smoking will replace this behaviour with another addiction. Our tendency to isolate and compartmentalize health promotion and treatment of illness may not represent optimal strategies for good health!

attention and resources onto short-term services. As a result, these short-term home care services are devouring the majority of home care resources and, in the process, long-term home care is being forgotten. The divide is increasing between medical services that are publicly funded through Medicare and social services.

Overall, health-care reform from the mid-1990s to the present appears to be a retrenchment back to a medical model of care and away from one based on a broader notion of health. Medicare remains focused on physician and acute hospital care to the exclusion of other services, including long-term home care in the community. These other services are devolving into a mixed mode of delivery, one that involves increasing privatization (see next section for an elaboration). This situation is not only contrary to the vision of health-care reform as originally conceived, but it is also counter to research demonstrating the cost- and care-effectiveness of long-term home care for an aging society. The ability of regionalization to solve these problems is questionable, given the exclusion of some of the most important aspects of the system. The question, as phrased by Hollander and colleagues (2007)—whose responsibility is it to pay for *social* services that are *medically* necessary?—is being answered de facto by the reforms taking place: it is the private responsibility of the individual. This answer reflects a return to the working assumption when the British North America Act was passed. At that time, individuals were held responsible for providing the contingencies of life for themselves and their families, which included heath care. Increasingly today, health care that is outside of medically defined Medicare is located within this domain known as **residual welfare**. We turn now to a discussion of one of the major reasons why this is occurring.

GLOBALIZATION AND CAPITALISM

The language we use when speaking of health care has been changing; the rhetoric of health-care reform is adopting the words of a market model. Perhaps the most obvious example of this change is the shift from being a patient to being a client or consumer of health-care services. Physicians and other fee-for-service providers, such as pharmacists, optometrists, and physiotherapists, have always operated within a market allocation model—they are paid (by clients or by private insurers) for providing services to clients who choose them over others available within the open market. Private insurers openly advertise for services not included in Medicare. Public debate concerning Canada's health-care system is typically phrased in terms of privatization. Because **privatization** can refer to anything that is not public, including private, not-for-profit health-care agencies, some consider **profitization** (the provision of health services as a profit-making business) a more appropriate term (Williams et al., 2001). Concern within Canada's health-care debate is centrally with the provision of health care for profit, not with private not-for-profit organizations. The pressures toward profitization within health care are hardly surprising, given that Canada is a capitalist country and is proximate to the large and powerful United States, which embraces capitalism to an even greater extent. The United States is one of the few industrialized countries of the world that does not have a universal, publicly financed medicare system.

The American style of free-market capitalism and the promotion of increased profitization characterize current trends toward globalization. Many countries have embraced **globalization**, or the internationalization of capital (Coburn, 2001, 2004), as a solution to their economic and financial crises. Indeed, in 1998, the WHO stated that countries resisting globalization 'will find themselves marginalized in the world community and in the world economy' (Navarro, 2002a). This international context includes threatened reductions to national credit ratings, higher interest rates, and/or withholding of business investments. The Canadian government responded by slashing expenditures, reducing deficits, and paying down the debt during the 1980s and 1990s. It reduced the power of the state and became more market oriented, introducing a business–state coalition to rationalize health care. It has been argued that part of the push toward globalization has come from American businesses located within a more or less saturated health-care business market looking beyond their borders for economic opportunities (Armstrong, 2001; McKee, 2001). Such organizations view Canada as a place to expand their investments, and they are doing so—trade between Canada and the United States has increased to the point where it now outstrips intra-Canada trade activity in virtually every region of the country (Mendelson and Divinsky, 2002). The North American Free Trade Agreement (NAFTA) allows them to argue for greater freedom to deliver health-care business in Canada.

In Canada, a neo-liberal political agenda is embracing global **capitalism**, in which the power and mobility of capital in production and financial markets seek to promote such things as profitization, deregulation and significant structural changes in national bureaucracies, decreases in welfare programs and public services, and the liberalization of trade and monetary policies to support market interests that favour high-income business sectors. A trickle-down effect from the top to the rest of the population, it is argued, will benefit everyone. Four beliefs characterize this neo-liberal ideology: public deficits are intrinsically negative; state regulation of the labour market is intrinsically negative; social protection guaranteed by the welfare state and its redistributive policies hinder economic growth; and the state should not intervene in regulating foreign trade or international financial markets (Navarro, 2002b). Therefore, Canada, like governments of other industrialized countries, has reframed its role from one of provider to one of partner or facilitator to other sectors. Its role is to complement and support the private sector rather than to act as 'big brother', setting limits on its activities (Meyer, 2000).

Hospitals became central to the new business approach to health care. This is not surprising given they are the largest expense within Canada's publicly funded health-care system and, as Rachlis and Kushner (1989) have pointed out, are about the only business that does not know what its product (healthy patients) costs to produce. Hospitals were restructured, their business focus (acute care) was more narrowly defined, surgical care was increasingly shifted to outpatient care provision, and nursing positions were reduced in number. In addition, lengths of stay were shortened and services were contracted out, not offered, or offered under the rubric of home care (such as rehabilitation services, prescription drugs, nursing care, and custodial care). It is important to note that when such services are moved outside the hospital, they no longer fall within Medicare and therefore lie outside of our universally insured and publicly provided health-care system.

Home care, as a service external to Medicare, is shifting to a mixed mode of managed competition; local health authorities purchase services from a mix of not-for-profit and for-profit service providers (usually on a 50/50 basis). Only a few provinces (Manitoba, Saskatchewan, and Quebec) still have publicly provided services. Such a mixed mode of service delivery is believed to keep the cost down through competition. However, the evidence does not support this assumption: for-profit firms are reportedly more likely to skimp on quality and to increase profits by selecting consumers who are in the least need—a practice known as cherry-picking (Bendick, 1989; Williams et al., 2001); care at private for-profit hospitals results in a higher risk-adjusted mortality rate than care at private not-for-profit hospitals; private for-profit hospitals have higher payments for care than private not-for-profit hospitals; in all sectors, services that are not profitable are cut and the not-for-profit, voluntary, and family sectors are left to fill the gaps; and there is downward pressure on wages and working conditions (Denton and Kusch, 2006; Devereaux et al., 2004). In many provinces, care assessment is provided at no cost to the individual. However, once individuals are deemed eligible for services, receipt is subject to income or means testing. Needed services are provided at no cost to individuals only if they cannot afford it themselves.

An important corollary of the profitization of home care is that multinational firms can buy for-profit home care agencies. When this occurs, profits more often than not leave the country. Under NAFTA, the Canadian government can allow for-profit firms entry into an area of the health-care field, but it cannot then return that area to public provision without providing compensation for lost future profits to those for-profit firms. This condition makes it virtually impossible to ever return to public care provision and is the reason why the Romanow Report (2002) devoted an entire chapter to the issue of globalization, urging the Canadian government to state in writing and in public at every opportunity that Canada's health care is excluded from all free trade agreements. Ralph Klein, former premier of Alberta, also gave the condition as his reason for cancelling his Third Way plan for greater privatization of health care in that province (Klein, 2005).

Importantly, for-profit health care is less expensive for governments but more expensive for consumers. Increased expenses derive both from business profits and from increased administrative overhead. Overhead costs for Medicare in Canada represent 1 per cent of total costs. Overhead costs for large American health maintenance organizations, private plans in Canada not covered under Medicare, and private prepayment in commercial health insurance carriers prior to Medicare are approximately 26 per cent. That is, public plans incur much lower overhead costs. Furthermore, in Canada, 100 per cent of the population is insured; in the United States, only 84 per cent of the population is insured. Yet, in Canada, the cost of health care per person is about half the cost in the United States (Marmor and Sullivan, 2000).

In addition, claims that the shift toward neo-liberalism will have a trickle-down effect within the economy and produce overall economic prosperity are not supported by the evidence. Rather, where profit shares and rates have increased, it has largely been the result of declines in wages rather than increased investment. All Organization for Economic Co-operation and Development (OECD) countries, including Canada, are witnessing increased unemployment and most increased salary differentials, decreased social expenditures, and a transfer of income from labour to capital (Navarro, 2002a). Part-time, home-based, and temporary work, self-employment, and outsourcing are all increasing, while working-class rights and unions are being undermined (Coburn, 2004). Importantly, countries with more redistributive policies and high trade-union density (such as Canada) show lesser wage and income inequalities than countries without these arrangements (such as the United States and the United Kingdom). The trends are still evident in these countries, but are less pronounced.

The situation is even worse for less developed countries. Anderson (2000) describes how loans given to less developed countries have harsh conditions attached for repayment that prevent those countries from investing in education, health care, and other welfare programs for their citizens. Employment conditions are exploitive, especially for women and children. Indeed, the globalization of market economies is increasing the feminization of poverty around the world.

The neo-liberal agenda is contrary to the vision of health-care reform that embraces an expansion of Medicare's mandate to include the social determinants of health, a broad definition of health beyond medicine, and health promotion. It represents a paradigm shift within Canadian society and its governments. Medicare is becoming more narrowly defined, thus increasing the territory for for-profit firms. This change is evident in the increased role for private clinics that, in the past, were restricted to specialized or elective services. They are now expanding to provide abortions, in vitro fertilization, and laser eye surgery. In other words, they are moving into the arena traditionally serviced by hospitals. The paradigm shift can also be seen in the narrowing of home care to short-term post-hospital services. (See Figure 5.1.)

Williams and colleagues (2001) refer to the current process as a **hollowing out** of Medicare. One result of this process is that many of the long-term home and community support services that seniors require are no longer available or are available only at a cost. Interestingly, proponents of profitization often use the older adult population and their increased medical use as support of their position—an example of **apocalyptic demography** at work. Yet the population that uses health-care services disproportionately, those aged 75 and older, will only grow from 5.8 per cent of the population in 2001 to 6.7 per cent in 2016. Even if we assume that they currently consume 50 per cent of health-care expenditures, their growth will add only about 1.1 per cent as a percentage of Gross Domestic Product. These statistics do not warrant the alarmist writings seen in the media (Mendelson and Divinsky, 2002).

The health-care reform process in Canada during the 1990s provided the opportunity for a broader, more appropriate, and more cost-effective health-care system. Simultaneously, it opened the door to a greater role for private interests and profitization amid an international climate favouring American-style global capitalism. The globalization of capital is drastically affecting

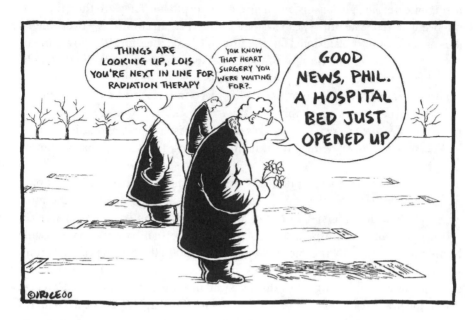

Source: Ingrid Rice, North Vancouver.

Canada's health-care system, despite the United Nations' Declaration of Human Rights (article 25) recognizing the right to health care as a human right, not a privilege. Health care for serious illnesses is a vital need, providing a moral argument for legislation to establish equal access to basic health care for all. Canadians are already convinced, as witnessed by the fact that there is strong grassroots support for Medicare, suggesting one reason why we are witnessing the hollowing out of Medicare rather than its outright demise. Restructuring and redefining acute care to serve only the most severely ill are presented as improved system efficiency even though the consequence is a Medicare system that is more medical than it was in the past. As Medicare is hollowed out, many of those who need health care the most (women, who experience more symptomatology than men; ethno-cultural minority groups, who tend to be economically disadvantaged and therefore also have greater illness needs; and seniors, who experience the most ill health and are the greatest users of our system) are defined as outside its protection.

Interestingly, there are other systems from which Canada could learn. For example, Asian countries provide an interesting contrast to health-care policy in Canada and other industrialized nations. By and large, developing countries have not established health-care systems built on medical foundations, as has Canada and most other industrialized countries. As their societies age and they become aware of the need for society-wide care, it is not clear that their economies can afford Western style Medicare, built upon the two most expensive forms of care (i.e., physicians and acute-care hospitals). They are therefore not intending to replicate our type of system. In many Asian countries, governments are eager to support traditional family care. In China, therefore, the government is embracing traditional notions of filial piety and children are explicitly taught that they should respect their parents and provide them with care when their health declines. Other older forms of filial piety emphasized this respect out of obligation; newer forms emphasize affection and reciprocity for the care received when they were younger. Nevertheless, it is family care that is promoted (Chappell, 2007c), with government providing formal support to family caregivers.

Japan stands as an exception among both industrialized and developing nations. Japan has officially embraced formal long-term home care as the most appropriate health-care system for an aging society. Japan has medical services (both physicians and hospitals), but its universal formal base is a nation-wide home care program. By the late 1990s and early 2000s, their home care program was launched with their Golden Plans and Social Care Insurance Schemes. As such, Japan is establishing a health-care system more consistent with Canada's vision for health-care reform than is Canada itself (Chappell, 2006b). The basis for the program was laid in the 1980s, by which time their public pension system had become widespread. Yamato (2006) reports that more Japanese adults prefer economic dependence on public pensions (46.3 per cent) than on children (7.9 per cent), the traditional values in their society. That is, despite their historical traditions of filial piety, they have embraced formal community care to support those with health needs and to support families caring for those in need.

This focus on community care is not to suggest that care of those who become ill or disabled does not also incorporate some historical roots (see Chapter 3). Nevertheless, Japan stands as an example that it is possible to develop universal health-care programs based on non-medical assumptions. Japan, like most Asian nations, has learned from the earlier experience of Western systems of health care and is moving in a different direction. To the extent that it does not have to deal with a medical (or other) system that is already in place with well-established powerful vested interests, it is easier for them to create alternate systems of care than it will be in Canada should we decide to travel this path.

OTHER VESTED INTERESTS: THE PHARMACEUTICAL INDUSTRY

Although much of the attention in health-care reform has focused on physicians and hospitals, and much of our concern has drawn attention to long-term home care for an aging population, the pharmaceutical industry has a major vested interest in the existing system. The **medical–industrial complex** encompasses the pharmaceutical industry because drugs and physicians are so closely linked—only physicians are allowed to prescribe drugs. Prescription drugs are excluded from Medicare unless provided within an acute-care hospital (payment arrangements for drugs prescribed outside of this setting vary from province to province). Access to pharmaceutical information has increased dramatically in recent years, with health-care workers, citizens, and governments deluged with volumes of often conflicting information. Back in the early 1990s, Lexchin (1993) estimated that 3,500 prescriptions were available to physicians with new information on side effects and drug-to-drug interactions, not to mention new drugs emerging continuously. Physicians rely on 'detail men' (drug company representatives) to stay current. Curiously, this is not considered a conflict of interest (Rachlis and Kushner, 1989; Segall and Chappell, 2000).

Despite all of this information, the Saskatchewan Commission on Medicare reports that physicians often prescribe poorly (Fyke, 2001). This finding includes prescribing antibiotics for viruses when they are ineffective, expensive drugs when cheaper drugs are just as effective, and multiple drugs that result in adverse reactions (an estimated 20 per cent of older adult hospital admissions are associated with adverse drug reactions). From a review of what is known about prescription drug use among older adults, Tamblyn and Perreault (2000) conclude that medications are both under- and over-prescribed for certain conditions, that there are errors in drug dose and therapy duration prescribed, and that there is suboptimal compliance. They also note that drug-related illness is the sixth leading cause of death in the United States. The area of prescription drugs is seen by some as a domain of self-care (previously exclusive to the private domain of families) that has been co-opted and exploited as an extension of medicine for the purposes of profit (Dean, 1981; Kickbusch, 1989).

Much of the attention now given to prescription medications by governments is a result of the dramatic and continuous increase in their costs. From 1987 to 1993, the average price of a prescription (excluding the dispensing fee) in Ontario rose by 93 per cent, from $12.48 to $24.09. The introduction of new patent medications was responsible for more than half of this increase. In 1987, Bill C-91 was introduced, extending the monopoly for new drugs coming on the market, abolishing compulsory licensing, and giving manufacturers (primarily multinational companies) 20 years of patent protection (Lexchin, 2001). Both NAFTA and the General Agreement on Tariffs and Trade (GATT) were used to help pass Bill C-91 and to eliminate competition from generic drugs (previously able to enter the market five to seven years after entry of the original product, and at substantially lower cost). Of note, the pharmaceutical industry invested heavily in Montreal at about this time; the Quebec government is an affiliate member of the Pharmaceutical Manufacturers Association of Canada (PMAC). The economic viability of the pharmaceutical industry therefore relates directly to Quebec's industrial strategy to develop the industry there and, according to Lexchin (2001), a threat to the industry could be used by separatists should the federal government position itself against PMAC.

In recent years, deductibles and patient co-payments for eligible Pharmacare programs have been increasing. Typically, they have been applied to groups differently. Older adults and those with very low incomes usually pay lower co-payments. In an effort to contain escalating costs, British Columbia introduced reference-based pricing, also practised in Germany. In this pricing structure, the cost of the cheapest of the most effective drugs with the least side effects, as decided by an expert panel, is reimbursed within the provincial drug plan. If it is considered medically necessary that a person receive a different, more expensive drug, physicians can request that the more expensive drug be reimbursed.

When reference-based pricing was being considered, PMAC responded by launching a public relations campaign, arguing that individuals would now receive the oldest and cheapest drugs, that provincial government economic concerns were driving the initiative over and above patient needs, that quality of care would be adversely affected, that worse health would result, that government bureaucrats were replacing physicians as medical decision-makers, and that the government did not consult on this policy (Brunt et al., 1998). The British Columbia government countered that the drug companies' campaign was motivated by their profit objective, that the reference-based pricing program represented good stewardship of threatened economic resources, and that the policy is both flexible and safe. Chappell and colleagues (1997) conducted a province-wide survey of older adults and reported strong support for the program—citizens felt that the media campaign launched by the pharmaceutical manufacturers reflected their self-interests. After the province implemented the program, PMAC sued for lost revenues. It lost its case and the subsequent appeal, and the Supreme Court of Canada denied permission for further appeal.

Despite the increasing costs of prescription drugs, the implementation of programs such as the one in British Columbia, and recommendations for action (see, for example, the National Forum on Health Report, 1997), it seems unlikely that Pharmacare will be added to Medicare. The Romanow Report (2002) made the following recommendations: two-year funding for the establishment of a Catastrophic Drug Transfer to fund a portion of increasing drug costs and to help reduce disparities in coverage from one jurisdiction to the next; a new National Drug Agency for the evaluation and approval of new prescription drugs, ongoing evaluation of existing drugs, negotiation and containment of drug prices, and the provision of objective information; and a National Prescription Drug Formulary. Discussions are now taking place among provincial and federal levels of government on coverage for catastrophic drugs and a national drug formulary.

CONSEQUENCES FOR INDIVIDUALS

Health-care policies impact and shape individual expectations and behaviours. Numerous examples of the consequences that society's structural arrangements have for each person and their comparative disadvantages for certain groups have been evident throughout this book. This section takes a closer look at the influence of health policy on care work and women. Individually and collectively, women have had little influence over when and how health-care reform occurs. Health-care reform's return to a medical model may result in less room for women's perspectives (among whom a more holistic approach to health care tends to prevail) (Armstrong and Armstrong, 1999). While we saw women's voices arguing for the return to a more natural approach to childbirth and to the treatment of diseases such as breast cancer, these remain more the exception than the rule.

It has been argued that women's traditional care work is neither recognized nor valued. Within market relations, care and nurturing are relevant only in relation to paid work and within this context are not highly valued. Care is gendered (female), familized (in the private domain) (Brown and Lauder, 2001), and simultaneously peripheral. As McDaniel (2002) notes, despite the lack of value and recognition accorded to women for their caring work, this work not only contributes but is also essential to the survival of a market economy. Workers come back to their families at the end of the day to recuperate and energize so that they can function effectively at their paid labour the next day. When they become sick or disabled, it is typically women who nurse them back to health so that they can rejoin the market economy. It is women who bear, raise, and socialize future generations of workers for the labour market.

As health-care system reform hollows out Medicare, reinforcing acute-care services as publicly funded while marketizing and commodifying long-term and social care, increased demand is placed on family members (primarily wives and daughters) to fill the gap. This is especially true for poorer families who cannot afford to purchase such services. For those who can afford the services, a market is created for the purchase of care (or the **commodification of care**). The vast majority of workers providing this care are women, especially among those who provide hands-on care (the home-care workers, the nurses' aids in hospitals and nursing homes) and receive low salaries, little training, and often no benefits or career trajectories. Importantly, the current trend toward a market approach to health care risks commodifying care relationships, which will likely cause an erosion of ties traditionally built on affection and obligation (McDaniel, 2002; Medjuck, Keefe, and Fancey, 1998).

One option that is consistent with the **marketization of care** is to pay family members for providing care. We see examples of this in Canada, but the practice is not widespread. As noted in Chapter 3, the Department of Veterans Affairs will sometimes pay family members for providing care. Within the disability movement, focusing primarily on those with lifelong disabilities, client-directed care is often possible. Clients are given a certain amount of money; they then decide who and when to hire. More commonly, the issue before policy makers is whether to provide services to caregivers directly (currently through the funding of respite care services so caregivers can have a break) or to provide care to the sick or disabled person, relieving the family member of providing that particular task.

These two options provide very different approaches to policy for informal caregivers. Pickard (2001), in her discussion of policy documents in the United Kingdom, labels them **carer break** and **carer blind** policies. The former focus on the well-being of the carer (relieving their burden), but do so in order that the caregiver can continue to provide care, with no intent to replace them. In a sense, they are viewed instrumentally in terms of the service they provide and can continue to provide. This is typically how caregivers are discussed within policy in Canada and other industrialized countries, if they are discussed at all. Such policies do not deal with situations when the interests of carers are in conflict with those of care receivers. For example, providing respite for the carer may not be the best alternative for the care receiver (such as when institutional respite is provided or a care attendant's presence in the home upsets the care recipient). Carer break policies also assume that the informal caregiver should continue providing care rather than providing options for relinquishing this role.

The latter, carer blind policy, is concerned not with relieving the caregiver but substituting for them and hence, at least partially, removing their responsibilities. Proponents of such an approach argue that these policies promote the independence and autonomy of the care receiver (assuming no cognitive impairment) rather than facilitating dependence on the caregiver. Inherent within this approach is an acceptance of the view that families, and women in particular, should be freed from obligations tied to the assumption that they will necessarily provide care and that they should be able to pursue other activities, including full-time labour force participation. Governments typically stay away from this discussion; concern with the increased costs of substituting informal care with formal services is sufficient to ensure that such an idea is not given serious consideration (Davies, Fernandez, and Saunders, 1998). Interestingly, Pickard and colleagues (2000) note that the costs estimated to fund carer blind services in the United Kingdom would be no more than the costs of providing two weeks of respite care for carers with heavy responsibilities. Both alternatives are considerably less costly than nursing home care.

These two policies are not, of course, mutually exclusive. Even if a carer blind policy was adopted, some families would maintain informal caregiving relationships and, among those who receive carer blind services, there may simultaneously be an informal caregiving relationship in certain areas, as occurs now. Indeed, Pickard (2001) argues that both types of policies are necessary to comprehensively address the needs of both caregivers and care recipients. She further suggests that policies in this area must address the interests of both parties more explicitly, including areas where the interests of one may conflict with those of the other. Germany is cited as an example of where such comprehensive policy exists for caregivers and care recipients. In Canada, carer blind policy is not being considered, as evidenced in a report for Health Canada by Keefe, Legare, and Carriere (2004). The policy directions they identify to support caregivers include caregiver assessments as part of home care policy, increasing caregiver services such as respite care, and expanding eligibility criteria to include friends and neighbours. There is no indication that governments are interested in re-drawing the boundaries between state and family care at the present time. The issue of caregiver policy options does, however, raise the issue of policies that support and facilitate individual agency.

ALLOWING FOR AGENCY

Can health-care policy that allows for and even promotes individual agency while not redefining it in terms of individual or family responsibility and a withdrawal of state support and services be devised? Aside from our individual choices about whether to visit a physician, which one to visit, or how much we comply with his or her orders, can policy embrace personal autonomy while simultaneously impacting our lives? It can be argued that there are options that allow for more agency and the facilitation of individual choice than is evident within our current structures. An alternative model that differs substantially from the current system is to be found within the health promotion perspective (discussed above).

Health-care systems could embrace self-care, without making excessive demands on the individual or blaming the victim if their health is not optimal. As noted by McCormack (2003), it is only after medicine rose to prominence that self-care became relegated to second-class importance within advanced industrialized societies. Historically, it was part of how societies functioned. But within the scientific era, rationality, technology, and materialism became valued over emotions. Scientifically trained health-care professionals became the experts, with their knowledge privileged over that of the individual. In the process, self-care was relegated to a less valued position behind formal services. The helping professions (such as social work, physiotherapy, psychology, child development, and community development) were well developed by the end of the 1970s. Professional human service workers had largely displaced lay persons as the preferred service providers. However, reform of the 1990s included a governmental shift in which responsibility started devolving back to the community, including to individuals themselves and to the not-for-profit sector (Gordon and Neal, 1997). The current attention paid to self-care has arisen within a context of privatization, profitization, and cost-efficiency for governments.

Embracing self-care provides both challenges and opportunities. The self-help/mutual-aid movement and a number of self-care initiatives have flourished. The women's movement, disease specific support groups, and grassroots wellness initiatives all promote autonomy and self-determination whether one is well or ill. Canada has a long history of involvement in promoting this perspective, one that dates back to the mid-1970s with the Lalonde report on health promotion. This working paper argued that health is influenced by a number of factors, including not only biological but also socio-environmental and lifestyle factors such as smoking and alcohol and drug consumption. It provided the basis for a number of major federal and provincial health promotion programs (primarily designed to increase our awareness of the health risks associated with behaviours such as smoking, drinking, nutrition, and fitness).

The Lalonde report was followed, in 1986, by *The Ottawa Charter for Health Promotion* (WHO, 1986), accompanied by the release of *Achieving Health for All: A Framework for Health Promotion* (Epp, 1986). The Epp report outlined various mechanisms by which the population's health could be improved: (1) self-care or the decisions individuals take in the interests of their own health; (2) mutual aid or the actions that people take to help one another; and (3) the development of healthy environments. The concepts of individual agency and empowerment are central to this approach; the purpose of health promotion is to enable people to gain greater control over the factors that influence their health (Green and Kreuter, 1990).

The community is where health promotion must take place. According to Epp, the three ways to implement this approach are fostering public participation, strengthening community services, and co-ordinating healthy public policy. Local communities (defined geographically and/or in terms of affinity) therefore have important roles to play. As well, local and provincial governments can provide leadership, financial and other resources, and formulate policy that will enhance the population's health (Segall and Chappell, 2000).

Although health promotion and disease prevention have continued to be of interest to policy-makers, particularly at the national level, limited resources have been directed towards community-based health promotion, prevention, and related activities such as health education, advocacy, and community development at the provincial level. Historically, health promotion strategies have focused on health education and media campaigns designed to disseminate informational materials (including pamphlets, health guides, videos, commercials, websites, etc.) to citizens through schools, libraries, community centres, health fairs and clinics, hospitals, and other community settings and events in order to enhance the public's knowledge and awareness.

As a result of this focus on personal agency, sociologists and others have frequently been critical of health promotion approaches and programs. One of their major criticisms has been the focus on individuals and their health-related behaviours as sources of health problems and the search for solutions in individual lifestyle change rather than in larger social forces that influence health (blaming the victim). In addition, while the conceptual frameworks of health promotion, population health, and the social determinants of health provide for self-care and individual agency, they all neglect to provide the mechanisms or roadmaps for implementing the idea. Within an existing system that privileges medical knowledge over lay knowledge and in which the former is not accessible to most citizens, how can the system incorporate self-care and individual agency? For laypersons to have more power in decision-making they require expert professionals to accurately convey the relevant health and illness knowledge important for them to make a decision. This is not a simple matter when such knowledge is often complex and differing individual values prioritize certain types of 'objective' knowledge over others. However, even within the current system, greater decision-making authority could be given to clients in instances where knowledge transmission is simple (for example, for the cold, flu, etc.) and more focus could be placed on teaching self-care skills to clients in home care. The system could, wherever possible, promote agency and individual choice.

Social Capital

One area where we see efforts to incorporate more complex understandings of the importance of people's everyday lives in promoting their health is **social capital**. The concept, recently popular in political circles, refers to a contextual level resource for individuals, one that derives from positive relationships and community involvement whereby norms of reciprocity, trustworthiness, and collective capacity emerge (Peterson, 2002). Social capital is said to be good for our health; some suggest that it is the mediating link between socio-economic status and health (Kawachi, 1999; Veenstra, 2002), as described in Chapter 2. Typically social capital is considered a community level factor that some (Lynch et al., 2000) argue thereby differs from the older concept of social support, an individual level factor (see Chapter 3). Others (Hyppa and Maki, 2003; Bolin et al., 2003) argue that it is individuals who build trust, participate in communities (i.e., create social capital), and benefit from it. Without individuals, there would be no social capital. Some, including Putnam (see Carpiano, 2006), define it at an individual level as patterns of interaction including trust and other values associated with these interactions.

Most conceptualizations of social capital follow from Putnam (1993, 2000) and include two central elements, one behavioural (social participation) and one attitudinal (interpersonal trust), in a reciprocal relationship. The relevance is twofold, whether this 'new' concept of social capital is related to individual and population health and, if so, whether the concept is related to health over and above its component parts (participation and trust). Research is inconclusive on whether the concept is related differently than when social participation and trust are considered separately—most of the research examines its component parts separately. That is, it does not combine them into an integrated social capital concept when examining its relationship to health (Ziersch, 2005). Whether social capital represents something distinct from participation and trust would seem to be a critical issue because the concept suggests that a person should be high on both social participation and interpersonal trust in order to be characterized as having high social capital. However, in many situations, there may be high participation accompanied by low trust or low participation and high trust (Lindstrom, 2004). Said differently, not all participation is associated with the high levels of trust—are these instances of social capital or not?

Edmondson (2003) argues that the reason empirical results are so inconclusive is because social capital takes different forms in different settings. Its changeable nature makes it elusive. We know little about how and when social participation results in trust and when it does not. Sometimes we resign from community committees (and therefore participate less) because we trust other members to make decisions consistent with their own values and desires. Sometimes we participate more when our level of mistrust is high (protests against government actions would be an example). In addition, high social capital in one arena might translate into low social capital in another (e.g., those embedded and with influence in the environmental movement may be unwelcome in circles unconcerned with pollution). And high social capital in one area may simply be unrelated to high social capital in other areas. That is, social capital in one context may not be in another.

Carpiano (2006) argues that many of the difficulties with the concept of social capital stem from the inconsistent and overlapping use of the term with its causes, correlates, and consequences. Focusing on neighbourhood social capital, he proposes a conceptual model that draws heavily on Bourdieu, rather than Putnam. For Carpiano, *structural antecedents* to neighbourhood social capital include, for example, the socio-economic conditions of the neighbourhood—structural antecedents are relevant for the type and strength of social ties and resources. In his view, *social cohesion* is distinct from social capital (contrary to Putnam) and refers to the patterns of social interaction and values that result in social capital and are intermediaries between structural antecedents and the resulting social capital. *Social capital*, again following Bourdieu, refers specifically to actual or potential resources embedded within neighbourhood social networks. *Outcomes of social capital* refer to goals or benefits for network members or the neighbourhood as a whole. Carpiano brings conceptual clarity to the discussion, but his model has yet to be empirically verified.

Irrespective of the difficulties, the concept of social capital is interesting because it embraces the notions of **relationality** and **sociality**, the inherent connectedness of each individual to the social where the individual and the collective are not separate but are meshed together. Indeed, Baron, Field, and Schuller (2000) suggest that policy interest in the concept represents an attempt to acknowledge and incorporate the interrelatedness of people that policy typically does not capture. One of the difficulties for policy makers is that social capital is inherently relational and, unlike resources (such as money) that operate between contexts, social support and social capital cannot exist without social context (Edmondson, 2003); it is therefore difficult to grasp, to measure, and to standardize policy relating to it. Governmental interest in social capital follows from a belief that it is related to enhanced public and individual health and can perhaps be used as a strategy for reducing societal inequalities. If there is a relationship though, we do not know the direction of causality. Do societies or groups with low social capital result in greater inequality or do greater inequalities within society result in low social capital?

Box 5.4
Examples of Health Canada Websites on Social Capital

Social Capital as a Health Determinant: How is it Defined? Health Policy Research Working Paper Series, Working Paper 02–07, March 2003: http://www.hc-sc.gc.ca/sr-sr/alt_formats/iacb-dgiac/pdf/pubs/hpr-rps/wp-dt/2003-0207-social-defin/2003-0207-social-defin_e.pdf.

Social Capital as a Health Determinant: How is it Measured? Health Policy Research Working Paper Series, Working Paper 02–08, March 2003: http://www.hc-sc.gc.ca/sr-sr/alt_formats/iacb-dgiac/pdf/pubs/hpr-rps/wp-dt/2003-0208-social-meas-mes/2003-0208-social-meas-mes_e.pdf.

'Social Capital and Health: Maximizing the Benefits', *Research and Science*: http://www.hc-sc.gc.ca/sr-sr/pubs/hpr-rpms/bull/2006-capital-social-capital/index_e.html.

'Example of a Conceptual Model for HHR Planning', appendix from *A Framework for Collaborative Pan-Canadian Health Human Resources Planning*: http://www.hc-sc.gc.ca/ahc-asc/alt_formats/ccs-smc/pdf/public-consult/col/hhr-rhs/PanCanHHR_Framework_sept.05_e.pdf.

'Population Health Approach: What's New?': http://www.phac-aspc.gc.ca/ph-sp/phdd/whatsnew.html.

Despite these questions, governments currently use policy to intervene in this area; such policies influence access to daycare, to public spaces, to educational programs, as well as to those that provide for support groups, community action, and town hall meetings and are related to the formation of social capital. Health Canada's (2006) article, 'Social Capital and Health: Maximizing the Benefits', notes that policy supportive of social capital simply refers to 'explicit attention to the role of social relationships in attaining policy objectives and, inversely, looking at the effects of policies on social relations'. Examples of Health Canada's interest in social capital appear in Box 5.4.

However, despite this interest in the concept, Canada's health (and other) policy has a long way to go before it could be claimed that it embraces the notion. And importantly, certain forms of social capital can undermine other types. As Edmondson (2003) points out, uniform organizational rules designed to apply the same standards to everyone are by design context free. Therefore, they do not allow for particularistic approaches. The old adage that equality does not mean sameness is less easily translated into bureaucratic policies than is uniformity. A key challenge raised by the social capital debate is how social policy can support values of appropriate universality while also allowing for and even facilitating particularistic and even individualistic contexts.

The concept of social capital also lays bare the difficulty with the fragmented system in place. Canada, like other industrialized countries, has ministries of health that are separate and distinct from ministries of education or of human resources, and so forth. Yet, as noted earlier, a holistic concept of health calls for a comprehensive approach to health promotion and to health care when illness strikes, an approach that necessarily cuts across ministries. A key question is how to reorganize governments so that they can cope with cross-cutting issues in a comprehensive way. For example, fast foods and soft drinks in schools are a health issue. Physical education in schools is a health issue. Availability of daycare, social support at work, and access to public spaces and to green spaces are all health issues. Governments will need to reorganize themselves to enable interaction around holistic issues such as heath care. While some *recognition* of the importance of concepts such as social capital is a first step, much more remains to be done. One area of promise is the notion of healthy communities.

Healthy Communities

The notion of healthy communities emerges within an area known as public health, an area distinct and separate from what we think of as the health-care system and associated services. **Public health** typically deals with concerns such as clean air and drinking water and proper sewage and sanitation systems. It also focuses on issues such as the re-emergence of possible disease epidemics following from recent SARS and West Nile Virus scares. The focus here on 'public' health diverts attention away from either medical or research elite experts to everyday people from varying backgrounds. It places emphasis on public assets including education, work, transportation, community life, and social cohesion—the **social determinants of health**. Healthy communities emphasize action over research, and partnerships and collaboration rather than top-down or authoritarian approaches.

Research in the area of population health has helped reinvigorate interest in the public health area. However, Canada's epidemiologists who initially brought attention to the importance of this area have been heavily criticized. Their work on the socio-economic status and health relationship, the social gradient, and what has become known as the **health inequality hypothesis**, is said to be rooted in a biomedical approach to health that views it as the absence of illness (Evans, 1994). Their work has also been criticized as lacking a values base and thereby ignoring issues related to equity, social justice, and participation; failing to make theoretical assumptions explicit (notably in relation to political and economic factors, the structural factors noted earlier); and lacking a critical analysis of societies (Raphael and Bryant, 2002).

Some, such as Raphael and Bryant (2002) consider the popularity of the population health perspective, especially among government departments, to be undesirable. In their view, it is supplanting a health promotion model (emanating from the WHO) that embraces a values-based approach. As noted earlier, the

WHO views health as a resource for daily living. Health promotion is considered an enablement process that assists people to increase their control over and to improve their health. Within this vision, healthy public policy, supportive environments, community action, and personal skills all promote health. Yet some proponents of a population health model also adhere to these tenets. Frank (1995), for example, argues that a population health perspective obliges us to exercise a critical analysis of the conditions of life as they influence the health of communities and to be involved in actions that will bring about change, a perspective consistent with a health promotion approach.

Others, such as Labonte and colleagues (2005), argue that the distinction is now moot and that the two perspectives (i.e., health promotion and population health) have in effect merged. Health promotion now typically incorporates population health promotion and population health researchers are more accepting of the tenets of this perspective. The federal government incorporates elements of both in their frameworks, including the goal of improving the health of the entire population, reducing health inequities among groups, and increasing collaborative action to effect change. Notwithstanding the movement towards merger by many, the originators of the population health model (largely epidemiologists and economists) tend not to examine structural relationships between capitalism, social inequalities, and health (Coburn et al., 2003). Such relationships can be considered the central domain of sociological thinking, a critical area where sociological thought has extended an important model.

Significantly, a population health approach presents us with the **health-care conundrum**: if health-care services do not create healthier people, but investments in education, the environment, housing, or other social determinants do, there would appear to be no need to increase funding to the health-care system. A health promotion perspective (and a combination of the two approaches or what Labonte and colleagues refer to as a **critical population health perspective**) allows for understanding social structures, economic relationships, and ideological assumptions, as well as how they create and perpetuate health disparities in order to improve equity in health. This approach allows for equal or greater funding to health care if needed or until such time as society has been re-organized to reduce existing disparities.

It is the action-oriented aspect of these approaches that directs attention to healthy communities. Dannenberg and colleagues define a **healthy community** as one that 'protects and improves the quality of life for its citizens, promotes healthy behaviours and minimizes hazards for its residents, and preserves the natural environment' (2003: 1500). Healthy communities speak to the involvement and empowerment of all people and all levels (micro, meso, and macro; individual, group, and community; municipal, provincial, and federal governments) comprehensively in establishing the health of the nation. They focus on the 'public' in public health, thereby embracing the principles of equity, collaboration, participation, and capacity-building, sometimes referred to as the **new**

public health (Raphael and Bryant, 2002). Building healthy communities means the involvement of all levels to bring about change (for example, changes in zoning laws to increase walking access and promote physical activity and improvements to parks and other public gathering places to encourage social activity). Strategies such as cleaning alleyways, reducing traffic speed, building traffic islands, and improving recreation facilities can increase social interaction, community participation, and sense of belonging, all of which must take residents' abilities and desires into account (Masotti et al., 2006).

CONCLUSIONS

In this chapter, you have learned about the construction of the Canadian health-care system. It was established primarily to treat ill health rather than to promote good health and prevent disease, and does so from a medical perspective premised on the view that all Canadians have the same right to medical care. As our knowledge evolved and Canadians came to understand that our health is more than the absence of disease, that there are many individuals and social factors that affect our state of health, and that many health-care professionals and non-professionals can contribute to our health, a new vision of what our health-care system should look like has emerged. That new vision is comprehensive in scope, is community based, and embraces both individual and structural factors as important for health.

However, the health-care reform process that began in the mid- to late 1990s and continues to this day, seems to be driven more by larger forces of globalization than by the vision that first provided the opportunity for change. Recent evidence suggests that reform is resulting in a more, not less, medically focused health-care system with increased privatization of services and little in the way of health promotion and disease prevention. The consequences for individual and population health may well be increased illness and increased disparity in the care received by citizens, varying by ability to pay. Nevertheless, there would appear to be an alternative available, namely a health-care system more consistent with the tenets of a social determinants health model that facilitates individual agency while also providing care to those in need.

Health-care policy has not been undergoing change in isolation, but reflects a larger picture. McDaniel (2006) describes the immediate post-World War II social contract as one in which Canadian governments focused on increasing citizens' economic security, expanding opportunities through education, and pooling risks. Medicare would appear to be a prime example of this more collective and protective orientation. In McDaniel's view, the past several years have witnessed a paradigm shift based on adaptation. Citizens are expected to adapt to change within a competitive environment where there are investments in human capital and individualized, privatized opportunity and risk. The massive restructuring of social policy in the 1990s is also evident in arenas outside of health care. For example, unemployment benefits dropped from covering 80 per cent of all unemployed in the 1970s and 1980s to covering only 40 per cent in 2000, with reduced benefit replacement. In terms of social assistance, average welfare incomes plummeted, and eligibility tightened and became contingent. What is happening in health-care policy, in other words, is part of a larger trend affecting social policy generally.

Social policy is socially constructed and can be constructed differently. As Navarro notes (2002b), structural arrangements created by those in power are resulting in increased inequalities that in turn result in poor health. Alternative structural arrangements can result in different consequences. Navarro (2002b) argues that two types of interventions, one in the labour market and one in the state, will reduce these escalating inequalities. One refers to the reduction of unemployment and the development of well-paid employment; the other refers to increased social cohesion through expansion of the welfare state (social expenditures on programs such as universal health care). Navarro's point is that structural arrangements emanate from power relations that maintain or change existing power relations, that the current ideology of neo liberalism is producing greater inequalities, that it need not do so, and that alternative arrangements are possible that will lead to greater equality and better health for populations. With data from most developed countries of the world, he shows how globalization of the world economy is not contrary to full-employment and social expenditures.

Questions for Critical Thought

1. Canadians often think we have universal health care because we have Medicare. Argue for or against this statement.
2. What relevance does American-style capitalism have for Canada's health-care system?
3. What effect is health-care reform having on Canada's system of formal health-care services?
4. What effect is health-care reform having on the health of Canadians? Explain your answer.
5. How could Canada's health-care system be restructured to promote agency and improve the health of the nation?

Suggestions for Further Reading

Chappell, N.L., B. Havens, M.J. Hollander, J. Miller, and C. McWilliam. 2004. 'Comparative Costs of Home Care and Residential Care', *The Gerontologist* 44, 3: 389–400.

Edmondson, R. 2003. 'Social Capital: A Strategy for Enhancing Health?', *Social Science & Medicine* 57, 9: 1723–33.

Navarro, V. 2002. 'Neo-liberalism, "Globalization", Unemployment, Inequalities, and the Welfare State', in V. Navarro, ed, *The Political Economy of Social Inequalities: Consequences for Health and Quality of Life*. Amityville, NY: Baywood Publishing Company, 33–107.

Penning, M.J., M.E. Brackley, and D.E. Allen. 2006. 'Home Care and Health Reform: Changes in Home Care Utilization in One Canadian Province, 1990–2000', *The Gerontologist* 46, 6: 744–58.

Veenstra, G. 2002. 'Social Capital and Health (Plus Wealth, Income Inequality and Regional Health Governance)', *Social Science and Medicine* 54, 6: 849.

Williams, A.P., R. Dever, P. Baranek, and A. Gildiner. 2001. 'From Medicare to Home Care: Globalization, State Retrenchment, and the Profitization of Canada's Health-care System', in P. Armstrong, H. Armstrong, and D. Coburn, eds, *Unhealthy Times: Political Economy Perspectives on Health and Care in Canada.* New York: Oxford University Press, 7–30.

Note

1. Short-term home care refers to services to a resident living in the community (i.e., not in an institution) that are received for no more than three or six (it varies by province) months. Long-term home care services are those received for more than three (or six) months. Services can include home nursing, home physiotherapy, and homemaking services. Usually the service comes to the person's home, although occasionally the individual goes to the service for a few hours as, for example, for adult daycare. In British Columbia the services include those referred to as home support services, whereas in other parts of the country and elsewhere they are known as home care services.

Chapter 6

Conclusions: The Sociology of Health and Health Care in the Future

Learning Objectives

In this chapter, you will learn that:

- Sedentary lifestyles and unhealthy environments threaten recent gains in life expectancy and improved health as the current university student generation ages through the life course.
- Increases in poverty and inequality threaten to undermine increases in the health of future populations, including both the economically advantaged and disadvantaged.
- Societal changes that are currently underway (such as increasing ethnic plurality, evolving gender roles, and abolishing mandatory retirement) will influence our health in unknown ways.
- Emphasis on self-care as well as new forms of informal care could increase as interest in consumerism and healthy lifestyles develops together with retrenchment back to traditional medical care within the public health-care system.
- Shifting health-care policies that narrow the scope of universal, publicly funded care to only physician and hospital care will widen the gap between the advantaged and disadvantaged in terms of receipt of services based on needs.
- Societal goals that emphasize the health, well-being, and quality of life of citizens rather than economic efficiency lead to an emphasis on health promotion and community development.
- A sociological perspective is well equipped to advance our understanding of health and health care as Canadian society changes.

To Summarize

We began this book with a brief introduction to understanding health and health care through a sociological lens. A short history of sociological thought in the area noted that, early on, sociologists focused on medicine, reflecting the esteem with which the medical profession was held within society as a whole at the time. Even as sociologists started adopting a more critical stance, the focus on medicine continued. They asked questions concerning power differentials between physicians and other health-care workers and about the quality of care delivered by for-profit agencies compared with not-for-profit and public agencies. The 1970s saw increased criticism both of the medical profession and the knowledge generated by sociologists. A broadening interest that included health as well as illness, alternative forms of care in addition to medicine, and macro societal perspectives as well as individual perspectives resulted in the emergence of a sociology of health and health care in the following decade. Today this area enjoys tremendous popularity as a substantive subfield within the discipline of sociology.

Not surprisingly, this large substantive area reflects the diversity of theoretical perspectives found in the discipline as a whole, ranging from macro structural perspectives such as structural functionalism and political economy to more micro social psychological approaches such as symbolic interaction and social constructionism. However, as we argued in Chapter 1, while major advances have been made in knowledge from macro, micro, and meso theoretical perspectives within sociology as well as within this sub-area, the integration of the different levels into a single theoretical approach has been less developed. Indeed, major tasks for sociology including the sociology of health and health care at the present time are to understand the interplay between social structure and individual agency rather than viewing them as separate dualisms. There are some recent theoretical developments that attempt to address these concerns. For example, life course and structuration theories represent efforts to link the two, but more theoretical development is needed. The challenge is great—to study both social structure and personal agency simultaneously is difficult indeed!

In order to convey the importance of both social structure and agency in relation to health and health care, the remaining chapters of this book discussed major topics within the sociology of health and health care (including health and illness, self and informal care, formal care, and health-care policy) from both perspectives. While some examples illustrate the connection between the two, existing studies overwhelmingly examine our health and health care from one perspective or the other, rather than linking the two. More is said about the need to integrate structure and agency later when discussing the future of this subfield.

We also drew attention to the concept of social inequality and its centrality for sociology in general and for the sociology of health and health care specifically. The unequal distribution of resources and rewards results in the unequal distribution of health and illness throughout the population. In turn, health itself is both a resource and reward while illness is not. Many structural inequalities (including class, gender, age, and race/ethnicity) have garnered the attention of sociologists and a relatively recent interest has developed in their intersections. This interest reflects the reality that each of us is situated differently with regard to these and other criteria and, as a result, many of us experience more than one inequality simultaneously, while others experience none at all.

In this concluding chapter, we revisit the topics previously examined and discuss future directions that are possible in terms of health status, self and informal care, formal care, and health-care policy. We also discuss future directions for sociological thought in order to gain new knowledge and understanding. Within these discussions, we demonstrate how the sociological study of health and health care involves asking questions and forming possible theories, rather than finding definitive answers and conclusions.

REVISITING HEALTH AND ILLNESS

We have seen that Canadians fare well in terms of their health compared with other countries, most notably in terms of physical health. Other aspects, including social and psychological domains, are much less studied and any comparative advantage Canada may have is less clear. It is also unknown whether the increases in longevity we have been experiencing over the last several decades are likely to continue and if so, for how long, at what pace, and in what social groups. Aside from any debates over the maximum length of life we are biologically capable of, a relevant question at the present time is whether the trend toward increased life expectancy will continue, will stabilize, or will begin to show decline. Nineteenth-century advances in public health (e.g., clean drinking water and sanitation measures) and standards of living are generally credited for the major increases in life expectancy found in Western societies, including ours. Yet continued progress in these areas is now being threatened. For example, air and water pollution are increasing; the gap between rich and poor is increasing in conjunction with the neo-liberal policies currently being enacted by various levels of government; and welfare measures that might have helped to lessen the negative impact of current reforms are being dismantled. As a result, in the not too distant future, the current university student generation may have to face the possibility of a shorter life expectancy than their parents.

However, if life expectancy does begin to decline, it will likely be minimal. Given that Canadians can now expect to live into their late seventies and eighties, it is probable that university student generations in the near future can still expect to live well into old age. That means that chronic conditions will no doubt characterize their later years. The increasing prevalence of obesity and its associated conditions (e.g., diabetes, heart disease) suggest that any gains made in recent years in pushing the onset of chronic illness to older ages may not continue. Sedentary lifestyles (of which sedentary workplaces form a large part), 'fast foods' with little nutritional value, and increasing air and water pollution pose threats to the relatively good health currently enjoyed by most Canadians. Whether today's young adults will reverse these trends is yet to be seen. While they can, to varying degrees, choose healthy eating and exercise habits, it will require active involvement in their communities and governmental policies, including international affairs, to ensure a healthy direction for the future. Will the increased recognition of healthy living translate into wider social changes, creating healthier communities and healthier generations of older adults?

As we have seen, socio-economic factors (such as unemployment rates, poverty rates, discriminatory practices) are critical influences on the health of the population. Consequently, as Evans (2006) notes, creating healthy environments requires more than individual choice. It requires collective choices about how much poverty is acceptable and how it will be addressed, as well as a culture of healthy living where the built environments in which we live encourage us to walk rather than drive and where fresh fruits and vegetables are available and accessible (and therefore not overly expensive). Recent decisions within some school districts to ban soft drinks and fast foods from schools are an example of what can be done. However, much more is required if fitness is to be a real public policy. It will require commitment, organization, regulation, and money. This argument does not mean that individuals should not make healthy choices within their own lives but highlights the need to also recognize the impact of social forces.

Society is by nature dynamic, however slowly and subtly. Changes are often visible only in hindsight. Yet we know, for example, that poverty (especially among single parents and their children) and inequality are on the increase in Canada. What does this mean for the future health of our population? Given that both poverty and inequality are associated with poorer health, the implications of such trends seem clear. Those directly and adversely affected will likely see their health decline and the need for health services increase. As well, there will be more of them within the population and therefore the overall health of the population will decline. And, since it is younger families who are among those most vulnerable to increasing poverty and inequality, these effects will be evident for many years to come.

What about those who are well off (in absolute or relative terms)? Recent research suggests that inequality per se is bad for our health and consequently affects all of us, not only those who are poor. While the by-products of poverty and inequality (such as increases in infectious disease, alcoholism, drug use, depression, suicides, crime, and violence) are visited most heavily on those who are most disadvantaged, they also have implications for the health of others in society. How does this occur? Although the pathways are not yet clearly established, acute infectious and untreated disease (such as tuberculosis and HIV) can easily spread beyond social-class borders. The same is true of chronic alcoholism, violence, and other social problems frequently linked to poverty and inequality. As Raphael (1999) informs us, Britain has been experiencing rapidly increasing inequality for decades, and recent statistics now reveal that the most well-off adult males and infants have death rates higher than the least well-off in Sweden. Notably, increasing inequality is not evident in Sweden.

The extent to which Canada is an ethnically diverse nation is striking when looking back only a few decades. For much of the baby boom generation, inter-ethnic marriages (especially between Caucasians and visible minorities) were rare. They are now relatively common. Ethnic foods, neighbourhoods, and celebrations are commonplace in Canada's urban centres. We know little about the extent and ways in which this increasing pluralism is changing the fabric of our society. For example, how are members of ethnic minority groups changed by living in Canada? How is Canadian society changed by their presence? Is racial tolerance increasing or are we finding different ways to discriminate against those we perceive to be different from ourselves? In Singapore, Prime Minister Yew's government mandated an ethnic mix within apartment blocks and condominiums because he wanted to prevent the ethnic hostility he had experienced first-hand when he was younger. He reasoned that if ethnic groups lived with one another, ethnic ghettoes would not form because people would learn from experience that those who are 'different' from themselves are not to be feared or hated (Yew, 2000).

The poor living conditions and poor health of Canada's Aboriginal populations is now well-documented, as is the fact that initiatives by the federal government have not solved these problems. More recent approaches that emphasize Aboriginal self-government and responsibility for their own communities is a promising direction, consistent with the tenants of empowerment (at the personal, organizational, and community levels) widely regarded as essential for good health. However, transference of responsibility must be accompanied by the resources necessary for self-sufficiency. These resources include material goods but, equally if not more importantly, the skills and knowledge necessary for decision-making within today's larger society. The extent to which Aboriginal peoples can succeed within Canadian society while also maintaining their traditional cultures is a question relevant to all ethnic and cultural groups.

Gender is also an important factor in discussing health and illness. With more women being employed, more men providing child care, and more couples sharing tasks, gender roles have begun to converge. The sociology of health and health care examines how this occurrence affects health and longevity, including whether men's and women's health will become more similar and whether men and women will retain distinct roles. Looking toward the future, we can ask the following questions: Will men and women always have distinct roles and/or distinct enactment of similar roles? Will it be possible to tease out the role of differential experiences as an influence on their health compared with biology? Will we also be able to examine the implications of sexual reassignment and gender-blending for health and if so, to be able to disentangle physiological from social causes?

It will be interesting to see how health changes as current and future generations age. For example, it has been suggested that the health and well-being of today's older adults is influenced not only by their recent experiences but also by the historical events of their past. Those currently in their mid-eighties and nineties were in their teens and young adult years during the Great Depression and World War II. Many participated in the war itself, while others lived through its effects (for example, as citizens of various European countries who moved to this country in the post-war years). How has this affected their current health and influenced their longevity? Are the long-term effects of such things as near starvation and poor nutrition, extreme stress of concentration camp experiences, lack of access to health services, and delays in education and occupational training being revealed in ill health in their old age? Along similar lines, how will recent events and experiences (such as 9/11 and threats of global terrorism, global warming, and the spread of HIV/AIDS) influence the health and well-being of today's young adults when they reach old age?

With mandatory retirement policies recently abolished in almost all Canadian provinces and territories, people will likely have more choice as to whether they are employed. Will this make a difference to their health and, if so, in what ways and for whom? Some will continue to work because they need the money; for them, having the option could be good for health. On the other hand, if current government programs are cut so that more people have to work longer, will this be good for their health? No doubt it will vary depending on social-class standing and the type of work involved. Professionals have always had more opportunity to continue work if they wished, even if it meant becoming a self-employed consultant rather than continuing as an employee.

The relationship between all of these factors and their affects on health and illness are other important issues within the sociology of health and health care. There is so much we have yet to learn! As we increasingly embrace the notion that our individual health behaviours (including diet, exercise, and stress) affect our health, how will it affect our interpretations and experiences? It could increase our guilt when we become ill; it could decrease our pleasure in many activities that we define as not optimal for health; it could increase the stress in our lives from ongoing attempts to make sense of the voluminous and contradictory 'evidence' about what is good for our health and what is not. Could such stress counterbalance any gains from healthier lifestyles? What, other than illness or dysfunction, creates awareness of our state of health? Is the current interest in healthy lifestyles facilitating a raised consciousness when we feel well, perhaps when we feel exceptionally well?

Finally, what changes are likely to take place in how we perceive and respond in times of illness? If, as Bury (2000) suggests, those experiencing illness and disabilities are becoming increasingly unwilling to accept a passive role and instead are embracing illness as a time for self-reflection, self-change, and social activism, where is this perspective heading? There are indications that it is consistent with contemporary neo-liberal agendas seeking to cut health-care costs through locating responsibility for illness care in the hands of individual citizens rather than state services. But what about those who are unaware or unable to assert an active role (e.g., young children, those in comas, individuals with cognitive impairments or disabilities)?

CHANGING SELF-CARE

Chapter 3 discussed self-care, the type of care that takes place when we are healthy and when we are ill. We learned that self-care involves both our health beliefs and our personal health behaviours, which are sometimes but not always or necessarily related to one another. Actions do not necessarily follow from our beliefs but often do. National surveys tell us that Canadians currently are aware of the importance of much healthy behaviour and many are changing their personal health practices for the better. The importance of not smoking, of not drinking and driving, or of using seat belts and fire detectors is more widely known than three decades ago. There is no reason to expect that the focus on quitting smoking or moderating alcohol consumption will decrease. However, with alarming increases in obesity, we might expect to see greater emphasis placed on lifestyle behaviours that can prevent this health risk. For example, we see people becoming more aware of their food intake, and this awareness will likely increase as will attention to physical exercise. Concern with air and water quality is likely to increase as well. Water and air filters in the home and citizen advocacy for greater pollution controls to be imposed by governments might be predicted.

The area of work–life balance is currently receiving much attention. There is increasing concern that a fast-paced technological age where computers, cell phones, and Blackberries ensure work never leaves our side may ultimately prove stressful and damaging to our health. This is likely to be an area of even heightened interest in the future, examining how we can be productive workers while also maintaining a healthy balance between different domains of our lives.

Not only are the effects of social factors an essential element of future health and health care, but the acceptance or rejection of our conceptual thinking is also important. For example, if the general susceptibility to ill-health hypothesis, which argues that some people are simply vulnerable to disease irrespective of the illness, is correct, new treatments and research will be needed. As we saw, even though the scientific community does not seem to be presently thinking in this direction, the general populace often speaks in these terms. We talk about people we know being prone to getting sick, having poor constitutions, or always being under the weather.

Another area of self-care that is likely to receive increased attention is the area of lifestyles. As we have learned, this common parlance is not easily translatable into what we actually do. This area is complex, far more so than common language suggests. We regularly talk about our lifestyles and label them as healthy or unhealthy, while in reality most of us engage in a combination of healthy and unhealthy behaviours. What we need to know is how our behaviours interact with one another to affect our health. Obtaining this knowledge is difficult because so many factors might be at play—what we consume, when and in what amounts; the types of physical activity we engage in, when, and how much; the air we breathe; the types and amounts of social supports and stresses in our lives; our biological makeup; our ability to relax; and many others. Not only must these factors be taken into account but their various combinations and interactions with one another must also be considered.

Our health practices often reflect personal agency, one that is enacted within structured contexts that both constrain and facilitate our actions. Although we maintain consistency with the literature in referring to these as structural 'determinants', they are more influences in that we are not suggesting a deterministic model. Our point is that both structure and agency are important. As noted in Chapter 1, we construct social structure—our actions and interactions change social structure. Simultaneously, structure impacts us. We have a primary interest in understanding how differential access to material living conditions and resources are relevant for self-care. Not unexpectedly, the relationships are complex, partly because of the multiple interactions noted above, partly because each individual is uniquely situated within differing social systems, and partly because individuals exercise agency. Because sociologists have tended to focus on one or a limited number of potential factors when studying any particular phenomenon, the result can be a lack of consistency from one study to the next.

Nevertheless, current knowledge is clear—there are a number of structural factors that are operative, including social class, gender, social support, and ethnicity. Those with higher socio-economic status are able to access more resources that facilitate their ability to adopt healthy behaviours (such as better food, recreational equipment and facilities, neighbourhoods with less traffic, better housing and more green space, and jobs with more flexibility). They are also more likely to be able to give priority to improving their own health and well-being rather than securing only the basic necessities of life. Women tend to report being less healthy than men except when it comes to mortality; men are likely to die before women. Women monitor their own as well as their families' health. However, married men are more likely to hold proactive health beliefs than unmarried men. Ethnic and racial differences in health beliefs and personal health practices are complicated and connected to cultural traditions and access to resources. Groups differ with regard to cultural practices (e.g., food and dietary preferences) and what is considered a healthy lifestyle. For example, Asian cultures, which emphasize holistic approaches to health, represent interesting contrasts with Western cultures in terms of health beliefs and consequent actions.

As previously mentioned, the Canadian population is becoming increasingly diverse as the years pass, evident in the array of ethnic foods, restaurants, and celebrations in all of Canada's major cities. This exposure to differing ideas together with a widespread increase in the availability of alternative forms of self-care (such as the popularity of personal trainers, fitness clubs, and hiking trails together with meditation, Traditional Chinese Medicine and Tai Chi) suggest that we will see increasing acceptance and use of a broader range of self-care strategies than in the past, raising questions about the boundaries between self and formal care. Can they be easily separated from one another? Often, we distinguish self-care from formal care based on whether the care is provided by the Canadian health-care system. Because most alternative therapies are not covered by provincial health insurance plans and the user must pay for them out of their own pocket or pay for extra insurance, does this constitute self-care? If someone hires a personal fitness trainer and thereby employs paid help, is this self- or formal care? Along similar lines, is Traditional Chinese Medicine (which is not covered) a form of self-care and conventional Western medicine (which is covered) formal care?

We are inherently social, interacting with many others in our daily lives. It is through these interactions that we form our beliefs about what makes us healthy and often bend to social pressure regarding the behaviours we engage in (whether we swim regularly, join certain clubs, and so on). Our social networks can influence us into engaging in risk-taking or harmful behaviour, such as smoking, excessive drinking, or driving when having consumed alcohol. They can also encourage healthy behaviours, such as exercising more, eating better, relaxing, or reducing stress. So far, most studies focus on the supportiveness of social networks. However, there is increasing interest in the negative aspects of interaction with others, particularly in social interactions that often, if not always, contain both positive and negative elements.

Indeed, the co-existence of positive and negative aspects of interaction is probably the norm. With regard to family life, for example, we typically focus either on the good or on the bad (primarily when it is extreme, such as in cases of abuse). Seldom do we balance our attention on multiple aspects. Yet families, marriages, friendships, and other relationships are almost never totally and only 'good'. A challenge for the future is to explore what aspects of interaction are defined as positive and how we cope with the negative aspects of relationships. When does the negative outweigh the positive sufficiently that we exit from them? Also, under what circumstances do some people tolerate more negative aspects? Women are widely reported to be more sociable than men. Does this mean they will tolerate more or less negativity in a relationship (and if so, in which types of relationships) or are they more likely to possess skills to prevent, mute, or transform negative aspects into something more positive?

Although such social factors affect both health and illness, we are often aware of them only when illness strikes. When illness strikes, we become aware of our (lack of) health. Typically, in the immediate aftermath of an illness, we are acutely aware of our good health and cherish its return. This awareness is usually short-lived—when we are healthy, we tend to take our good health for granted. However, when illness occurs, we typically know we are sick (though not always, such as in many cases of high blood pressure). While many studies tell us about illness experiences, there has been a relative lack of focus on the organization of care from the ill person's point of view (such as how they experience the fragmentation of services, how they feel about the options for accessing health information by telephone or through the Internet and how structural constraints impinge on their lives).

More and more, individuals are viewed as partners in their care, an involvement that contrasts with earlier times when we were told to follow doctors' orders and it was assumed that the individual had little to contribute. Today, it is increasingly accepted that lay knowledge is relevant to the recovery and/or adaptation process, while health-care professionals hold other relevant specialized knowledge. We know little about whether and how the two can best be integrated to result in optimal care for the sick person. A sociological perspective would predict that interactions between health-care professionals and ill persons will differ depending on social class, race, gender, and other social factors, but we know little about this variation and how to ensure no one is disadvantaged. With retrenchment of Canada's public health-care system back to physician and acute hospital care, the future is likely to see more and more sick people going without, especially when care falls outside of traditional Western medicine. This is occurring at a time when alternative forms of care are gaining credibility with the general public.

We know little about how communications and other technological innovations affect how we care for ourselves when sick, how we interact with health-care professionals, and how much we adhere to physician directives. While much information is now accessible, we suffer from overload not only of the information itself but also from multiple sources whose validity is not always easy to assess. Nevertheless, we now often visit our physicians armed with suggestions and questions obtained from the Internet or other sources. Little is known about the extent to which this practice is advantageous and the circumstances under which it is harmful. For example, do we respond differently to this information depending on the culture we are embedded in? We know that different ethnic groups often have different health beliefs and self-care practices but know almost nothing about the impact of the information age on them, nor on diversity within a group. For example, second- and third-generation Punjabi, Filipino, or Japanese Canadians typically do not face the same language barriers as their first-generation counterparts.

Self-care has always been the major form of care for the vast majority of us, whether in sickness or in health. No doubt it will remain so. The current popularity of alternative forms of care (such as massage therapy, herbal remedies, and yoga) and belief in the importance of everyday living for our health suggest self-care may be even more important in the future than it has been in the past.

Heightened awareness of potential health benefits and harmful effects that may result from everyday activities is leading many to consciously choose eating, exercise, and recreation with health effects in mind. As this trend continues, it will be important to not blame the victim when someone becomes sick. We must also be conscious that self-care activities (including tanning, surgical interventions such as face lifts and breast implants, or the use of Viagra) are increasingly embraced, not necessarily for reasons of improving physical health but for purposes of self-esteem and body enhancement. Moreover, these practices are major sources of profitization. Finally, notwithstanding any effects our individual choices may have, it is equally important to understand that our agency is exercised within structural constraints and facilitators. It should also be noted that while this book has focused on sociological perspectives incorporating agency and social structure, genetics, biology, and psychological traits are also relevant and influence the individual in the areas of health and illness.

RELYING ON OTHERS

After self-care, informal care is the second most prevalent form of care in our society. When we become ill, others (our family and friends) help out, typically without being paid. Similarly, when one of our family members or friends becomes ill, we help them. This practice is not likely to change. We are social by nature, living with and among others and forming into small units. Family structures are changing and becoming more diverse. In addition to traditional nuclear families, we now acknowledge single-parent, gay, lesbian, blended, extended, and unrelated families. Yet the caring functions of families do not appear to be changing. The vast majority of all families care about and for one another when the need arises. The future, though, may hold some differing caregiving arrangements than are prevalent today, as gaps in need are filled with creative solutions. For example, we can imagine the possibility of more men, more sisters and brothers, and more groups of unrelated individuals providing more hands-on and emotional care than was evident in the past. As long as the healthcare system continues to be retrenched, these arrangements will become increasingly necessary for recovery and functioning.

We do not know how these differing arrangements will affect the care provided or the relationships evident between care providers and recipients. At the present time, men and siblings are less likely to be primary caregivers than are wives and daughters. If it becomes commonplace for others to also become primary caregivers, will the dynamics of caring change? If a role is expected, the recipient and others (such as other family members) might be less appreciative of what is provided, perhaps resulting in fewer rewards and increased burden for the caregiver. Alternatively, perhaps the role itself will intensify the bond between the caregiver and the recipient, potentially increasing feelings of closeness. Perhaps in some situations the role may be performed more instrumentally, more business-like, and with less emotional attachment. Finally, perhaps there will be more sharing of responsibilities. Currently, there tends to be one primary caregiver—what is the likelihood that it will become commonplace for caregiving to be a multi-person role?

If the trend towards dual working couples continues, the management of a full-time job and caregiving will continue to be a challenge. It is also possible that, as the demands for more self-care increase, we will be less able to provide care for others. We can imagine self-care accompanied by technological monitoring devices that tell a health-care worker when they should visit us in our home. Will there be a resurgence of not-for-profit voluntary agencies to fill the gap, perhaps drawing on a growing senior population in their retirement years? These voluntary agencies may differ from those of the past. Perhaps there will be fewer church- and occupation-based societies and more interest-based and needs-based groups that form specifically to fill a societal need in assisting others.

Challenges for the sociologist are to identify and examine trends and dominant forms of social interaction and to reveal the diversity within the population. In other words, who among us and under what circumstances engage in what types of caregiving? How is the experience constructed differentially and what works for whom under what circumstances? It is easy to ask the questions but not so easy to answer them because of the complexity of social interaction, with its multi-faceted layering of influences interacting with one another. While not simple, this challenge is part of the fascination of sociology—trying to understand people, their interactions, and the social structures they create.

As long as the neo-liberal emphasis on individual responsibility (often equated with a rhetoric of personal agency and empowerment) maintains dominance and is accompanied by declining availability and accessibility to formal care, there will be increased demands on family and friends for caregiving. Without the resources to purchase needed care, individuals are left to fend for themselves the best they can or to rely on family members, friends, and/or voluntary organizations in times of need. Those demands will continue to be differentially distributed with the weight of the pressure felt by those with the greatest needs and the fewest resources. Often these groups are one and the same—those with the greatest needs have the fewest resources available to meet them. The result is inequity in the receipt of care, the distribution of responsibilities for care, and health consequences. Although social scientists have shown that better social program provisions (characteristic of a Welfare State) are good for our health, the current trend is in the opposite direction. Given the dominance of global capitalism at the present time, it is difficult to envision a reversal in the near future.

Social class intersects with factors such as gender, race, and ethnicity. Women (especially those who were previously married) and racial and ethnic minorities are more likely to have lower incomes than men and non-minority group members. However, we do not have a good understanding of these intersections. In other words, how is it different to be a poor East-Indian female than it is to be poor but male and Caucasian or middle class or East Indian and male? The disjuncture between economic disadvantage and social support is especially fascinating. Ethnic minority groups seem to have at least as good if not better family relationships and resources for care provision than non-minority groups. We do not know whether ethnic minority groups offer more or better care than others. When speaking of non-minority groups, it is important to remember that they are not a homogeneous group but show tremendous diversity as well. As Canadian society becomes increasingly diverse, at what point is it still meaningful to speak of certain citizens as members of ethnic minority groups? As cultures blend, what does caregiving look like, and for whom? Are we able to adapt best practices from different cultures for a composite of optimal caregiving at least in some circumstances?

HEALTH-CARE SERVICES IN THE FUTURE

As we have learned, medicine's rise to prominence within the health-care system is relatively recent. And already there are threats to this privileged position. On the one hand, the corporatization of medicine together with managerialism pose difficult challenges for the profession's autonomy. On the other hand, recent attempts to restrict physicians' earning power in Canada have met with little success. Furthermore, changes due to health-care reform are protecting physician and hospital care (a major arena of physicians' work) as the centrepieces of the country's publicly funded, universal health-care system. At least thus far, the profession of medicine appears to be retaining a large part of its autonomy and dominance. While the Canadian public heralds Medicare as part of the country's core identity, the current direction of reform suggests neoliberal thinking about privatization is barking at the door. How long Canada can resist such pressures, particularly those from the United States, is yet to be seen.

There is much discussion about the need to reform medical practice (to include salaried rather than fee-for-service practitioners and multidisciplinary teams of care providers in which the physician represents but one of several specializations). Although there are areas in the country where such reforms have occurred, there have not been major moves in these directions. In the future, we could see general practitioners becoming salaried while specialists continue working on a fee-for-service basis. We could see health-care teams emerge where the physician is the lead or is first among equals. One notion often discussed in the context of lowering costs for physician care is to assign some physician work to nurses who, when properly trained, are just as capable of carrying out these tasks. Arguments in favour of this nurse-practitioner strategy come from developing countries and from northern regions within Canada, where physician shortages have long meant that nurses routinely perform medical procedures that they have been forbidden from doing where physicians are more readily available.

Nurses' work is closely tied to that of physicians. As physicians' work changes so too does that of nurses. While the profession is currently undergoing many changes to its training (including an increased focus on research, regarded as important to their claims for professional autonomy), nurses do not generally practise independently but remain responsible for implementing physicians' orders. Nevertheless, university-based schools of nursing are now graduating research-trained nurses, many with PhDs. As well, the federal government has recently completed a multi-year program that specifically funded research on nursing, and all provinces are acutely aware of nursing shortages that are projected to become even worse as many nurses begin to retire. These trends suggest change is likely.

The nurse-practitioner model, noted above, wherein experienced nurses receive Master's level training to undertake some of the tasks routinely performed by physicians is gaining popularity. In Canada, nurse practitioners are now being trained to carry out such tasks as routine physical examinations and referrals to specialists. They are being trained to work with patients requiring lower levels of care, either alongside or independently of physicians. In this division of labour, general practitioners see patients who are more ill and require more complex care. Nurse practitioners give nursing greater autonomy as a profession and have the added advantage of cost savings (since they are less expensive than physicians) for governments. They can be considered a potential threat to general practitioners but need not be if a satisfactory division of labour can be negotiated. This model has been operating successfully in the United States for several years. However, their health-care system differs from ours; they have fewer general practitioners (but more specialists) per capita than does Canada.

Another threat to the profession of medicine's dominance is the aging of the population itself. As it has become normal to live to older age and the baby boom generation begins to swell in numbers in their later years, there will be an expanded market search for alternative forms of care that may work better for chronic conditions than conventional medicine. Whether it is chiropractic care, naturopathy, or some other form of complementary and alternative medicine (CAM), people tend to seek out such forms of care when their ailment is not improving despite repeated visits to their medical doctor. The demographic shift toward an aging population suggests complementary and alternative practitioners may become increasingly popular in the years to come.

Beliefs that health is more than the absence of disease and that health care constitutes more than medical care are increasing. In this sense, increasing interest in alternative forms of care is at odds with the recent direction of health reform. Despite increasing coverage during the 1970s and 1980s, alternative forms lost much of the ground they had gained during cost-cutting health reforms implemented during the 1990s. This change means that people will have to pay out of their own pockets for these services, pay for private insurance that will cover such services, or receive such coverage through employment-related health plans. Those with fewer resources will go without. CAM services are not likely to be covered under the provisions of Canada's public health-care system anytime soon. Will interest in and use of CAM be maintained or continue to grow despite recent coverage withdrawals or will use decline? Given that those who are able to access CAM tend to have higher education and income levels and to live in urban areas, it is possible that two increasingly separate systems of care will result: a publicly supported medical care system for those of lower socio-economic standing; and a more pluralistic (publicly and privately supported) system that includes medical care and other treatment options for those at higher levels.

It is also interesting to consider recent trends in CAM popularity. CAM use is increasing in conjunction with shifts toward an economic model of care, one that emphasizes consumerism and corporatization within health care. Yet the philosophy of care that CAM represents and which is often given as a reason for its use emphasizes notions of holistic health (incorporating mind, body, and spirit), patient-centred care, and more open and democratic patient–practitioner relationships, all of which appear to be more consistent with a humanistic than an economic model. If these shifts toward economic models of care continue, at least two possible results are possible. CAM use may become increasingly separated from its philosophical roots. Alternatively, consumers may embrace the vision of care originally attached to CAM, either reconciling the two forms or rejecting links to consumer and corporate models.

An examination of health-care settings also highlights the dynamic nature of society. Having achieved remarkable stature as the major setting within which physicians' work is carried out, hospital costs have been skyrocketing. This increase is due to a number of factors, including the increasing costs associated with ensuring continued access to the latest technological advances in medicine. In order to contain these costs, changes that attempt to restrict hospital physicians' scope of practice more narrowly to *acute care* are underway. Long-stay patients awaiting placement in nursing homes or other settings are being defined as no longer appropriate recipients of hospital care. As a result, lengths of stay are shortening. In some rural areas, where hospitals may have been built for political and employment reasons (such as to ensure equitable access and employment in rural areas) and have been chronically underutilized (such as in many parts of rural Saskatchewan), entire hospitals have been closed. Thus, the current trend could lead to hospitals providing acute care only, turning those who require other forms of care away. Will this result in hospitals moving away from the centre to the periphery of our health-care system? If so, what are the implications of such a move for doctors, patients, and our health-care system as a whole? Given that hospitals are currently the only care settings protected under the terms of the Canada Health Act, placing more restrictions on the care they deliver means that more types of care become susceptible to profitization.

All other health-care settings are excluded from the provisions of the Canada Health Act and therefore vary from one province or territory to another and are vulnerable to profitization. As we have learned, many provinces are increasing the proportion of privately owned and operated, for-profit nursing homes. One of the arguments behind this trend is that competition increases the efficiency of public and not-for-profit nursing homes. But research reveals that quality of care is generally better in public homes. The popularity of the neo-liberal agenda suggests that it is unlikely that this trend will reverse in the near future. Given a growing elderly population and therefore a likely need for more nursing homes in the near future, this issue is of immediate importance. Even if community care is enhanced (see below), the continued role of nursing homes for those with greater health-care need is predictable.

There is widespread recognition of the importance of home and communi-ty care for a cost-effective and appropriate health-care system for an aging soci-ety such as ours. Yet need has not increased the prominence of these types of care within the Canadian health-care system. In fact, current trends suggest that such care is being transformed into a more narrowly focused medical support system designed to provide post-hospital care rather than long-term care for the chronically ill. This finding poses a problem, especially for a cost-efficient health-care system for an aging society. Those with resources will be able to pur-chase needed insurance or pay for assistance and treatment outright. However, if current trends continue, those who are chronically ill and who do not have the resources (either monetary or social support) to secure private care will go with-out needed care. As a result, the poor, older adults, single parents, and members of ethnic minority groups will shoulder a disproportionate share of the negative consequences. In addition to being inequitable, this narrow focus may backfire. For example, those with chronic illnesses and disabilites who are unable to obtain necessary care will probably enter the expensive medical care system sick-er through emergency rooms, thereby increasing the cost to the system and experiencing poorer quality of life. Whenever governments move toward an individualistic private model for health services, it is those without resources who bear the brunt of added cost.

Finally, what will the future hold for people's health-care experiences and abilities to participate actively in their own care? As Potter and McKinlay (2005) suggest, we may see the continuation of trends toward medical consumerism and corporatization, enabling patients to gain the knowledge necessary to make informed decisions regarding treatment options and to challenge their physi-cians. Alternatively, we may witness the emergence of a model of care in which sustained and personal relationships between patients and health-care providers are to be replaced by brief instrumental encounters, such as those between a cab driver or sales clerk and their customers, that operate within a medical market-place and offer numerous services provided by competing providers for care.

In this regard, one question that needs to be asked is what we mean when we refer to patient (or consumer) agency, empowerment, and involvement in care. Are we referring to patient control over decision-making? Certainly, as consumers, we do not have input into decisions about the products being offered for sale or their cost. Instead, we are empowered to make decisions regarding whether to purchase a given product, where we will purchase it, and at what cost. If this is the type of empowerment that is being offered, to what extent is medical consumerism a positive direction for patients? Is the desire for agency a desire for personal control over decisions or is it a desire for active involvement in patient–provider relationships that are supportive, characterized by mutual respect, and offer access to information, two-way communication, and participatory decision-making?

HEALTH-CARE POLICY: IS THERE AN ALTERNATIVE?

While sociologists typically focus attention on policy as a structural factor with consequences for individuals, it is also important to remember that it is people who create policy. It is, of course, people with certain social-class backgrounds, in certain positions, and with certain types of power who make the decisions that ultimately form social policies. And in a capitalist society, those who control resources, especially monetary ones, have great influence. Lavis (2002) reports that civil servants who work in Canadian finance departments have little knowledge of the social determinants of health, have little interest in learning more about them, and do not see the need for more population health research. Finance is the only department in which a majority of workers believe that improved economic prosperity is more important than reducing inequalities in order to improve health. These findings are consistent with Evans's (2001) argument that those who negotiate trade agreements on behalf of the country and who are typically trained in economics, tend to think in terms of efficiencies rather than equity. Trade agreements and other economic policies greatly influence health care. Yet, when it is those trained in finance and not in broader social perspectives who are largely responsible for creating social policy, it is little wonder that its relevance and consequences for the health of citizens hold little sway.

The consequences of emphasizing economic efficiency over equity are clear in current government policies to reform health care. Within health-care reform, home and community care are seen primarily as strategies to ensure economic efficiency by reducing labour and increasing profits. Curbing expensive institutional care, especially hospital care, is also a solution of choice. Since those who are sick or disabled prefer to remain in their own homes, care at home is also promoted on humanitarian grounds. As noted in earlier chapters, governments have interpreted this preference to mean increased demands for family care rather than a reason to resource community programs adequately.

When formal community care is promoted, as Aronson and Neysmith (1996) elaborate, it is as a cost-effective alternative to hospital care. This type of care is low-paid work requiring minimal preparation or supervision, an extension of women's 'natural' nurturing work. Thus, it is devalued. Home care work is another example of intersecting structural constraints. Such workers are most

**Box 6.1
The Canadian Association of Retired Persons
First Report Card on Home Care in Canada**

The Canadian Association for Retired Persons (CARP) issued its first report card on home care in Canada in 2001. CARP's mandate is to promote the rights and quality of life for older adults—those aged 50 years and older. The report card was developed by Karen Parent and Malcolm Anderson of Queen's University for CARP. It assigned the following grades:

Strategic Direction	D
Funding	C
Human Resources	E
Service Delivery	D
Caregivers	D
Data	B
Knowledge About Home Care	B

Key: E = negative change; D = no change; C = insufficient change; B = positive change

Recommendations included

- develop home care by design not by default;
- develop sustainable funding by federal, provincial, and territorial governments;
- involve regional and local governments as well as the public at large;
- develop national standards, uniform guidelines, and common national definitions; and
- address human resource issues for paid and family caregivers.

Source: Karen Parent, Malcolm Anderson, William Gleberzon, and Judy Cutler. 2003. 'CARP's Report Card on Home Care by Default Not by Design'. Available at: http://www.carp.ca. Reproduced with the permission of CARP, Canada's Association for the Fifty-Plus.

often women from lower socio-economic backgrounds with few marketable skills. Increasingly, they also come from ethnic minority groups. These workers represent and reflect the low status accorded the work of caring for the sick and disabled (who are often older adults and women) in our society. Adequate training, pay, hours of work, benefits, and recognition that human service work is valuable represent a more equitable alternative. Box 6.1 features the first report card developed by the Canadian Association for Retired Persons (CARP), which grades different components of Canadian home care and includes recommendations for 'home care by design not by default'.

When the health, well-being, and quality of life of citizens rather than economic efficiency are regarded as the goals, a different path becomes evident.

Attention is then focused on the provision of basic needs (for example, food, shelter, education, clean water, income) and not just those who are privileged; social equity; economic development without adverse environmental, social, and health effects; ecological sustainability at all times (including during population growth and increased consumption); supportive social networks, community capacity, and a civic society; a culture of peace and non-violence; and democratic governance. As Hancock (1996, 1999) notes, this focus will require a change in societal values from economic to human development, followed by a transformation in the organization of our communities and society as a whole.

There is growing awareness that economic development is not inherently beneficial and that a country's Gross Domestic Product (GDP) is not necessarily an indicator of human (and social) progress. An alternative measure is the Genuine Progress Indicator (Talberth et al., 2006). It includes non-monetary community-building, child-rearing, homemaking and food-growing contributions while deducting ecological, social, and human costs of economic activity in measuring progress. According to the GPI, the United States' participation in these practices declined after the mid-1970s, even though the GDP increased. Consistent with this approach, Hancock (1999) argues that interaction between three spheres (social well-being, ecosystem health, and economic activity) determines the level of human development within society. The overlap between them indicates our need for social equity, sustainability, and community livability.

The model posited by Hancock assumes that economic activity that does not support social well-being and ecosystem health is undesirable. In order to achieve such a goal and thereby create healthy public policy, health must be put on the social and political agendas of all levels of public policy. **Healthy public policy** is concerned not only with changing diets but also with food security, not only with preventing motor vehicle accidents but also with creating car-free cities, not only about promoting physical fitness but also about promoting active living, and not only about preventing violence but also about creating safe cities to live in. Importantly, it is about more than making medical care more cost-efficient and about much more than the health-care system. From a sociological perspective it places major emphasis on communities (therefore on the meso rather than micro level) including households, city blocks, neighbourhoods, and 'villages' within towns and cities. See Figure 6.1 for Walker's (2004) schematic of the conditions necessary for **social quality**—'the extent to which individuals are able to participate in the social and economic life of their communities under conditions that enhance their well-being and individual potential'.

The concept of community is central in a health promotion perspective that incorporates the social determinants of health. **Community** is often conceptualized as having ties to geography as it is spatially or locality based. Chaskin and colleagues (2001) note that it is recognized by characteristics associated with its physical location or appearance, based on the assumption that location and proximity affect our lives. Others, such as Rubin and Rubin (2001), conceptualize

Figure 6.1   The Conditions for Social Quality

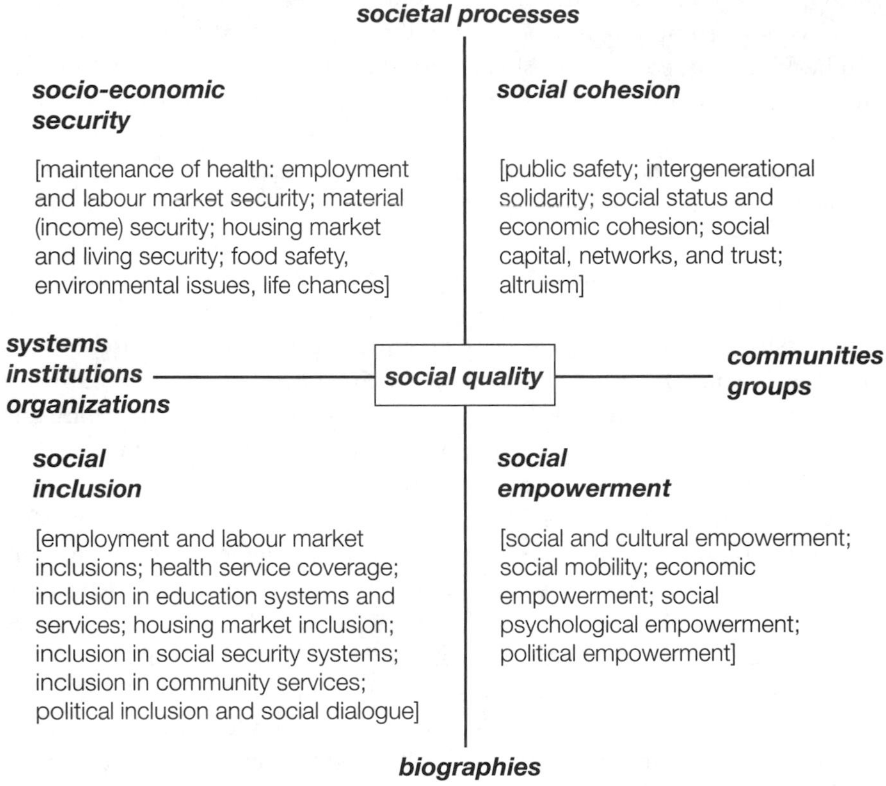

societal processes

socio-economic security

[maintenance of health: employment and labour market security; material (income) security; housing market and living security; food safety, environmental issues, life chances]

social cohesion

[public safety; intergenerational solidarity; social status and economic cohesion; social capital, networks, and trust; altruism]

systems
institutions ——————
organizations

social quality

—————— *communities*
groups

social inclusion

[employment and labour market inclusions; health service coverage; inclusion in education systems and services; housing market inclusion; inclusion in social security systems; inclusion in community services; political inclusion and social dialogue]

social empowerment

[social and cultural empowerment; social mobility; economic empowerment; social psychological empowerment; political empowerment]

biographies

Source: A. Walker. 2004. 'Reexamining the Political Economy of Aging: Understanding the Structure/ Agency Tension', in J. Baars et al., eds, *Aging, Globalization, and Inequality: The New Critical Gerontology*. New York: Baywood Pub. Co., 59–80. © Baywood Publishing Company, Amityville, NY, 2006. Reproduced with permission.

community as primarily relational with psychological characteristics (such as feelings of affinity, similarity, and belonging) assuming primary importance. And indeed, some conceptualizations of community combine the two components. The World Health Organization (WHO) (1998), for example, defines a community in terms of a sharing of a common culture, values, norms, and/or identity among a group of people who often live in a given geographic area.

We know more about adverse health effects than we do about sustainable communities (see Srinivasan, O'Fallon, and Dearry, 2003, for a discussion of urban design, the built environment, and health). However, the current rise in popularity of terms such as sustainable, livable, collaborative, safe, and smart growth communities (replacing earlier references to healthy communities; see Wolff, 2003) reflects increased awareness that when we are speaking about health and healthy places to live, we are talking about much more than what was encompassed by traditional notions of health. We are talking about all of the multiple intersecting facets of our lives, the crux of which are power relations. That is why **critical** or **reflective knowledge** that addresses the role that societal structures and power relations play in promoting inequalities and disenabling people is so important. Wolff (2003) maintains that only when we, as people residing in communities, have the power to change or not change those communities will we have sustainability. (See Box 6.2 for an example of a community arts centre as a health strategy.)

National and international policies also impact communities and individuals. In a unique comparison of Canada and the United States, Siddiqi and Hertzman (2007) reveal how policy decisions and population health trends evolve over years and even decades at a slow pace to nevertheless eventually create large differences between countries. More specifically, they examined how spending on social programs leads to more evenly distributed national incomes, thereby resulting in better population health. In other words, social programming does not have an impact on health that is independent or different from the effect of income distribution (the gap between the rich and poor). Instead, it affects the distribution of income, thereby demonstrating the combined effect of the two on health.

Siddiqi and Hertzman studied the period from 1950 to the present, examining several health outcome indicators (including gender-specific life expectancy, adult and infant mortality), labour market indicators (unemployment rate, purchasing power, adjusted GDP per capita, worker protection, female labour force participation), poverty/income distributions (Gini coefficient, post tax/transfer change in income inequality, income share, child poverty rates), and societal values (postmaterialist index, social trust). Their findings revealed that the gradual development of public provisions is in effect the development of a social infrastructure that is related to better health. Both absolute wealth and the actual amount spent on health care are unrelated to health outcomes. To cite the authors:

> In Canada, the history is one of a more muted response (than the United States) to the Great Depression, but a gradual phasing in of national hospital and unemployment insurance, old age pensions, physician coverage. Federal–provincial social assistance transfers, increasing secondary and tertiary education subsidies, and increasingly 'progressive' labour legislation after World War II that caught up with, then surpassed, the American programs by the 1970s and were not eroded, at least to the same degree, thereafter . . . Canada invests far more than the United States in 'bread and butter' infrastructure such as high-quality public transit, public education, community centres, child care facilities, public recreational facilities, medical facilities, and well-maintained parks. (2007: 599–600)

In Chapter 5 we talked about Canada needing to state emphatically that the Free Trade Agreement does not apply to our health-care services. Recognizing

Box 6.2
A Community Arts Centre as a Health Promotion Strategy

A community arts centre was established in a relatively disadvantaged area (with the help of well-to-do pockets of residents) of a medium-sized Canadian city for value-added to more traditional health promotion initiatives such as physical activity and community gardens activities. Community residents themselves requested one, noting that it would bring residents together and be positive for youth; that is, it would enhance a sense of community. It was housed in a heritage, brick-annex building adjacent to an elementary school in the area that had been unused for many years. The arts centre is a multi-level endeavour: individuals gain skills and many participate as teachers and volunteers; at the interpersonal level there is interaction that involves the exchange of social support; at the organizational level the school's capacity increases; at the community level the entire area gains a resource; and at the policy level decision-makers are involved (e.g., to lease the building).

The centre helps coalesce community. A community health festival was held on the property of the arts centre and adjacent school, bringing many agencies together. For example, traditional carving and drum-making classes attracted First Nations participants of all ages from the area and forged links with agencies that serve this population. Links were also forged with other cultural groups: a local restaurant hosted a fundraiser for bursaries and other materials for the arts centre; other businesses then began donating to the centre. The centre also helped build constitutive capacity as a symbol of positive rather than negative change within the area. In contrast to recent negative developments such as the closing of an area school and cuts in government services, the arts centre reflects positive energy. Participant feedback suggests they valued the centre as a place where they felt comfortable, could learn at affordable prices, and felt safe and encouraged. Community leaders saw the advantage of building relationships among people, a gathering place that facilitates community connection, as a 'resource which has the potential to strengthen a sense of community, using art as a way to promote a more creative, safer, and stronger community' (school principal).

The arts centre provides an opportunity to build community capacity through positive involvement that celebrates individual and community assets through creativity and connection. That is, although the arts are seen by many as valuable in their own right, they are typically viewed as peripheral to the social infrastructure of the community rather than integral to enhancing individual well-being and facilitating the development of community and hence ultimately our health.

Source: A.J. Carson, N.L. Chappell, and C.J. Knight. 2006. 'Promoting Health and Innovative Health Promotion Practice through a Community Arts Centre', *Health Promotion Practice: A Journal of Health Promotion/Health Education Applications* 10, 10: 1–9. Copyright © 2007 Society for Public Health Education. Reprinted by permission of SAGE Publications, Inc.

the importance of international relations to the everyday health of Canadians, Mendelson and Divinsky (2002) go further, arguing that international economic agreements will benefit Canada most if they are democratic and respect each

country's values. They argue that Canada should be a leader in seeking to establish international agreements based on the principles of fairness and equity.
Important questions for sociologists to address regarding this matter include
how to create healthy communities given the role of differing levels of government, the increasing importance of international relations, and the historic role
of economic efficiency over human development in these deliberations.

SOCIOLOGICAL ADVANCES

What about the sociology of health and health care in the future? Clearly, it can
enlighten us on many issues, including those raised above and many more. As
time marches on, sociologists will study many aspects of health and care from
social psychological and social structural lenses. While they will do so among different age groups throughout the life span, they can also do more. As we began
arguing in Chapter 1, it is time for the discipline as a whole, and the sub-discipline
that is our interest, to begin integrating the micro and macro. This is not to say
that sociologists should not also continue conducting studies from exclusively
social psychological or exclusively structural perspectives. Knowledge is generated from the depth allowed in such studies and by focusing on specific age groups.
However, we need to add to this insightful work more integrated approaches, for
they are in many ways two sides of the same coin (Layder, 1994).

One of the reasons why so few studies encompass the entire life span relates
to the time and costs involved. Ideally, answering questions about the aging
process requires longitudinal prospective (forward looking) research designs.
That is, it requires us to study people from birth (or before) and follow them
throughout their lives. Setting aside the issue of how many people we would
need to study, such research would literally take a lifetime to complete. This is
why so-called lifespan studies often compare different age groups at one point
in time and then draw conclusions about how earlier behaviour affects later
behaviour. These studies are valuable provided we understand their limitations
and that they are not conclusive (perhaps confounding age and cohort effects).

We also need to start thinking in terms of the life course and asking lifespan
questions. For example, over the course of our lives, what combinations of good
and not so good eating habits are harmful to our health and are there certain
periods when they are more harmful than at others? How are men's and
women's responses to stress similar as well as different over the lifespan and is
there greater convergence during certain periods? What are the cumulative
effects of lifelong discrimination on ethnic minorities? As you can see, lifespan
questions are also more complicated to answer than those phrased in terms of a
single point in time.

Sociology has much to bring to such questions, even though epidemiologists have been at the forefront of research on the effects of early childhood
experiences on later adult health. For example, Halfon and Hochstein (2002)
present a Life Course Health Development framework, devised to explain how

health trajectories develop over a person's lifetime. They define health development as a 'lifelong adaptive process that builds and maintains optimal functional capacity and disease resistance' (437). Their framework combines the social
with the biological but with a major physiological emphasis. Within a focus on
how the body functions and adapts, this framework accepts that there are multiple contexts of health development. They include genetic endowment (our
biology), physical environmental factors (such as the availability of resources,
food, clear air, and pathogen exposure), social environmental factors (such as
income, economic resources, and connectedness), family environment (family
structure, resources, and support), psychological environmental factors (stress
and behavioural response patterns), cultural and policy environments (norms,
values, and policies), and the health-care system (access, organization, and quality). Notice the overlap of many sociological concepts—the environmental factors and family environment are both part of cultural environments, for
example. These contexts are seen as dynamic; their influence varies throughout
the life course. The focus though is on health *development* rather than health
outcomes such as disease, disability, and mortality.

However, epidemiologists have directed less attention to other segments of
the life course (such as the effects of teenage life experiences on young adult
health or the effects of young adulthood experiences on middle- or later-life
health). More importantly from a sociological viewpoint, they tend to examine
associations between variables without examining the broader structures (such
as capitalism and neo-liberalism) that produce them. Questions about why
observed relationships occur, their consequences, and what can be done to
change the situation are given scant attention. Lack of attention to agency at
both the micro and meso levels (that is, at how individuals and organizations
can change their local environments to influence the income–health relationship) is especially noticeable.

Attention to the critical roles played by both structural forces and individual agency is a primary strength of a sociological perspective. Historically these
have been twin but separate strengths. It is time to focus on integrating social
psychological and social structural perspectives. As we saw in Chapter 1, there
are examples of efforts to integrate at the theoretical level; however, more theoretical work is needed. The gap is even larger at the empirical level—the doing
of sociology. There are several reasons for this absence, not the least of which is
ongoing debate within sociology regarding the legitimacy of integrating different research methodologies. Another reason is simply the practical difficulty of
undertaking studies that include both and do so while doing both perspectives
justice (e.g., not making one more important or central than the other).

Studying the health of ethnic minority groups is an example. It is too difficult to include all ethnic minority groups in Canada within such studies, so specific groups must be chosen. Selecting one simplifies matters. In order to study
the importance of both structural factors and agency to their health requires

macro level data on larger societal factors and the barriers and facilitators that policies, geography, monetary costs, transportation systems, and so forth present for that ethnic minority group. These factors include the educational system, employment practices that might discriminate against (e.g., language requirements) or work for (e.g., affirmative action programs) this group, welfare programs that might or might not discriminate against the group (e.g., residency requirements), as well as other possible macro forces. One would also want to collect data on the interpretive experiences of members of the minority group within the education, employment, and welfare systems in addition to their perceptions of the discrimination they and other members of their families or the wider community have experienced.

Let's say we study this group at one point in time. Once we have collected all of these data (having made decisions about what group to include, how many people to sample, where to sample, whether to include a comparison group of Caucasian Canadians and/or another ethnic minority group, and how and what kinds of information to collect), how do we then put it all together and make sense of it? We have the means to analyze the individual data and we have the means to analyze group level data, but how do we relate the two? Certainly, procedures exist. For example, depending on the type and quantity of data, one might conduct textual analyses and relate experiences of minority group members with various characteristics of the places where they live. Alternatively, given sufficient numbers of both individuals and locations, one might conduct statistical analyses (such as multi-level modelling) that take these different levels of data (individual level and community level) into account. At this point we have not yet begun to place our research within a lifespan perspective or to introduce multiple time periods into our analyses.

Despite the complexities involved, there are steps we can take toward a more integrated approach. For example, when conducting social psychological studies, we can include a discussion of the potential structural factors at play. When conducting studies with a structural focus, we can recognize the potential influence of individual and group experience and consider (if not measure) possible avenues for change (i.e., for agency). In recognition that each of our methods provides a certain type of information but none provides all, the use of more than one methodology (known as **triangulation**) is becoming increasingly popular. Often, several social psychological or several more structural methodologies are employed but we can envision implementing triangulation, or **mixed methods**, in order to collect both types of data. Increasingly, graduate students today, in contrast to those in sociology 20 years ago, want to learn both qualitative and quantitative methodologies and many different theoretical orientations. They often speak of their belief that there is no single correct theoretical perspective or single methodological approach but rather, that the discipline requires the strengths and insights that can be garnered from all approaches. This perspective bodes well for the future of the discipline.

Questions for Critical Thought

1. Do you believe the health of Canadians will improve over the next 50 years? Why or why not?
2. What new social arrangements might evolve in the future for people to care for one another?
3. How can we construct a society so that social well-being, rather than economic efficiency, is enhanced?
4. How are individual agency and social structure inevitably intertwined in our lives?
5. Why is sociology especially well-equipped to advance knowledge in the area of health and health care?

Suggestions for Further Reading

Evans, R.G. 2006. 'Fat Zombies, Pleistocene Tastes, Autophilia, and the Obesity Epidemic', *Healthcare Policy* 2, 2: 18–26.

Hancock, T. 1999. 'Health Care Reform and Reform for Health: Creating a Health System for Communities in the 21st Century', *Futures* 31, 5: 417–36.

Siddiqi, A., and C. Hertzman. 2007. 'Towards an Epidemiological Understanding of the Effects on Long-Term Institutional Changes on Population Health: A Case Study of Canada versus the USA', *Social Science & Medicine* 64: 589–603.

Walker, A. 2004. 'Reexamining the Political Economy of Aging: Understanding the Structure/Agency Tension', in J. Baars, D. Dannefer, C. Phillipson, and A. Walker, eds, *Aging, Globalization, and Inequality: The New Critical Gerontology.* New York: Baywood Pub. Co., 59–80.

Wister, A.V. 2005. *Baby Boomer Health Dynamics: How Are We Aging?* Toronto: University of Toronto Press.

Suggested Websites

ACADEMIC ASSOCIATIONS

American Sociological Association (Section on Medical Sociology)
http://www.asanet.org/cs/root/leftnav/sections/section_pages/section_on_medical_
sociology

Canadian Association on Gerontology
http://www.cagacg.ca/

Canadian Association for Health Services and Policy Research
http://www.cahspr.ca/

Canadian Sociological Association/La Société Canadienne de Sociologie
http://www.csaa.ca/

Canadian Mental Health Association
http://www.cmha.ca/bins/index.asp

Canadian Public Health Association
http://www.cpha.ca/

European Society for Health and Medical Sociology (ESHMS)
http://www.eshms.org/AboutEshms.htm

European Sociological Association (Research Network in Sociology of Health and Illness)
http://www.valt.helsinki.fi/esa/medsoc.htm

International Sociological Association (Research Committee of Health)
http://www.isa-sociology.org/rc15.htm

Society for the Social History of Medicine (SSHM)
http://www.sshm.org/intro.html

Academic Journals

Canadian Journal of Public Health
http://www.cpha.ca/english/cjph/cjph.htm

Disability & Society
http://www.tandf.co.uk/journals/carfax/09687599.html

Health: An Interdisciplinary Journal for the Social Study of Health, Illness and Medicine
http://hea.sagepub.com/

Health and Place
http://www.elsevier.com/wps/find/journaldescription.cws_home/30519/description#description

Health Policy
http://www.elsevier.com/wps/find/journaldescription.cws_home/505962/description#description/

Health Reports
http://www.statcan.ca/english/ads/82-003-XPE/

Health Services Research
http://www.blackwellpublishing.com/journal.asp?ref=0017-9124&site=1

Health Sociology Review
http://hsr.e-contentmanagement.com/

International Journal of Health Service
http://www.baywood.com/journals/previewjournals.asp?id=0020-7314

International Journal of Self Help and Self Care
http://www.baywood.com/journals/previewjournals.asp?id=1091-2851

International Journal for Equity in Health
http://www.equityhealthj.com/home/

Journal of Aging and Health
http://jah.sagepub.com/

Journal of Health & Social Behavior
http://www.asanet.org/cs/root/leftnav/publications/journals/journal_of_health_and_social_behavior/homepage

Medical Sociology online (MSo)
http://www.medicalsociologyonline.org/

Social History of Medicine Journal
http://shm.oxfordjournals.org/archive/

Social Science & Medicine
http://www.elsevier.com/wps/find/journaldescription.cws_home/315/description#description

Social Theory & Health
http://www.palgrave-journals.com/sth/index.html

Sociology of Health & Illness
http://www.blackwellpublishing.com/journal.asp?ref=0141-9889&site=1

Canadian Governmental, Health Information, Policy, and Research Sites

Canada Health Act
http://laws.justice.gc.ca/en/C-6/index.html?noCookie

Canada's Health Care System
http://www.hc-sc.gc.ca/hcs-sss/index_e.html

Canadian Association for Community Care
http://www.cacc-acssc.com/

Canadian Centre for Policy Alternatives
http://www.policyalternatives.ca/

Canadian Foundation for Women's Health
http://www.cfwh.org/

Canada Health Infoway
http://www.infoway-inforoute.ca/

Canadian Healthcare Association
http://www.canadian-healthcare.org/

Canadian Health Network (CHN)
http://www.canadian-health-network.ca

Canadian Health Services Research Foundation (CHSRF)
http://www.chsrf.ca/

Canadian Institute for Advanced Research (CIAR)
http://www.ciar.ca/

Canadian Institute of Child Health (CICH)
http://www.cich.ca/

Canadian Institute for Health Information (CIHI)
http://secure.cihi.ca/cihiweb/dispPage.jsp?cw_page=home_e

Canadian Institutes of Health Research (CIHR)
http://www.cihr-irsc.gc.ca/e/193.html

Canadian Interprofessional Health Collaborative
http://www.cihc.ca/

Canadian Policy Research Networks
http://www.cprn.com/

Canadian Society for International Health
http://www.csih.org/en/index.asp

The Canadian Women's Health Network
http://www.cwhn.ca/indexeng.html

Government of Canada Policy Research Initiative
http://policyresearch.gc.ca/page.asp?pagenm=root&langcd=E

Health Canada
http://www.hc-sc.gc.ca/

Public Health Agency of Canada
http://www.phac-aspc.gc.ca/

Institute for Work and Health
http://www.iwh.on.ca/about/about.php

Women's Health Research Network
http://www.whrn.ca/

INTERNATIONAL GOVERNMENTAL, HEALTH INFORMATION, POLICY AND RESEARCH SITES

Council on Health Research for Development
http://www.cohred.org/main/

European Observatory on Health Systems and Policies
http://www.euro.who.int/observatory

Foundation for Women's Health Research and Development
http://www.forwarduk.org.uk/about

Global Forum for Health Research
http://www.globalforumhealth.org/Site/001__Who%20we%20are/001__History.php

International Society for Equity in Health
http://www.iseqh.org/

National Institutes of Health (US)
http://www.nih.gov/

Pan American Health Organization
http://www.paho.org/

World Health Organization
http://www.who.int/en/

HEALTH CARE CONSUMER SITES

Alliance for Natural Health
http://www.alliance-natural-health.org/

The Canadian Caregiver Coalition (CCC)
www.ccc-ccan.ca

Canadian Consumer Information Gateway
http://consumerinformation.ca/

Canadian Home Care Association
http://www.cdnhomecare.ca/

Caregiver.com
http://www.caregiver.com/index.asp

Caregiver Network Inc. (CNI)
www.caregiver.on.ca

Consumers Association of Canada
http://www.consumer.ca/

Family Caregiver Alliance (US)
www.caregiver.org

Healthfinder.gov (US)
http://www.healthfinder.gov/

Health Internet
http://www.health.gov.bc.ca/exsites/

Mental Health Support Network of Canada
http://mdm.ca/cmhsn/index.htm

National Center for Complementary and Alternative Medicine (NCCAM) (US)
http://nccam.nih.gov/

National Family Caregivers Association (US)
www.thefamilycaregiver.org

National Self-Help Clearinghouse (US)
http://www.selfhelpweb.org/

Quality End-of-Life Care Coalition of Canada (QELCCC)
http://www.chpca.net/qelccc.htm

World Institute of Natural Health Sciences
http://www.winhs.org/

OTHER SITES OF INTEREST

People's Health Movement
http://www.phmovement.org/

Social Science Information System (SocioSite Project, Sociology of Health)
http://www.sociosite.net/topics/health.php

Sociologists without Borders
http://www.sociologistswithoutborders.org/

Glossary

acculturation A process of cultural transformation that takes place as a result of contact between different cultures.

age effect Changes that occur as we age.

apocalyptic demography The argument that a demographic trend, such as population aging, has extreme negative consequences for society.

baby boomers People born between 1946 and 1964.

bi-culturalism The hybridizing or blending of two cultures, typically the donor culture and receiving culture when referring to a cultural minority group; also referred to as trans-national identities.

biographical disruption A concept introduced by Bury (1982) to refer to events, such as chronic illness, within an individual's biography or life history that disrupt everyday life and the assumptions on which it is based.

biomedical model A model that views health and health care from the perspectives of biology and medicine. A major assumption within this model is that disease can be explained by deviations from normal biological functioning and that health consequently represents the absence of disease.

black feminists Feminists who politicize their situatedness in relation to oppressive hierarchies of socio-relationality, balancing gender and race consciousness.

blaming the victim Accusing the sufferer, in this case someone with health problems, as responsible for the problems he or she has. It includes a lack of recognition that larger societal forces may also be at play.

boomerang kids Adult children who have moved out of the parental home and then move back in.

burden The physical, psychological, emotional, social, and/or financial problems resulting from caring for a person who is impaired. Burden can be objective and/or subjective.

capitalism The power of capital in production and financial markets that seeks to promote profitization, deregulation, and significant structural changes in national bureaucracies, including welfare programs and public services, while also seeking the liberalization of trade and monetary policies to support market interests that favour high-income business sectors.

caregiving Assisting another person when his or her health fails and that person is unable to continue his or her daily life without assistance. Caregiving is a special type of social interaction and social support.

carer blind policies Policies that provide options so that care being provided by an informal caregiver might be replaced by formal services.

carer break policies Policies that focus on the well-being of the caregiver seeking to relieve their burden so that the individual can continue to provide care.

chiropractic A system of care that focuses on the relationship between bodily structure (primarily that of the spine) and function as it affects health.

chronic conditions Health problems that are expected to persist over time (e.g., one year or more).

cohort effect An effect that results from the fact that historical events differentially affect people of different ages (i.e., cohorts).

collaborative models of care Based on collaboration among care providers, these models typically involve multidisciplinary and/or interdisciplinary teams of health-care providers that are interdependent and share power and responsibilities for care.

complementary and alternative medicine (CAM) A label often used to refer to various forms of health care considered to lie outside the realm of conventional Western medicine. Complementary medicine refers to those forms of care provided together with conventional medicine, while alternative medicine refers to care used instead of conventional medical care.

compositional differences Differences in the social characteristics of individuals located within different social groups.

compression of morbidity hypothesis Proposed by James Fries (1980), holds that the future will see the period of morbidity experienced prior to death become shorter and, increasingly, people will live a relatively healthy life until they die, usually in very old age.

conflict and power approaches Theoretical approaches that focus on the societal level with a concentration on competing interest groups. Society is considered characterized by groups with different levels of access to power and associated resources and hence emphasize power relations within social political and economic structures.

consumerism A model that emphasizes the rights and power of consumers. According to Freidson (2001), it represents one of three sources of control over work.

convoy of social support The large number of social relationships we accumulate throughout our lives, depicting the dynamic nature of social interaction over time.

corporatization A process of increasing corporate ownership and control (privatization).

critical or reflective knowledge Concerned with the role that societal structures and power relations play in promoting inequalities and disenabling people.

critical population health perspective A theoretical approach that allows for understanding how social structures, economic relationships, and ideological assumptions create and perpetuate health disparities.

deprofessionalization A process of professional status decline and loss by a professional group (e.g., physicians).

differential exposure hypothesis Attributes group differences in health status (such as gender differences) to differences in their exposure to the conditions that influence health (such as poverty, stress, etc.).

differential vulnerability hypothesis Attributes group differences in health status to differences in their reactions to the conditions that influence health.

disability Difficulties in functioning that are attributed to individual impairments (medical model) or to processes of social exclusion (social model).

'doctor–nurse game' Developed by Stein (1967) to refer to what he saw as a standard pattern of doctor–nurse interactions that allowed both to contribute to patient care but also ensured that physicians appeared superordinate and nurses subordinate.

dramaturgical analysis Analyzes life as a stage with ordinary people enacting social roles in scripted performances that change depending on the context.

duality The view that structure and agency are two ways of considering the same phenomenon, namely social action (see Giddens).

epidemiological transition A shift in patterns of disease and mortality in a country that is associated with development; particularly, a shift away from the acute infectious diseases that are characteristic of underdeveloped societies to the chronic non-infectious diseases characteristic of modernization and advanced levels of development.

equity of care Within health care, the ability of the health-care system to provide services across groups in accordance with their needs for care. Horizontal equity means treating those who have the same level of need the same, while vertical equity refers to treating those who have different levels of need differently.

feminist theorizing Theoretical approaches that take gender inequalities as their point of departure, viewing gender as a fundamental organizing principle of society.

feminization of aging Refers to the increasing concentration of women within the older adult population.

fictive kin Refers to individuals who are not related by birth or marriage, but who are socially defined as having kinship ties (such as when a close family friend is considered a member of the family and referred to as an aunt or uncle).

field A concept employed by Bourdieu to refer to the arena in which we perform our social actions, consisting of a system of social positions.

fundamental cause explanation Developed by Link and Phelan (2000) to refer to the importance of social factors (including resources such as knowledge, money, power, prestige, or social connections) that have persistent effects on health even when the specific circumstances through which they influence health (e.g., specific risk or protective factors) change.

gender An array of socially constructed roles and relationships, personality traits, attitudes, behaviours, values, and relative power and influence ascribed to the two sexes on a differential basis.

gender conflict approaches Approaches that emphasize structural inequalities and issues of power and conflict taking gender inequalities as their point of departure.

gendered ageism A term used to refer to the combined effects of sexism and ageism.

general symptomatology Common health concerns that each of us experiences from time to time, such as coughing and feeling tired.

Generation X People born between 1961 and 1974.

Generation Y People born in 1975 or later.

globalization The process of internationalization, or reaching around the world.

habitus Bourdieu's concept, referring to a lasting and acquired system of dispositions (habitual schemes of thought in action).

health belief model A theoretical model that focuses on the subjective decision-making process that influences health behaviours. This model posits that people are motivated to act if they perceive the severity of the disease and their susceptibility to getting sick as greater than their risk if they do not take any particular action.

health-care conundrum If health-care services do not create healthier people but investments in education, the environment, housing, and other social determinants do, there would appear to be no need for increasing funding to the health-care system.

health inequality hypothesis Refers generally to the empirical relationship between socio-economic status and health.

health promotion perspective An approach that recognizes the social determinants of health.

healthy community A community that facilitates quality of life for its residents, minimizes aspects that may have negative consequences for its residents, promotes healthy living, and protects the natural environment.

healthy immigrant effect Recent immigrants tend to have good health and, in fact, tend to be in better health than non-immigrants.

healthy public policy Governmental policy characterized by a concern for health.

hollowing out In this instance, refers to the gradual transfer of services that at one time were included within provincial health-care programs over to the private sector and away from public coverage.

homeopathic medicine, or homeopathy A form of alternative medicine in which small, highly diluted quantities of medicinal substances are given to cure symptoms. The same substances, if given at higher or more concentrated doses, would cause those symptoms.

horizontal shrinkage Each generation contains fewer members.

host response, or general susceptibility The notion that we have a general vulnerability to all illnesses per se, rather than to one particular illness.

human agency Actions and decisions that are reflective of meaningful choice.

illness The personal or subjective experience of disease by an individual—how he or she perceives, lives with, and responds to symptoms and disabilities (Eisenberg, 1977).

illness behaviour Self-care that is a response to symptoms.

impairment Biological dysfunction.

incidence The number of new cases of a specific disease or health problem within a particular population during a specified period of time, calculated by dividing the number of new cases of a disease reported within the population of interest during a given period of time by the total number of people considered to be at risk.

infant mortality rate The number of deaths of infants under the age of one for every 1,000 live births in a population during a given year.

informal care Assistance provided to an individual who cannot carry out those activities for themselves; that is, the assistance is required and it is primarily unpaid.

insider perspective Focuses directly on people's subjective experiences within the contexts of their everyday lives; it can be contrasted with the perspective of an 'objective' outside observer.

institutional racism Polices and practices embedded within societal institutions serving to disadvantage individuals from particular racial or ethnic groups.

interiorization of race In this context, refers to a significant growth in the size and diversity of racial minorities in Western countries.

intersectionality Refers to the idea that multiple forms of oppression (including those based on class, gender, age, race, and ethnicity) interact to create a broader system of inequality in society.

labelling theory Concerned with the implications of labelling processes, and especially negative or stigmatizing labels, on individual self-concept, behaviour, etc.

laissez-faire racism Refers to an ideology of equality for all, but within unequal class-based systems so that people believe they are not being racist.

Lesbian, Gay, Bisexual, and Transsexual (LGBT) **studies** Studies that advance the interests of these groups and contribute culturally and intellectually to their movements.

life course perspective Focuses on both biography and history plus the intersections of the two within social structure, attempting to link both micro and macro levels.

life expectancy Refers to the average number of years that individuals at a given age can expect to live before death; it is usually, but not necessarily, measured from birth.

life stage principle The impact of a transition or event depends on when it occurs in a person's life.

lifestyle Refers to a grouping of behaviours that are believed to affect our health negatively or positively. Empirical research to date has been unable to successfully demonstrate that our health behaviours cluster in a coherent fashion.

linked lives The notion that lives are interdependent or meshed with those of multiple others.

lived body Structure and the experiencing body are intertwined.

managerialism A model of work based on the application of business management techniques, emphasizing the power of managers over work. According to Freidson (2001), it represents one of three sources of control over work.

marketization of care The act or process of providing care for payment.

Marxist theory A conflict perspective focusing on class structures and economic inequalities in the production and distribution of the treatment of illness. Capitalism and the pursuit of profit is considered responsible for negative health effects on the working class.

materialist approach Draws attention to the role of the material (or structural) conditions (such as economic standing) in influencing various outcomes, such as health.

medical gaze A term used by Michel Foucault (1973) to refer to the power of medicine to create a discourse on its subject matter (the human body) and to define how people should understand, regulate, and experience their bodies (e.g., as separate from their minds; see Lupton, 1997: 99).

medical–industrial complex All aspects of the medical industry and all aspects of the pharmaceutical industry that are related to medicine.

medicalization Refers to the process wherein various areas of life come under the purview of medical science and consequently under medical authority and control (see Zola, 1983).

medical sociology Sociological study of relationships between social factors and health and health care, viewed from a medical perspective.

medical support system In this instance, refers to home care services that serve primarily to support a medical system and not other aspects of health such as a social system of care.

mixed methods Involve the use of more than one methodological approach and could include qualitative and quantitative methods, more than one qualitative method, or more than one quantitative method.

moral career A concept used by Erving Goffman (1961) to refer to the progressive changes that take place in individuals' self-images and identities as they move through various societal institutions over the course of their lives, including mental hospitals and other 'total institutions'.

morbidity Refers to the level of disease within a given population at a particular point in time and tends to be assessed in terms of incidence and prevalence.

mortality rates The number of deaths (in general, disease-specific) in a particular population during a given period of time.

mortification of the self A process (characterized by humiliation, degradation) in which one's prior conception of oneself is gradually undermined. It is a process that Goffman (1961) associates with institutionalization.

multiple jeopardy Refers to the idea that experiencing multiple forms of inequality will compound the difficulties associated with experiencing fewer forms. Related notions include 'double jeopardy' (the combined effects of two forms of inequality) and 'triple jeopardy' (the combined effects of three sources of inequality).

naturopathic medicine, or naturopathy A form of alternative medicine that uses various therapies (such as nutrition, dietary supplements, exercise, and homeopathy) to support the natural power of the body to establish, maintain, and restore health.

neo-materialist approach Directs attention to the effects of societal infrastructure (e.g., health, education, and social services) as well as individual material resources as determinants of health.

new public health A healthy community approach or public health perspective that incorporates principles such as equity and collaboration.

new racism See **laissez-faire racism**.

participatory action research (PAR) Approaches that have an interest in involving research participants within the research enterprise, with a goal to assist in restructuring local power arrangements.

period effect A historical event that affects persons of all ages in a similar manner.

personal determinants of health Our health beliefs and our personal health behaviours.

personal health behaviours A wide range of activities undertaken in an effort to maintain good health.

political economy perspective An approach that assumes that experiences of health and illness are inextricably shaped by larger socio-political and economic contexts.

population health perspective A broad approach that examines the health of large groups of people (i.e., populations) rather than the individual and that incorporates broad social structural factors as affecting population health.

post-structural approach As used here, refers to Foucault's perspective that injects notions of agency or sovereign power to overcome determinism.

potential years of life lost (PYLL) The total number of years of potential life that are lost when a person dies prematurely, generally defined as dying before the age of 75.

power/knowledge A concept used by Michel Foucault (1972, 1982) to refer to the inseparability of power and knowledge.

prevalence The total number of cases of a disease or health problem within the population during a specified time period.

privatization The act or process of changing from public (governmental) to private ownership.

professional dominance A concept, used to refer to the power of professionals (e.g., medical authorities) to control their own work (autonomy) as well as the work of others operating in the same sphere (dominance).

profitization The act or process of profit making.

proletarianization A process, linked to capitalism, through which non-proletarian workers (e.g., medical and other professionals) gradually lose control over the terms and conditions of their work, thereby becoming part of the proletariat.

psychosocial comparison approach People's perceptions of their situations compared to others (such as perceived economic deprivation compared to others) in influencing various outcomes such as health.

public health Any health concerns, such as clean air and drinking water, that relate to the population as a whole or large segments of the population.

public policy Policy created by governments.

queer theory A search for an essentiality beneath the dominant narratives of identity; an attempt to argue for and expose multiple subjectivities experienced at the local level.

race relations problematic The reification of race or race relations by using the terms that tend to imply race as biologically based when science has rejected this notion.

regionalization The act or process of moving toward a regional level of government.

relationality The inherent inter-connectedness of the individual and the social.

residual welfare Health care outside of medically defined medicare.

restorative self-care, or sick role behaviour Personal actions that are oriented toward becoming well or adjusting to chronic illness or disability and encompassing the management of activities when ill.

salvaged self According to Charmaz (1987), emerges in situations in which people who are ill try to retain a past identity associated with their previously healthy selves.

sandwich generation, hidden victims, 'generation-in-the-middle' Middle-aged children providing care to older adults, typically their parents. The notion suggests that these middle-aged children experience multiple demands in their lives.

self-care Any form of caring behaviour that we ourselves initiate.

self-care model Any model that considers the layperson as the centre of health care and therefore as the primary provider of health care.

sense of coherence Comprehensibility (a belief that the world is ordered, consistent, and predictable), manageability (a sense of confidence in our ability to cope with life's problems), and meaningfulness (a belief that areas of life make sense to us emotionally and are worth commitment).

serial caregiving Refers to situations in which care providers experience raising their children, followed by caring for thier parents, and then caring for their partners, rather than providing all of this caring simultaneously.

sex Biological characteristics such as anatomy and physiology distinguishing males and females.

sickness The socially defined actions taken by a person as a result of illness or disease (e.g., taking medication, visiting the doctor, resting in bed, or staying away from work).

sick role Institutionalized behavioural expectations associated with being sick.

social capital A contextual level resource for individuals deriving from positive relationships and community involvement containing norms of reciprocity, trustworthiness, and collective capacity.

social causation A focus on the role of social factors in influencing various outcomes (e.g., the impact of poverty on health).

social closure The process through which powerful groups (e.g., the medical profession) are able to maintain their privileged access to status and resources and to exclude others from gaining access.

social connectiveness How associated we are with others; frequently includes being in contact with friends and relatives, being married, and being involved in groups.

social constructionist sociology A focus on how people interpretively produce and organize their lives as they make everyday experiences meaningful.

social determinants of health The social factors (such as income, gender, race, ethnicity, and social support) that are said to influence health.

social determinants of health perspective See **population health perspective**.

social ecology An approach that posits a set of principles for examining inter-dependencies between individual and aggregate manifestations of health.

social integration and isolation The existence or quantity of relationships.

sociality See **relationality**.

social model of disability Argues that disability is not a characteristic of individuals, but is socially constructed and results from the exclusion that people with impairments face in being able to participate fully in social life.

social policy A plan intended to influence and determine decisions and actions with respect to social affairs.

social psychological approaches Approaches that share an interest in social interaction and the belief that we construct meaning and interpret the world through our social interactions.

social quality In this context, refers to Walker's notion about the extent to which people can participate in the social and economic life of their communities, or an understanding of the conditions that enhance people's well-being and individual potential.

social selection An argument that draws attention to the importance of individual characteristics for determining social group membership (e.g., poor health leads to poverty); it is typically contrasted with a social causation argument (e.g., poverty leads to poor health).

social support The functional content of social relationships such as emotional concern, instrumentality, and information.

sociological perspective A perspective that addresses interactions in relationships between individuals; between individuals and groups, communities, or larger social structures; and between different social structures.

sociology in medicine Sociological research on questions of interest to, and often defined by, the medical profession.

sociology of medicine The study of medicine, its workers, and its methods of delivery, often from a critical approach.

stigma An attribution that discredits the value of a person (see Goffman, 1963).

stress process model A model that views stress as a process involving various sources of stress (stressful life events, on-going strains, etc.), mediating resources (coping skills, social support, etc.), and health outcomes.

structural functionalism A perspective that views society as consisting of a number of social institutions (social structures) that are interdependent and, when functioning properly, ensure social order and stability.

structurally embedded Refers to the notion that social relations are situated within social structures that influence their position (including their access to resources, etc.).

structuration The reciprocal relationship between structure and systems.

structuration theory Associated with Giddens, a theoretical approach attempting to link structure and agency using the concept of duality.

supernormal social identity Refers to an identity founded on extraordinary achievement wherein those who are chronically ill compete with and try to outperform those who are not ill, despite the limitations of their illness (see Charmaz, 1987).

symbolic interaction A theoretical perspective arguing that our interactions with others continuously create and re-create reality.

symbolic violence The imposition of ways of thinking and perceiving onto others who interpret these ways of thinking as correct.

total institutions Settings within which people live or work, are isolated from the wider society for a significant period of time, and where all aspects of their lives are formally administered or controlled. Examples include nursing homes, mental hospitals, and prisons (see Goffman, 1961).

upstream factors Refers to psycho-social and environmental factors that influence health.

vertical extension Several generations of one family alive at one time.

Veteran Generation People born before 1946.

vision for health-care reform An image of how the health-care system should, or could, look.

References

Ali, J. 2002. 'Mental Health of Canada's Immigrants', *Health Reports* 13: 1–11.

Allan, D.E., and M. Penning. 2001. *An Early Look at Regionalization in British Columbia: Regional Equity or Equality?* Paper presented at the Annual Meeting of the International Association of Gerontology, Vancouver, BC.

Allen, D. 2002. 'Doing Occupational Demarcation: The Boundary Work of Nurse Managers in a District General Hospital', in A.M. Rafferty and M. Traynor, eds, *Exemplary Research for Nursing and Midwifery*. London: Routledge, 205–30.

Allen, W.R., and A.Y. Chung. 2000. '"Your Blues Ain't Like My Blues": Race, Ethnicity and Social Inequality in America'. *Contemporary Sociology* 29, 6: 796–805.

Alter, D.A., C.D. Naylor, P.C. Austin, and J.V. Tu. 2002. 'Biology or Bias: Practice Patterns and Long-Term Outcomes for Men and Women with Acute Myocardial Infarction', *Journal of the American College of Cardiology* 39: 1909–16.

Anderson, J. 2000. 'Gender, "Race", Poverty, Health, and Discourses of Health Reform in the Context of Globalization: A Post-Colonial Feminist Per- spective in Policy Research', *Nursing Inquiry* 7, 4: 220–29.

———, S. Wiggins, R. Rajwani, A. Holbrook, C. Blue, and M. Ng. 1995. 'Living with a Chronic Illness: Chinese Canadian and Euro- Canadian Women with Diabetes— Exploring Factors that Influence Management', *Social Science Medicine* 41, 2: 181–95.

Anderson, R., G.E. Barnes, D. Patton, T. Perkins. 1999. 'Personality in the Development of Substance Abuse', *Personality Psychology in Europe* 7: 141–58.

Annandale, E. 1998. *The Sociology of Health and Medicine: A Critical Introduction*. Oxford: Blackwell.

Antonovsky, A. 1979. *Health, Stress and Coping*. San Francisco: Jossey-Bass.

———. 1987. *Unraveling the Mystery of Health: How People Manage Stress and Stay Well*. San Francisco: Jossey-Bass.

Antonucci, T.C. 1985. 'Personal Characteristics, Social Support and Social Behaviour', in R.H. Binstock and E. Shanas, eds, *Handbook and the Social Sciences*, 2nd edn. New York: Van Nostrand Reinhold, 94–129.

Arber, S., J. McKinlay, A. Adams, L. Marceau, C. Link, and A. O'Donnell.

2006. 'Patient Characteristics and Inequalities in Doctors' Diagnostic and Management Strategies Relating to CHD: A Video-Simulation Experiment', *Social Science & Medicine* 62, 1: 103–15.

Armstrong, P. 2001. 'Science, Enterprise and Profit: Ideology in the Knowledge-Driven Economy', *Economy and Society* 30, 4: 524–52.

————, and H. Armstrong. 1999. 'Women, Privatization and Health Care Reform: The Ontario Scan (Working Paper #10)'. Health Reform Reference Group, Centres of Excellence for Women's Health Program, Women's Health Bureau. Toronto: The National Network of Environments and Women's Health, York University.

————, ————, and D. Coburn. 2001. *Unhealthy Times: Political Economy Perspectives on Health and Care in Canada*. Don Mills, ON: Oxford University Press.

Aronson, J. 2002. 'Elderly People's Accounts of Home Care Rationing: Missing Voices in Long-Term Care Policy Debates', *Ageing & Society* 22: 399–418.

————. 2006. 'Silenced Complaints, Suppressed Expectations: The Cumulative Effects of Home Care Rationing', *International Journal of Health Services* 36, 3: 535–56.

————, M. Denton, and I. Zeytinoglu. 2004. 'Market-Modeled Home Care in Ontario: Deteriorating Working Conditions and Dwindling Community Capacity', *Canadian Public Policy* XXX, 1: 111–25.

————, and S.M. Neysmith. 1996. '"You're Not Just in There to Do the

Work": Depersonalizing Policies and the Exploitation of Home Care Workers' Labor', *Gender & Society* 10, 1: 59–77.

————, and ————. 2001. 'Manufacturing Social Exclusion in the Home Care Market', *Canadian Public Policy* 27, 2: 151–65.

Asada, Y., and G. Kephart. 2007. 'Equity in Health Services Use and Intensity of Use in Canada', *BMC Health Services Research* 7, 41.

Ashworth, C.D., P. Williamson, and D. Montano. 1984. 'A Scale to Measure Physician Beliefs about Psychosocial Aspects of Patient Care', *Social Science & Medicine* 19: 1235–8.

Asvali, J. 1986. 'Forward-Medical Sociology and the WHO's Programme for Europe', *Social Science & Medicine* 22: 113.

Atchley, R.C., and A. Barusch. 2004. *Social Forces and Aging—An Introduction to Social Gerontology*, 10th edn. Belmont CA: Wadsworth/Thomson Learning.

Backett, K., C. Davison, and K. Mullen. 1994. 'Lay Evaluation of Health and Healthy Lifestyles: Evidence from Three Studies', *The British Journal of General Practice: The Journal of the Royal College of General Practitioners* 44, 383: 277–80.

Bajekal, M., D. Blane, I. Grewal, S. Karlsen, and J. Nazroo. 2004. 'Ethnic Differences in Influences on Quality of Life at Older Ages: A Quantitative Analysis', *Ageing and Society* 24, 5: 709–28.

Baker, C., and P. Stern. 1993. 'Finding Meaning in Chronic Illness as the Key to Self-Care', *Canadian Journal of Nursing Research* 25: 23–36.

Bakker, I. 1998. *Unpaid Work and Macroeconomics: New Discussions, New Tools for Action*. Ottawa: Status of Women Canada.

Ballinger, G., J. Zhang, and V. Hicks. 2001. *Home Care Estimates in National Health Expenditures*. Ottawa: Canadian Institute for Health Information.

Barnes, C., G. Mercer, and T. Shakespeare. 1999. *Exploring Disability Studies*. Cambridge: Polity.

Barnes, G.E., M.D. Barnes, and D. Patton. 2005. 'Prevalence and Predictors of "Heavy" Marijuana Use in a Canadian Youth Sample', *Substance Use and Misuse* 40: 1849–63.

———, R.P. Murray, D. Patton, P.M. Bentler, and R.E. Anderson. 2000. *The Addiction Prone Personality*. New York: Kluwer Academic/Plenum Publishers.

Baron, S., J. Field, and T. Schuller. 2000. *Social Capital: Critical Perspectives*. Oxford: Oxford University Press.

Barot, R. 2006. 'Reflections on Michael Banton's Contribution to Race and Ethnic Studies', *Ethnic and Racial Studies* 29, 5: 785–96.

Barrett, R., C.W. Kuzawa, T. McDade, and G.J. Armelagos. 1998. 'Emerging and Re-Emerging Infectious Diseases: The Third Epidemiologic Transition', *Annual Review of Anthropology* 27: 247–71.

Bastiaens, H., P. Van Royen, D.R. Pavlic, V. Raposo, and R. Baker. 2007. 'Older People's Preferences for Involvement in Their Own Care: A Qualitative Study in Primary Health Care in 11 European Countries', *Patient Education and Counseling* 68, 1: 33–42.

Beck, A.H. 2004. 'The Flexner Report and the Standardization of American Medical Education', *The Journal of the American Medical Association* 291: 2139–40.

Beeney, L.J., and S.M. Dunn. 1990. 'Knowledge Improvement and Metabolic Control in Diabetes Education: Approaching the Limits?', *Patient Education Counseling* 16: 217.

Bendick, M., Jr. 1989. 'Privatizing the Delivery of Social Welfare Services: An Ideal to Be Taken Seriously', in S.B. Kamerman and A.J. Kahn, eds, *Privatization and the Welfare State*. Princeton, NJ: Princeton University Press, 97–120.

Bengtson, V.L., G.H. Elder, and N.M. Putney. 2005. 'The Lifecourse Perspective on Aging: Linked Lives, Timing, and History', in M.L. Johnson, ed, *The Cambridge Handbook of Age and Ageing*. Cambridge: Cambridge University Press, 493–501.

———, L. Lawton, and M. Silverstein. 1994. 'Affection, Social Contact and Geographic Distance between Adult Children and Their Parents', *Journal of Marriage and the Family* 56, 1: 57–68.

Benoit, C. 1998. 'Rediscovering Appropriate Care: Maternity Traditions and Contemporary Issues in Canada', in D. Coburn, C. D'Arcy, and G.M. Torrance, eds, *Health and Canadian Society: Sociological Perspectives*. Toronto: University of Toronto Press: 359–78.

———, D. Carroll, and A. Millar. 2002. 'But Is it Good for Non-Urban Women's Health? Regionalizing Maternity Care Services in British Columbia', *Canadian Review of*

Sociology and Anthropology 39, 3: 373–95.

————, S. Wrede, I. Bourgeault, J. Sandall, R. de Vries, and E.R. van Teijlingen. 2005. 'Understanding the Social Organization of Maternity Care Systems: Midwifery as a Touchstone', *Sociology of Health & Illness* 27, 6: 722–37.

Benrud, L.M., and D.M. Reddy. 1998. 'Differential Explanations of Illness in Women and Men', *Sex Roles* 38: 5–6.

Berkman, L.F., and S.L. Syme. 1979. 'Social Networks, Host Resistance, and Mortality: A Nine-Year Follow-Up Study of Alameda County Residents', *American Journal of Epidemiology* 109, 2: 186–204.

Berta, W., A. Laporte, and V. Valdmanis. 2005. 'Observations on Institutional Long-Term Care in Ontario: 1996–2002', *Canadian Journal on Aging* 24, 1: 71–84.

————, ————, D. Zarnett, V. Valdmanis, and G. Anderson. 2006. 'A Pan-Canadian Perspective on Institutional Long-Term Care', *Health Policy* 79, 2–3: 175–94.

Blais, R., and A. Maïga. 1999. 'Do Ethnic Groups Use Health Services like the Majority of the Population? A Study from Quebec, Canada', *Social Science & Medicine* 48: 1237–45.

Blando, J.A. 2001. 'Twice Hidden: Older Gay and Lesbian Couples, Friends, and Intimacy', *Generations* 25: 87–89.

Blau, Z.S., G.T. Oser, and R.E. Stephens. 1979. 'Aging, Social Class, and Ethnicity: A Comparison of Anglo, Black, and Mexican-American Texans', *Pacific Sociological Review* 22, 4: 501–25.

Blaxter, M., and L. Patterson. 1982. *Mothers and Daughters: A Three Generational Study of Health Attitudes and Behaviour*. London: Heinemann Educational Books.

Blumer, H. 1969. *Symbolic Interactionism: Perspective and Method*. New York: Prentice Hall.

Bolaria, B.S. 2002. 'Sociology, Medicine, Health, and Illness: An Overview', in B.S. Bolaria and H.D. Dickinson, eds, *Health, Illness and Health Care in Canada*, 3rd edn. Scarborough, ON: Nelson Thomson Learning, 3–19.

Bolin, K., B. Lindgren, M. Lindstrom, and P. Nystedt. 2003. 'Investments in Social Capital—Implications of Social Interactions for the Production of Health', *Social Science & Medicine* 56: 2379–90.

Bonilla-Silva, E. 2000. '"This is a White Country": The Racial Ideology of the Western Nations of the World-System', *Sociological Inquiry* 70, 2: 188–214.

Bonner, T.N. 1995. *Becoming a Physician: Medical Education in Great Britain, France, Germany and the United States, 1750–1945*. Oxford: Oxford University Press.

Boon, H., J.B. Brown, A. Gavin, M.A. Kennard, and M. Stewart. 1999. 'Breast Cancer Survivors' Perceptions of Complementary/Alternative Medicine (CAM): Making the Decision to Use or Not to Use', *Qualitative Health Research* 9: 639–53.

Bourdieu, P. 1977. *Outline of a Theory of Practice*. Cambridge: Cambridge University Press.

————. 1984. *Distinction: A Social Critique of the Judgment of Taste*. London: Routledge.

Bourgeault, I.L. 2000. 'Delivering the "New" Canadian Midwifery: The Impact on Midwifery of Integration into the Ontario Health Care System', *Sociology of Health & Illness* 22, 2: 172–96.

———, and C. Benoit. 2004. 'Reconceiving Midwifery', in I. Bourgeault, C. Benoit, and R. Davis-Floyd, eds, *Reconceiving Midwifery: The New Canadian Model of Care*. Montreal: McGill-Queen's University Press.

———, S. Lindsay, E. Mykahalovsky, P. Armstrong, H. Armstrong, J. Choiniere, J. Lexchin, S. Peters, and J. White. 2004. 'At First You Will Not Succeed: Negotiating Care in the Context of Health Reform', *Research in the Sociology of Health Care* 22: 261–76.

———, and G. Mulvale. 2006. 'Collaborative Health Care Teams in Canada and the USA: Confronting the Structural Embeddedness of Medical Dominance', *Health Sociology Review* 15: 481–95.

Broese van Groneau, M.I. 2003. 'Unequal Chances for Reaching "A Good Old Age": Socioeconomic Health Differences among Older Adults from a Life Course Perspective', *Tijdschr Gerontol Geriatr* 34, 5: 196–207.

Brown, E.R. 1979. *Rockefeller Medicine Men: Medicine and Capitalism in America*. Berkeley, CA: University of California Press.

Brown, P. 2000. *Perspectives in Medical Sociology*, 3rd edn. Prospect Heights, IL: Waveland Press, Inc.

———, and H. Lauder. 2001. *Capitalism and Social Progress: The Future of Society in a Global Economy*. Houndmills, UK: Palgrave.

Browne, I., and J. Misra. 2003. 'The Intersection of Gender and Race in the Labor Market', *Annual Review of Sociology* 29: 487–513.

Broyles, R.W., P. Manga, D.A. Binder, D.E. Angus, and A. Charette. 1983. 'The Use of Physician Services under a National Health Insurance Scheme', *Medical Care* 21: 1037–54.

Brunt, J.H., N.L. Chappell, N. Maclure, and A. Cassels. 1998. 'Assessing the Effectiveness of Government and Industry Media Campaigns on Seniors' Perceptions of Reference-Based Pricing Policy', *Journal of Applied Gerontology* 17, 3: 276–95.

Bryden, K. 1974. *Old Age Pensions and Policy Making in Canada*. Montreal: McGill-Queen's University Press.

Buckley, N.J., F.T. Denton, A.L. Robb, and B.G. Spencer. 2005. 'Socio-Economic Influence on the Health of Older People: Estimates Based on Two Longitudinal Surveys', *Canadian Public Policy* 22: 59–83.

Bunton, R., and A. Petersen. 1997. 'Introduction: Foucault's Medicine', in A. Petersen and R. Bunton, eds, *Foucault, Health and Medicine*. London: Routledge, 1–11.

Burnette, D., A.C. Mui, and B.D. Zodikoff. 2004. 'Gender, Self-Care and Functional Status among Older Persons with Coronary Heart Disease: A National Perspective', *Women & Health* 39, 1: 65–84.

Bury, M. 1982. 'Chronic Illness as Biographical Disruption', *Sociology of Health & Illness* 4: 167–82.

———. 2000. 'On Chronic Illness and Disability', in C.E. Bird, P. Conrad, and A.M. Fremont, eds, *Handbook of Medical Sociology*. Upper Saddle River, NJ: Prentice Hall, 173–83.

Buske, L. 2000. 'Pulse: Availability of Services in Rural Areas', *Canadian Medical Association Journal* 162, 8: 1193.

Butler, R., and S. Bowlby. 1997. 'Bodies and Spaces: An Exploration of Disabled People's Experiences of Public Space', *Environment and Planning D: Society and Space* 15, 4: 379–504.

Butters, J., and P.G. Erickson. 2003. 'Meeting the Health Care Needs of Female Crack Users: A Canadian Example', *Women and Health* 37, 3: 1–17.

Cahill, S., K. South, and J. Spade. 2000. *Outing Age: Public Policy Issues Affecting Gay, Lesbian, Bisexual and Transgender Elders*. Washington, DC: Policy Institute of the National Gay and Lesbian Task Force.

Calasanti, T. 2004. 'New Directions in Feminist Gerontology', *Journal of Aging Studies* 18, 1: 1–121.

Callahan, J.L. 2004. 'Reversing a Conspicuous Absence: Mindful Inclusion of Emotion in Structuration Theory', *Human Relations* 57, 11: 1427–48.

Calnan, M. 1987. *Health and Illness: The Lay Perspective*. London: Tavistock.

Canadian Association of Naturopathic Doctors (CAND). 2007. 'Questions: Education and Regulation'. Available at: http://www.cand.ca/index.php?40. Accessed 12 December 2007.

Canadian Fitness and Lifestyle Research Institute. 2004. *Socio-Demographic and Lifestyle Correlates of Obesity*. Ottawa: Canadian Institute for Health Information.

Canadian Health Services Research Foundation (CHSRF). 2005. 'A Parallel Private System Would Reduce Waiting Times in the Public System', *Mythbusters*. Available at: http://www.chsrf.ca/mythbusters/pdf/myth17_e.pdf. Accessed 12 June 2007.

Canadian Institute of Advanced Research (CIAR). 1991. *The Determinants of Health*. Toronto: Canadian Institute for Advanced Research.

Canadian Institute for Health Information (CIHI). 2000. *Health Care in Canada—First Annual Report*. Ottawa: Canadian Institute for Health Information.

———. 2001. *Health Care in Canada*. Ottawa: Canadian Institute for Health Information.

———. 2004a. *Canadian Population Health Initiative: Improving the Health of Canadians*. Ottawa: Canadian Institute for Health Information.

———. 2004b. *Health Personnel Trends in Canada, 1993–2002*. Ottawa: Canadian Institute for Health Information.

———. 2005a. *Canada's Health Care Providers—2005 Chartbook*. Ottawa: Canadian Institute for Health Information.

———. 2005b. *Exploring the 70/30 Split: How Canada's Health Care System is Financed*. Ottawa: Canadian Institute for Health Information.

———. 2006a. *Drug Expenditure in Canada:1985 to 2005*. Ottawa: Canadian Institute for Health Information.

———. 2006b. *Full-Time Equivalent Physicians Report: Fee-for-Service Physicians in Canada, 2004–05*.

Ottawa: Canadian Institute for Health Information.

———. 2006c. *Health Care in Canada*. Ottawa: Canadian Institute for Health Information.

———. 2006d. *How Healthy are Rural Canadians? An Assessment of Their Health Status and Health Determinants*. Ottawa: Canadian Institute for Health Information.

———. 2007. *Public-Sector Expenditures and Utilization of Home Care Services in Canada: Exploring the Data*. Ottawa: Canadian Institute for Health Information.

———. 2005. *Gender and Sex-Based Analysis in Health Research: A Guide for CIHR Researchers and Reviewers*. Ottawa: Canadian Institutes of Health Research.

Canadian Institute of Health Research (CIHR). 2007. *CIHR Guidelines for Health Research Involving Aboriginal People*. Ottawa: Canadian Institutes of Health Research.

CIHR Institute of Musculoskeletal and Skeletal Health and Arthritis. 'Overall Prevalence of Chronic Conditions by Category, Canada 2001'. Available at: http://www.cihr-irsc.gc.ca/e/18976.html. Accessed 14 December 2007.

Canadian Nurses Association. 2005. 'Primary Health Care: A Summary of the Issues'. Ottawa: Canadian Nurses Association.

Canadian Population Health Initiative (CPHI). 2005. *Select Highlights on Public Views of the Determinants of Health*. Ottawa: Canadian Institute for Health Information.

Canadian Sickness Survey. 1960. *Illness and Health Care in Canada*. Ottawa: The Queen's Printer.

Carpiano, R.M. 2006. 'Toward a Neighbourhood Resource-Based Theory of Social Capital for Health: Can Bourdieu and Sociology Help?', *Social Science & Medicine* 62: 165–75.

Carson, A.J., N.L. Chappell, and C.J. Knight. 2006. 'Promoting Health and Innovative Health Promotion Practice through a Community Arts Centre', *Health Promotion Practice: A Journal of Health Promotion/Health Education Applications* 10, 10: 1–9.

Casey, M.M., K.T. Call, and J.M. Klingner. 2001. 'Are Rural Residents Less Likely to Obtain Recommended Preventive Healthcare Services?', *American Journal of Preventive Medicine* 21, 3: 182–8.

Cecile, M.T., G. van Wijk, H. Huisman, and A. Kolk. 1999. 'Gender Differences in Physical Symptoms and Illness Behavior: A Health Diary Study', *Social Sciences & Medicine* 49, 8: 1061–74.

Chafetz, J.S. 1997. 'Feminist Theory and Sociology: Underutilized Contributions for Mainstream Theory', *Annual Review of Sociology* 23: 97–120.

Chan, B., and M. Barer. 2000. 'Access to Physicians in Underserved Communities in Canada: Something Old, Something New'. Paper presented at the meeting of the 8th International Medical Workforce Conference, Sydney, Australia.

Chappell, N.L. 1983. 'Informal Support Networks among the Elderly', *Research on Aging* 5, 1: 77–99.

———. 1992. *Social Support and Aging*. Toronto: Butterworths.

———. 1993a. 'Implications of Shifting Health Care Policy for Caregiving in

Canada', *Journal of Aging and Social Policy* 5, 1–2: 39–55.

———. 1993b. 'The Future of Health Care in Canada', *Journal of Social Policy* 22, 4: 487–505.

———. 1994. 'Health Care in Canada', in D.G. Gill and S.R. Ingman, eds, *Eldercare, Distributive Justice and the Welfare State*. Albany: State University of New York Press, 233–54.

———. 1995. 'Policies and Programs for Seniors in Canada', *World Review of Sociology* 1: 17–35.

———. 2003. 'Correcting Cross-Cultural Stereotypes: Aging in Shanghai and Canada', *Journal of Cross-Cultural Gerontology* 18, 2: 127–47.

———. 2006. 'Lessons to be Learned form Aging in Japan—Will Canada Benefit from or Misuse Them?' Invited presentation at the 2006 International Conference hosted by Japan Studies Association of Canada, Kamloops, BC.

———. 2007a. *Aging in Contemporary Canada*, 2nd edn. Toronto: Pearson Educational.

———. 2007b. 'Aging among Chinese Canadian Immigrants—Reflections', *Reading Sociology Canadian Perspectives*. Don Mills, ON: Oxford University Press, 159–62.

———. 2007c. 'Ethnicity and Quality of Life', in Heidrun, Mollenkopf, and Walker, eds, *Quality of Life in Old Age—International and Multi-Disciplinary Perspectives*. New York: Social Indicators Research Series, Springer Publishing.

———. 2008. 'The Future of Aging in Health Care', in D. Cloutier-Fisher, H. Foster, and D. Hultsch, eds, *Vulnerability and Resilience in Health and Aging*. Victoria, BC: Canadian Western Geographical Services, Western Geographical Press.

———, L.M. Funk, A.J. Carson, P. MacKenzie, and R. Stanwick. 2006. 'Multilevel Community Health Promotion: How Can We Make it Work?', *Community Development Journal* 41, 3: 352–66.

———, E. Gee, L. McDonald, and M. Stones. 2003. *Aging in Contemporary Canada*. Toronto: Prentice Hall.

———, B. Havens, M.J. Hollander, J. Miller, and C. McWilliam. 2004. 'Comparative Costs of Home Care and Residential Care', *The Gerontologist* 44, 3: 389–400.

———, and K. Kusch. 2007. 'The Gendered Nature of Filial Piety—A Study among Chinese Canadians', *Journal of Cross-Cultural Gerontology* 22, 1: 29–45.

———, and D. Lai. 1998. 'Health Care Service Use among Chinese Seniors in British Columbia, Canada', *Journal of Cross-Cultural Studies* 13: 21–37.

———, and R. Litkenhaus. 1995. 'Informal Caregivers to Adults in British Columbia'. Joint Report of the Centre on Aging, University of Victoria and the Caregivers Association of British Columbia.

———, L. MacDonald, and M. Stones. 2007. *Aging in Contemporary Canada*, 2nd edn. Toronto: Pearson Educational.

———, M. Maclure, H. Brunt, J. Hopkinson, and J. Mullett. 1997. 'Seniors' Views of Medication Reimbursement Policies: Bridging Research and Policy at the Point of Policy Impact', *Canadian Journal on Aging* (Spring Supplement): 114–31.

————, and M. Penning. 2005. 'Family Caregivers in the Context of Health Reform', in M. Johnson, ed, *The Cambridge Handbook of Age and Aging*. Cambridge: Cambridge University Press, 455–62.

————, and R.C. Reid. 2002. 'Burden and Well-Being among Caregivers: Examining the Distinction', *The Gerontologist* 42, 6: 772–80.

Charmaz, K. 1983. 'Loss of Self: A Fundamental Form of Suffering in the Chronically Ill', *Sociology of Health & Illness* 5: 168–95.

————. 1987. 'Struggling for a Self: Identity Levels of the Chronically Ill', *Research in the Sociology of Health Care* 6: 283–321.

————. 1991. *Good Days, Bad Days: The Self in Chronic Illness and Time*. New Brunswick, NJ: Rutgers University Press.

————. 1994. 'Identity Dilemmas of Chronically Ill Men'. *The Sociological Quarterly* 35, 2: 269–88.

Chaskin, R.J., P. Brown, S. Venkatesh, and A. Vidal. 2001. *Building Community Capacity*. New York: Aldine de Gruyter.

Chen, J., E. Ng, and R. Wilkins. 1996. 'The Health of Canada's Immigrants in 1994–95', *Health Reports* 7, 4: 33–45.

Chen, S. 1997. 'Being Chinese, Becoming Chinese-American: The Transformation of Chinese Identity in the United States, 1910–1928'. PhD Dissertation. Salt Lake City: University of Utah.

Chiu, L., L. Balneaves, M.C. Barroetavena, R. Doll, and A. Leis. 2006. 'Use of Complementary and Alternative Medicine by Chinese Individuals Living with Cancer in British Columbia', *Journal of Complementary and Integrative Medicine* 3, 1: 1–19.

Chodos, H., and B. Curtis. 2002. 'Pierre Bourdieu's "Masculine Domination": A Critique', *The Canadian Review of Sociology and Anthropology* 39, 4: 397–412.

Chui, T. 2003. *Longitudinal Study of Immigrants to Canada: Process, Progress, and Prospects* (Catalogue no. 89-611). Ottawa: Statistics Canada.

Ciambrone, D. 2001. 'Illness and Other Assaults on Self: The Relative Impact of HIV/AIDS on Women's Lives', *Sociology of Health & Illness* 23: 517–40.

Clarke, J.N. 2008. *Health, Illness, and Medicine in Canada*, 5th edn. Don Mills, ON: Oxford University Press.

Coburn, D. 1993. 'State Authority, Medical Dominance and Trends in the Regulation of the Health Professions: The Ontario Case', *Social Science & Medicine* 37: 841–50.

————. 1999. 'Professional Autonomy and the Problematic Nature of Self-Regulation: Medicine, Nursing, and the State', in D. Coburn, S. Rappolt, I. Bourgeault, and J. Angus, eds, *Medicine, Nursing and the State*. Aurora, ON: Garamond Press, 25–53.

————. 2001. 'Health, Health Care, and Neo-Liberalism', in P. Armstrong, H. Armstrong, and D. Coburn, eds, *Unhealthy Times. Political Economy Perspectives on Health and Care in Canada*. Don Mills, ON: Oxford University Press, 45–65.

————. 2004. 'Beyond the Income Inequality Hypothesis: Class, Neo-Liberalism, and Health Inequalities', *Social Science & Medicine* 58, 1: 41–56.

————. 2006. 'Medical Dominance Then and Now: Critical Reflections', *Health Sociology Review* 15: 432–43.

————, and C.L. Biggs. 1986. 'Limits to Medical Dominance: The Case of Chiropractic', *Social Science & Medicine* 22, 10: 1035–46.

————, K. Denny, E. Mykhalovskiy, P. McDonough, A. Robertson, and R. Love. 2003. 'Population Health in Canada: A Brief Critique', *American Journal of Public Health* 93, 3: 392–96.

————, G.M. Torrance, and J.M. Kaufert. 1983. 'Medical Dominance in Canada in Historical Perspective: The Rise and Fall of Medicine?', *International Journal of Health Services* 13, 3: 407–32.

Cohen, M., J. Murphy, K. Nutland, and A. Ostry. 2005. *Continuing Care Renewal or Retreat? BC Residential and Home Health Care Restructuring 2001–2004.* Vancouver: Canadian Centre for Policy Alternatives.

Cohen, S., and L.S. Syme. 1985. *Social Support and Health.* New York: Academic Press.

Coleman, E., N. Strapko, M. Zubrzycki, and C.L. Broach. 1993. 'Social and Psychological Needs of Lesbian Mothers', *Canadian Journal of Human Sexuality* 2, 1: 13–17.

Collins, P.H. 1990. *Black Feminist Thought: Knowledge, Consciousness, and the Politics of Empowerment.* Boston: Unwin Hyman.

Connidis, I.A. 1994. 'Growing Up and Old Together: Some Observations on Families in Later Life', in V. Marshall and B. McPherson, eds, *Aging: Canadian Perspectives.* Peterborough, ON: Broadview, 195–205.

Conrad, P. 1975. 'The Discovery of Hyperkinesis: Notes on the Medicalization of Deviant Behaviour', *Social Problems* 23: 12–21.

————. 1992. 'Medicalization and Social Control', *Annual Review of Sociology* 18: 209–32.

————, and R. Kern. 1986. 'General Introduction', in P. Conrad and R. Kern, eds, *The Sociology of Health & Illness: Critical Perspectives*, 4th edn. New York: St. Martin's Press, 1–6.

Coombs, M., and S.J. Ersser. 2004. 'Medical Hegemony in Decision-Making—A Barrier to Interdisciplinary Working in Intensive Care?', *Journal of Advanced Nursing* 46, 3: 245–52.

Cooper-Patrick, L., J.J. Gallo, J.J. Gonzales, H.T. Vu, N.R. Powe, and C. Nelson. 1999. 'Race, Gender, and Partnership in the Patient–Physician Relationship', *Journal of the American Medical Association* 282: 583–9.

Corker, M., and T. Shakespeare. 2002. 'Mapping the Terrain', in M. Corker and T. Shakespeare, eds, *Disability/Postmodernity: Embodying Disability Theory.* London: Continuum, 1–17.

Coyte, P. 2000. *Home Care in Canada: Passing the Buck.* Toronto: University of Toronto Home Care Evaluation and Research Centre.

————, and P. McKeever. 2001. Submission to the Standing Committee on Social Affairs, Science and Technology. Toronto: Home and Community Care Evaluation and Research Centre, University of Toronto.

Cranswick, K. 2003. 'Caring for an Aging Society', *General Social Survey, Cycle 16* (Statistics Canada Catalogue no. 89-582-XWE). Ottawa: Statistics Canada.

Crompton, S. 2000. '100 Years of Health', *Canadian Social Trends*, Statistics Canada, Catalogue no. 11-008.

Crossley, N. 2001. 'Embodiment and Social Structure: A Response to Howson and Inglis', *The Sociological Review* 49, 3: 318–26.

Cujec, B., H. Quan, Y. Jin, and D. Johnson. 2004. 'The Effect of Age upon Care and Outcomes in Patients Hospitalized for Congestive Heart Failure in Alberta, Canada', *Canadian Journal on Aging* 23, 3: 255–67.

D'Arcy, C. 1998. 'Social Distribution of Health among Canadians', in D. Coburn, C. D'Arcy, and G.M. Torrance, eds, *Health and Canadian Society: Sociological Perspectives*, 3rd edn. Toronto: University of Toronto Press, 73–101.

Dannenberg, A.L., R.J. Jackson, H. Frumkin, R.A. Schieber, M. Pratt, C. Kochtitzky, et al. 2003. 'The Impact of Community Design and Land-Use Choices on Public Health: A Scientific Research Agenda', *American Journal of Public Health* 93, 9: 1500–08.

Davies, B., J.-L. Fernandez, and R. Saunders. 1998. *Community Care in England and France: Reforms and the Improvement of Equity and Efficiency*. Aldershot, UK: Ashgate.

Deacon, A., and K. Mann. 1999. 'Agency, Modernity and Social Policy', *Journal of Social Policy* 28, 3: 413–35.

Dean, K. 1981. 'Self-Care Responses to Illness: A Selected Review', *Social Science & Medicine* 151: 673–87.

Deber, R., L. Narine, P. Baranek, N.K. Sharpe, R. Zlotnik-Shaul, P. Coyte, G. Pink, and P. Williams. 1998. 'The Public–Private Mix in Health Care', *Canada Health Action: Building on the Legacy*. Ottawa: National Forum on Health, 423–546.

De Coster, C., S. Bruce, and A. Kozyrskyi. 2005. 'Use of Acute Care Hospitals by Long-Stay Patients: Who, How Much, and Why?', *Canadian Journal on Aging* 24 (Supplement 1): 97–106.

Denton, M., and K. Kusch. 2006. 'Well-Being throughout the Senior Years: Issues Paper on Key Events and Transitions in Later Life'. Prepared for the Expert Roundtable on Seniors in Ottawa.

———, S. Prus, and V. Walters. 2004. 'Gender Differences in Health: A Canadian Study of the Psychosocial, Structural and Behavioural Determinants of Health', *Social Science & Medicine* 58: 2585–2600.

———, and V. Walters. 1999. 'Gender Differences in Structural and Behavioral Determinants of Health: An Analysis of the Social Production of Health', *Social Science & Medicine* 48: 1221–35.

Department of National Health and Welfare and Dominion Bureau of Statistics. 1960. *Illness and Health Care in Canada—Canadian Sickness Survey, 1950/51*, Cat no. 82-518. Ottawa.

DesMeules, M., J. Gold, A. Kazanjian, D. Manuel, J. Payne, B. Vissandjee, et al. 2004. 'New Approaches to Immigrant Health Assessment', *Canadian Journal of Public Health* 95, 3: 122–6.

Devereaux, P.J, D. Heels-Ansdell, C. Lacchetti, T. Haines, K.E.A. Burns, D.J. Cook, et al. 2004. 'Payments for Care at Private For-Profit and Private Not-for-Profit Hospitals: A Systematic Review and Meta-Analysis', *Canadian*

Medical Association Journal 170, 12: 1817–24.

Diamond, T. 1992. *Making Gray Gold*. Chicago: University of Chicago Press.

———. 1996. 'Social Policy and Everyday Life in Nursing Homes: A Critical Ethnography,' in P. Brown, ed, *Perspectives in Medical Sociology*. Prospect Heights, IL: Waveland Press, 684–702.

———. 2000. 'Nursing Homes as Trouble,' in J. Gubrium and J. Holstein, eds, *Aging and Everyday Life*. Blackwell Publishing, 401–12.

Dill, A.E.P. 1990. 'Transformations of Home Care, The Formal and Informal Process of Home Care Planning,' in J.F. Gubrium and A. Sankar, eds, *The Home Care Experience, Ethnography and Policy*. London: Sage, 227–51.

Doucet, A. 2006. '"Estrogen-Filled Worlds": Fathers as Primary Caregivers and Embodiment,' *Sociological Review* 54, 4: 696–716.

Dubos, R. 1959. *The Mirage of Health*. Garden City, NY: Doubleday.

Dunlop, S., P.C. Coyte, and W. McIsaac. 2000. 'Socio-Economic Status and the Utilization of Physicians' Services: Results from the Canadian National Population Health Survey,' *Social Science & Medicine* 51, 1: 123–33.

Dunn, E.M., T. Burbine, A.C. Bowers, and S. Tantleff-Dunn. 2001. 'Moderators of Stress in Parents of Children with Autism,' *Community Mental Health Journal* 37, 1: 39–52.

Dunn, J.R., and I. Dyck. 2000. 'Social Determinants of Health in Canada's Immigrant Population: Results from the National Population Health Survey,' *Social Science & Medicine* 51: 1573–93.

Eales, K., N. Keating, and B. Prior. 2002. 'Sustaining Care at Home in Small Rural Communities'. Final Report submitted to the New Rural Economy project. Edmonton, AB: Department of Human Ecology, University of Alberta.

Edmondson, R. 2003. 'Social Capital: A Strategy for Enhancing Health?', *Social Science & Medicine* 57, 9: 1723–33.

Eisenberg, L. 1977. 'Disease and Illness: Distinctions between Professional and Population Ideas of Sickness', *Culture, Medicine and Psychiatry* 1: 9–23.

Elder, G.H. Jr. 1975. 'Age Differentiation and the Life Course', *Annual Review of Sociology* 1: 165–90.

———, ed. 1985. *Life Course Dynamics: Trajectories and Transitions, 1968–1980*. Ithaca, NY: Cornell University Press.

———. 2000. 'The Life Course', in E.F. Borgatta and R.J.V. Montgomery, eds, *The Encyclopedia of Sociology, Vol. 3*, 2nd edn. New York: Wiley, 1615.

Engelhardt, H.T. 1974. 'The Disease of Masturbation: Values and the Concept of Disease', *Bulletin of the History of Medicine* 48: 244–5.

Engels, F. 1958 [1848]. *The Condition of the Working Class in England*, trans. O.W. Henderson and W.H. Chaloner. Stanford, CA: Stanford University Press.

Entwistle, J., and A. Rocamora. 2006. 'The Field of Fashion Materialized: A Study of London Fashion Week', *Sociology* 40, 4: 735–51.

Epp, J. 1986. *Achieving Health for All: A Framework for Health Promotion*. Ottawa: Minister of National Health and Welfare.

Esmail, N. 2007. 'Complementary and Alternative Medicine in Canada:

Trends in Use and Public Attitudes', *Public Policy Sources* 87: 1–53.

Esposito, L., and J.W. Murphy. 2000. 'Another Step in the Study of Race Relations', *The Sociological Quarterly* 41, 2: 171–87.

Estes, C.L. 1991. 'The New Political Economy of Aging: Introduction and Critique', in *Critical Perspectives on Aging: The Political and Moral Economy of Growing Old*. New York: Baywood Press, 19–36.

———. 2005. 'Women, Ageing and Inequality: A Feminist Perspective', in M.L. Johnson, ed, *The Cambridge Handbook of Age and Ageing*. Cambridge: Cambridge University Press, 552–59.

Evans, R.G. 1994. 'Health Care as a Threat to Health: Defense, Opulence, and the Social Environment', *Daedalus* 123, 4: 21–42.

———. 2001. 'Ideology, Religion, and the WTO', in A. Ostry and K. Cardiff, eds, in *Trading Away Health? Globablization and Health Policy*. Report from the 14th Annual Health Policy meetings.

———. 2006. 'Fat Zombies, Pleistocene Tastes, Autophilia and the "Obesity Epidemic"', *Healthcare Policy* 2, 2: 18–26.

———, and G.L. Stoddart. 1990. 'Producing Health Consuming Health Care', *Social Science & Medicine* 31, 12: 1347–63.

Eyles, J., M. Brimacombe, P. Chaulk, G. Stoddart, T. Pranger, and O. Moase. 2001. 'What Determines Health? To Where Should We Shift Resources? Attitudes towards Determinants of Health among Multiple Stakeholder Groups in Prince Edward Island,

Canada', *Social Science & Medicine* 53, 12: 11611–19.

Farley, C., S. Haddad, and B. Brown. 1996. 'The Effects of a 4-Year Program Promoting Bicycle Helmet Use among Children in Quebec', *American Journal of Public Health* 86, 1: 46–51.

Featherstone, M., M. Hepworth, and B.S. Turner. 1991. *The Body: Social Process and Cultural Theory*. London: Sage.

Few, A.L. 2007. 'Integrating Black Consciousness and Critical Race Feminism into Family Studies Research', *Journal of Family Issues* 28, 4: 452–73.

Findlay, D., and L. Miller. 2002. 'Through Medical Eyes: The Medicalization of Women's Bodies and Women's Lives', in B.S. Bolaria and H.D. Dickinson, eds, *Health, Illness and Health Care in Canada*, 3rd edn. Scarborough, ON: Nelson Thomson Learning, 276–306.

Fine, B. 1996. 'Feminism, Objectivity and Economics' (Book Review). *Economica v.* 63: 704–06.

Flack, M. 2000. 'Working the Family In: A Case Study of the Determinants of Employees' Access to and Use of Alternative Work Arrangements, and Their Home-to-Work Spillover', *The Humanities and Social Sciences* 60, 11: 4200A–01A.

Flexner, A. 1910. *Medical Education in the United States and Canada*. Carnegie Foundation for Higher Education.

Foote-Ardah, C.E. 2003. 'The Meaning of Complementary and Alternative Medicine Practices among People with HIV in the United States: Strategies for Managing Everyday Life', *Sociology of Health & Illness* 25, 5: 481–500.

Forbes, W.F., J.A. Jackson, and A.S. Kraus. 1987. *Institutionalization of the Elderly in Canada*. Toronto: Butterworth.

Foster, K. 2006. 'Mind the GAP', *Carleton University Magazine* (Spring): 14–17.

Foucault, M. 1972. *The Archaeology of Knowledge*, trans. A.M. Sheridan Smith. London: Tavistock.

———. 1973. *The Birth of the Clinic: An Archaeology of Medical Perception*. London: Tavistock.

———. 1977. *Discipline and Punish: The Birth of the Prison*. London: Allen Lane.

———.1979. *The History of Sexuality, Volume 1: An Introduction*. London: Allen Lane.

———. 1982. 'The Subject and Power', in H.L. Dreyfus and P. Rabinow. *Michel Foucault: Beyond Structuralism and Hermeneutics*. Hemel Hempstead: Harvester Wheatsheaf.

———.1984. 'Space, Knowledge and Power', in P. Rabinow, ed, *The Foucault Reader*. New York: Pantheon, 239–56.

———.1985. *The History of Sexuality, Volume 2. The Use of Pleasure*. New York: Random House.

Fox, N.J. 1993. 'Discourse, Organization and the Surgical Ward Round', *Sociology of Health & Illness* 15, 1: 16–42.

———.1997. 'Is There Life after Foucault? Texts, Frames and Differends', in A. Petersen and R. Bunton, eds, *Foucault, Health and Medicine*. London: Routledge, 31–50.

Frank, A.W. 1993. 'The Rhetoric of Self-Change: Illness Experience as Narrative', *The Sociological Quarterly* 32, 1: 39–52.

———. 1997. 'Illness as Moral Occasion: Restoring Agency to Ill People', *Health* 12: 131–48.

———. 1998. 'Stories of Illness as Care of the Self: A Foucauldian Dialogue', *Health* 2, 3: 329–48.

Frank, J. 1995. 'Why Population Health?', *Canadian Journal of Public Health* 86: 162–4.

Frank, R. 2002. 'Homeopath and Patient—A Dyad of Harmony? Patterns of Communication, Sources of Conflict and Expectations in Homeopathic Physician–Patient Relationship', *Social Science & Medicine* 55: 1285–96.

Frederick, J., and J. Fast. 1999. 'Eldercare in Canada: Who Does How Much?', *Canadian Social Trends* 54 (Fall): 26–32.

Freidson, E. 1970a. *Profession of Medicine*. New York: Dodd Mead.

———. 1970b. *Professional Dominance: The Social Structure of Medical Care*. Chicago: Aldine.

———.1984. 'The Changing Nature of Professional Control', *Annual Review of Sociology* 10: 1–20.

———.1985. 'The Reorganization of the Medical Profession', *Medical Care Research and Review* 42, 1: 11–35.

———. 2001. *Professionalism, the Third Logic: On the Practice of Knowledge*. Chicago: University of Chicago Press.

———. 2003. 'Comments on JHPPL Review Symposium', *Journal of Health Politics, Policy and Law* 28, 1: 168–72.

French, D.P., E. Maissi, and T.M. Marteau. 2004. 'The Purpose of Attributing Cause: Beliefs about the Causes of Myocardial Infarction', *Social Sciences & Medicine* 60, 7: 1411–21.

Freund, P.E.S., and M.B. McGuire. 1999. *Health, Illness and the Social Body: A Critical Sociology*, 3rd edn. Upper Saddle River, NJ: Prentice Hall.

Frideres, J.S. 2002. 'Overcoming Hurdles: Health Care and Aboriginal Peoples', in B.S. Bolaria and H.D. Dickinson, eds, *Health, Illness, and Health Care in Canada*. Scarborough, ON: Nelson Thomson Learning, 144–66.

Fries, J.F. 1980. 'Aging, Natural Death, and the Compression of Morbidity', *New England Journal of Medicine* 303: 130–5.

———. 2000. 'Compression of Morbidity in the Elderly', *Vaccine* 18: 1584–89.

Frolich, K.L., E. Corin, and L. Potvin. 2001. 'A Theoretical Proposal for the Relationship between Context and Disease', *Sociology of Health & Illness* 23, 6: 776–97.

Funk, L.M. 2002. 'Autonomy, in Context: Understanding Preferences for Decision-Making Involvement among Long-Term Care Residents'. MA thesis, University of Victoria.

Fyke, K. 2001. *Caring for Medicare. Sustaining a Quality System*. Regina, SK: Commission on Medicare, Government of Saskatchewan, 72.

Gage-Rancoeur, D.M., and M.A. Purden. 2003. 'Daughters of Cardiac Patients: The Process of Caregiving', *Canadian Journal of Nursing Research* 35, 2: 90–105.

Galabuzi, G.E. 2004. 'Social Exclusion', in D. Raphael, ed, *Social Determinants of Health: Canadian Perspectives*. Toronto: Canadian Scholars' Press, 235–51.

———. 2006. *Canada's Economic Apartheid: The Social Exclusion of Racialized Groups in the New Century*. Toronto: Canadian Scholars' Press.

Gantz, S.B. 1990. 'Self-Care: Perspectives from Six Disciplines', *Holistic Nursing Practice* 4, 2: 1–12.

Ganz, P.A. 1992. 'Treatment Options for Breast Cancer—Beyond Mere Survival', *New England Journal of Medicine* 326, 17: 1147–9.

Gee, E.M., B.A. Mitchell, and A.V. Wister. 1995. 'Returning to the "Parental Nest": Exploring a Changing Canadian Life Course', *Canadian Studies in Population* 22: 121–44.

George, L.K., and L.P. Gwyther. 1986. 'Caregiver Well-Being: A Multidimensional Examination of Family Caregivers of Demented Adults', *The Gerontologist* 26: 253–9.

Giddens, A. 1979. *Central Problems in Social Theory: Action, Structure, and Contradiction in Social Analysis*. Berkeley, CA: University of California Press.

———. 1984. *The Constitution of Society: Outline of the Theory of Structuration*. Cambridge: Polity Press.

Goffman, E. 1959. *The Presentation of Self in Everyday Life*. New York: Doubleday.

———. 1961. *Asylums: Essays on the Situation of Mental Patients and Other Inmates*. New York: Anchor Press.

———. 1963. *Stigma: Notes on the Management of Spoiled Identity*. Englewood Cliffs, NJ: Prentice Hall.

Goldner, M. 2004. 'The Dynamic Interplay between Western Medicine and the Complementary and Alternative Medicine Movement: How Activists Perceive a Range of Responses from Physicians and Hospitals', *Sociology of Health & Illness* 26, 6: 710–36.

Goldscheider, F.K., and L. Lawton. 1998. 'Family Experiences and the Erosion of Support for Intergenerational

Coresidence', *Journal of Marriage and the Family* 60, 3: 620–32.

Goodman, R. 2000. 'Bridging the Gap in Effective Program Implementation: From Concept to Application', *Journal of Community Psychology* 3: 309–21.

Gordon, J., and R. Neal. 1997. 'Voluntary Non-Profit Organizations: A New Research Agenda', *Society/Société* (Newsletter of the Canadian Sociology and Anthropology Association) 21, 1: 15–19.

Gorey, K.M., E.J. Holowaty, E. Laukkanen, G. Fehringer, and N.L. Richter. 1998. 'The Association of Socioeconomic Status with Cancer Incidence in Toronto, Ontario: Possible Confounding of Cancer Mortality by Incidence and Survivorship', *Cancer Prevention & Control* 2: 236–41.

Gough, I. 2000. 'Welfare Regimes in East Asia'. Social Policy and Development Centre, Paper no. 4, University of Bath. Available at: http://www.bath. ac.uk/Faculties/HumSocSci/IFIPA/ GSP.

Goulet, D. 2003. 'Last Resort: Hospital Care in Canada'. Available at: http://www.musee-mccord.qc.ca/ scripts/printtour.php? tourID=VQ_ P2_10_EN&Lang=1. Accessed 7 April 2007.

Graham, H. 2000. 'Socio-Economic Change and Inequalities in Men and Women's Health in the UK', in E. Annandale and K. Hunt, eds, *Gender Inequalities in Health*. Buckingham, UK: Open University Press, 90–122.

Graham, K., and D. Vidal-Zeballos. 1998. 'Analysis of Use of Tranquillizers and Sleeping Pills across Five Surveys of the Same Population (1985–1991): The Relationship with Gender, Age, and Use of Other Substances', *Social Science & Medicine* 46, 3: 381–95.

Gramsci, A. 1977. *Selections from Political Writings, 1910–1920*. London: Lawrence and Wishart.

Gray, E.D. 1994. 'Coping with Autism: Stresses and Strategies', *Sociology of Health & Illness* 16, 3: 275–300.

———. 2002. 'Ten Years On: A Longitudinal Study of Families with Children with Autism', *Journal of Intellectual & Developmental Disability* 27, 3: 215–22.

Gray, R.E., M. Greenberg, M. Fitch, N. Parry, M.S. Douglas, and M. Labrecque. 1997. 'Perspectives of Cancer Survivors Interested in Unconventional Therapies', *Journal of Psychosocial Oncology* 5, 3/4: 149–71.

Grayson, J.P. 2002. 'The Academic Legitimization of Chiropractic: The Case of CMCC and York University', *Journal of the Canadian Chiropractic Association* 46, 4: 265–79.

Green, C.A., and C.R. Pope. 1999. 'Gender, Psychosocial Factors and the Use of Medical Services: A Longitudinal Analysis', *Social Science & Medicine* 48, 10: 1363–72.

Green, L.W., and M.W. Kreuter. 1990. 'Health Promotion as a Public Health Strategy for the 1990s', *Annual Review of Public Health* 11: 319–34.

Gubrium, J.F., and J.A. Holstein. 1997. *The New Language of Qualitative Method*. New York: Oxford University Press.

——— and ———, eds. 2000. *Aging and Everyday Life*. Oxford: Blackwell Publishing.

Gurung, R.A.R., E. Taylor, and T.E. Seeman. 2003. 'Accounting for Changes in Social Support among

Married Older Adults: Insights from the MacArthur Studies of Successful Aging', *Psychology and Aging* 18, 3: 487–96.

Gustafson, E. 1972. 'Dying: The Career of the Nursing Home Patient', *Journal of Health and Social Behavior* 13, 3: 226–35.

Hagestad, G.O., and D. Dannefer. 2001. 'Concepts and Theories of Aging: Beyond Microfication in Social Science Approaches', in R.H. Binstock and L.K. George, eds, *Handbook of Aging and the Social Sciences*, 5th edn. San Diego, CA: Academic Press, 3–21.

Halfon, N., and M. Hochstein. 2002. 'Life Course Health Development: An Integrated Framework for Developing Healthy Policy and Research', *The Millbank Quarterly* 80, 3: 433–80.

Hancock, T. 1996. 'Healthy Sustainable Communities: Concept, Fledgling Practice and Implications for Governance', *Alternatives Journal* 22, 2: 18.

———. 1999. 'Health Care Reform and Reform for Health: Creating a Health System for Communities in the 21st Century', *Futures* 31, 5: 417–36.

Harding, J.S., A.H. Leighton, D.B. Madding, and A.M. MacMillan. 1963. *The Character of Danger: Psychiatric Symptoms in Selected Communities*. New York: Basic Books.

Harrington, C. 1996. 'The Nursing Home Industry: Public Policy in the 1990s', in P. Brown, ed, *Perspectives in Medical Sociology*. Prospect Heights, IL: Waveland Press, 515–34.

Harris, D., and S. Guten. 1979. 'Health-Protective Behavior: An Exploratory Study', *Journal of Health and Social Behavior* 20 (March): 17–29.

Harris, P.B., and J. Bichler. 1997. *Men Giving Care: Reflections of Husbands and Sons*. New York: Garland Publishing, Inc.

Hartley, H. 2002. 'The System of Alignments Challenging Physician Professional Dominance: An Elaborated Theory of Countervailing Powers', *Sociology of Health & Illness* 24, 2: 178–207.

Haug, M.R. 1973. 'Deprofessionalization: An Alternate Hypothesis for the Future', *Sociological Review* Monograph 20: 195–211.

———. 1988. 'A Re-Examination of the Hypothesis of Physician Deprofessionalization', *The Milbank Quarterly* 66 (Supplement 2): 48–56.

———, and B. Lavin. 1983. *Consumerism in Medicine: Challenging Physician Authority*. Beverly Hills, CA: Sage.

Hay, D.I. 1994. 'Social Status and Health Status: Does Money Buy Health?', in B.S. Bolaria and R. Bolaria, eds, *Racial Minorities, Medicine and Health*. Black Point, NS, and Saskatoon, SK: Fernwood Publishers and University of Saskatchewan, 9–51.

Health Canada. 1990. *Report on Home Care*. Ottawa: Health Services and Promotion Branch.

———. 1997. *Canadians and Healthy Eating: How Are We Doing?* Nutrition Highlights, *National Population Health Survey*, 1994–95.

———. 1998. 'Taking Action on Population Health: A Position Paper for Health Promotion and Programs Branch Staff'. Available at: http://www.phac-aspc.gc.ca/ph-sp/phdd/pdf/tad_e.pdf . Accessed 4 December 2006.

———. 1999a. *Home Care in Canada*. Available at: http://www.hc-sc.gc.ca/hcs-sss/pubs/care-soins/1999-home-domicile/introduction_e.html. Accessed 8 April 2007.

———. 1999b. *Physical Activity of Canadians. National Population Health Survey Highlights, Cycle 2, 1996/97*. Ottawa, ON.

———.1999c. *Statistical Report on the Health of Canadians* (Statistics Canada Catalogue no. 82-570-XIE). Ottawa: Minister of Public Works and Government Services Canada.

———. 2000. *Statistical Profile on the Health of First Nations in Canada*. Available at: http://www.hc-sc.gc.ca/fnih-spni/pubs/gen/stats_profil_e.html. Accessed 4 December 2006.

———. 2004. 'Aboriginal Health'. Available at: http://www.hc-sc.gc.ca/ahc-asc/media/nr-cp/2004/2004_60bk3_e.html. Accessed 24 February 2006.

———. 2005a. *Canada's Health Care System*. Available at: http://www.hc-sc.gc.ca/hcs-sss/pubs/care-soins/2005-hcs-sss/del-pres_e.html#1. Accessed 7 April 2007.

———. 2005b. *First Nations Comparable Health Indicators*. Available at: http://www.hc-sc.gc.ca/fnih-spni/pubs/gen/2005-01_health-sante_indicat/index_e.html. Accessed 4 December 2006.

———. 2006a. 'First Nations and Inuit health: HIV and AIDS'. Available at: http://www.hc-sc.gc.ca/fnih-spni/dis-eases-maladies/aids-sida/index_e.html. Accessed 1 January 2007.

———. 2006b. *Healthy Canadians: A Federal Report on Comparable Health Indicators 2006*. Available at: http://www.hc-sc.gc.ca/hcs-sss/pubs/care-soins/index_e.html. Accessed 1 January 2007.

———.2006c. 'Social Capital and Health: Maximizing the Benefits', *Health Policy Research* 12: 1–3.

Health Statistics Division. 2000. 'Taking Risks/Taking Care'. *Health Reports: How Healthy are Canadians?* (Statistics Canada Catalogue no. 82-003). 12, 3: 11–20.

Heinz, W.R., and H. Kruger. 2001. 'Life Course: Innovations and Challenges for Social Research', *Current Sociology* 49, 2: 29–45.

Hendricks, J. 2003. 'Structure and Identity—Mind the Gap: Toward a Personal Resource Model of Successful Aging', in S. Biggs, A. Lowenstein, and J. Hendricks, eds, *The Need for Theory*. Amityville, NY: Baywood Publications, 63–87.

Hertzman, C., C. Power, S. Matthews, and O. Manor. 2001. 'Using an Interactive Framework of Society and Lifecourse to Explain Self-Rated Health in Early Adulthood', *Social Science & Medicine* 53, 12: 1575–85.

Herzlich, C. 1973. *Health and Illness*. London: Academic Press.

———, and J. Pierret. 1987. *Illness and Self in Society*. Baltimore: Johns Hopkins University Press.

Hesmondhalgh, D. 2006. 'Bourdieu, the Media and Cultural Production', *Media, Culture & Society* 28, 2: 211–31.

Hewa, S. 2002. 'Physicians, Medical Profession, and Medical Practice', in B.S. Bolaria and H.D. Dickinson, eds, *Health, Illness, and Health Care in Canada*. Toronto: Nelson Thomson Learning, 55–81.

Hicks, M.H., and M.S. Lam. 1999. 'Decision-Making within the Social

Course of Dementia: Accounts by Chinese-American Caregivers', *Culture, Medicine and Psychiatry* 23: 415–52.

Hindmarsh, J., and A. Pilnick. 2002. 'The Tacit Order of Teamwork: Collaboration and Embodied Conduct in Anaesthesia', *Sociological Quarterly* 43, 2: 139–64.

Hinton, W.L., K. Fox, and S. Levkoff. 1999. 'Exploring the Relationships among Aging, Ethnicity and Dementing Illness', *Culture, Medicine and Psychiatry* 23, 4: 403–13.

Hofmann, B. 2002. 'On the Triad of Disease, Illness and Sickness', *Journal of Medicine and Philosophy* 27, 6: 651–73.

Hollander, M.J. 2001. *Final Report on the Comparative Cost Analysis of Home Care and Residential Care Services*. A report prepared to the Health Transition Fund, Health Canada.

———, and N.L. Chappell. 2001. *Final Report on the Comparative Cost Analysis of Home Care and Residential Care Services*. A report prepared for the Health Transition Fund, Health Canada.

———, ———, M.J. Prince, and E. Shapiro. 2007. 'Providing Care and Support for an Aging Population: Briefing Notes on Key Policy Issues', *Healthcare Quarterly* 10, 3: 34–45.

———, and P. Pallan. 1995. 'The British Columbia Continuing Care System: Service Delivery and Resource Planning', *Aging: Clinical and Experimental Research* 7, 2: 94–109.

Holstein, J.A. 1990. 'Describing Home Care: Discourse and Image in Involuntary Commitment Proceedings', in J. Gubrium and A. Sankar, eds, *The Home Care*

Experience. Newbury Park, CA: Sage, 209–26.

Honjo, K., A. Tsutsumi, I. Kawachi, and N. Kawakami. 2006. 'What Accounts for the Relationship between Social Class and Smoking Cessation? Results of a Path Analysis', *Social Science & Medicine* 62, 2: 317–28.

House, J.S. 2001. 'Understanding Social Factors and Inequalities in Health: 20th Century Progress and 21st Century Prospects', *Journal of Health and Social Behavior* 43: 125–42.

———, and R.L. Kahn. 1985. 'Measures and Concepts of Social Support', in S. Cohen and S.L. Syme, eds, *Social Support and Health*. Orlando, FL: Academic Press, 83–108.

Howson, A., and D. Inglis. 2001. 'The Body in Sociology: Tensions Inside and Outside Sociological Thought', *The Sociological Review* 49, 3: 297–317.

Hubka, D. 2003. 'Closing the Gaps in Aboriginal Health'. Available at: http://www.hc-sc.gc.ca/sr-sr/pubs/ hpr-rps/bull/2003-5-aboriginal- autochtone/method_e.html. Accessed 24 February 2006.

Hughes, B., and Paterson, K. 1997. 'The Social Model of Disability and the Disappearing Body: Towards a Sociology of Impairment', *Disability and Society* 12, 3: 325–40.

Hughes, D. 1988. 'When Nurse Knows Best: Some Aspects of Nurse/Doctor Interaction in a Casualty Department', *Sociology of Health & Illness* 10, 1: 1–22.

Hughes, S.L., A. Giobbie-Hurder, F.M. Weaver, J.D. Kubal, and W. Henderson. 1999. 'Relationship between Caregiver Burden and

Health-Related Quality of Life', *The Gerontologist* 39, 5: 534–45.

Humpel, N., A.L. Marshall, E. Leslie, A. Bauman, and N. Owen. 2004. 'Changes in Neighborhood Walking are Related to Changes in Perceptions of Environmental Attributes', *Annals of Behavioral Medicine* 27, 1: 60–7.

Humphries K.H., and E. van Doorslaer. 2000. 'Income-Related Health Inequality in Canada', *Social Science & Medicine* 50: 663–71.

Hunt, A. 1998. 'The Great Masturbation Panic and the Discourses of Moral Regulation in Nineteenth- and Early Twentieth-Century Britain', *Journal of the History of Sexuality* 8, 4: 575–615.

Hyppa, M.T., and J. Maki. 2003. 'Social Participation and Health in a Community Rich in Stock of Social Capital', *Health Education Research* 18, 6: 770–9.

Ikels, C. 1998. 'The Experience of Dementia in China', *Culture, Medicine and Psychiatry* 22: 257–83.

———. 2002. 'Constructing and Deconstructing the Self: Dementia in China', *Journal of Cross-Cultural Gerontology* 17: 233–51.

Illich, I. 1975. *Medical Nemesis: The Expropriation of Health*. London: Calder and Boyers.

———.1976. *Limits to Medicine. Medical Nemesis: The Expropriation of Health*. London: Marion Boyars Publishers Ltd.

Iversen L., P.C. Hannaford, D.B. Price, and D.J. Godden. 2005. 'Is Living in a Rural Area Good for Your Respiratory Health? Results from a Cross-Sectional Study in Scotland', *Chest* 128, 4: 2059–67.

Jefferis, B., C. Power, and C. Hertzman. 2002. 'Birth Weight, Childhood Socioeconomic Environment, and Cognitive Development in the 1958 British Birth Cohort Study', *British Medical Journal* 325, 7359: 305–11.

Jenish, D., 'Chronic Fatigue Syndrome Recognized', *Maclean's*. 4 May 1998, 60–1.

Jennings, B. 2006. 'The Politics of End-of-Life Decision-Making: Computerized Decision-Support Tools, Physicians' Jurisdiction and Mortality', *Sociology of Health & Illness* 28, 3: 350–75.

Kaminsky, L., and D. Dewey. 2001. 'Sibling Relationships of Children with Autism', *Journal of Autism & Developmental Disorders* 31, 4: 399–410.

Kane, R.A., A.L. Caplan, E.K. Urv-Wong, I.C. Freeman, M.A. Aroskar, and M. Finch. 1997. 'Everyday Matters in the Lives of Nursing Home Residents: Wish for and Perception of Choice and Control', *Journal of the American Geriatrics Society* 45, 9: 1086–93.

Kane, R.L., J.G. Evans, and D. MacFayden. 1990. *Improving the Health of Older People: A World View*. World Health Organization Report. Geneva: World Health Organization.

Katz, P.P. 1998. 'Education and Self-Care Activities among Person with Rheumatoid Arthritis', *Social Science & Medicine* 46, 8: 1057–66.

Kaufert, P.A, and P. Gilbert. 1986. 'Women, Menopause, and Medicalization', *Culture, Medicine and Psychiatry* 10: 7–21.

Kawachi, I. 1999. 'Social Capital and Community Effects on Population and Individual Health', *Annals of the New York Academy of Sciences* 896: 120–30.

————, S.V. Subramanian, and N. Almeida-Filho. 2002. 'A Glossary for Health Inequalities', *Journal of Epidemiology and Community Health* 56: 647–52.

Keating, N., J. Fast, J. Frederick, K. Cranswick, and C. Perrier. 1999. *Eldercare in Canada: Content, Context and Consequences* (BR. 89-570-XPE). Ottawa: Statistics Canada.

Keefe, J., J. Legare, and Y. Carriere. 2004. 'Projecting the Future Availability of Informal Support and Assessing its Impact on Home Care Services'. Executive Summary, Submitted to Health Canada in Fulfillment of Contribution Agreement #6603-03-2000/2590175.

————, and K. Side. 2003. *Net Loss Population Settlement Patterns and Maintenance of Rural Health Status: A Case Study in Atlantic Canada.* (Technical report to the Strategic Initiative in Rural Health: Diagnostic and Integrative Projects). Halifax: Mount Saint Vincent University.

Kelly, M., and B. Charlton. 1995. 'The Modern and the Post-Modern in Health Promotion', in R. Burrows and S. Nettleton, eds, *The Sociology of Health Promotion*. London: Routledge, 78–90.

————, and D. Field. 1996. 'Medical Sociology, Chronic Illness and the Body', *Sociology of Health & Illness* 18, 2: 241–57.

Kelley-Moore, J.A., and K.F. Ferraro. 2004. 'The Black/White Disability Gap: Persistent Inequality in Later Life?', *Journal of Gerontology: Social Sciences* 59B, 1: S34–43.

Kelner, M., B. Wellman, S. Welsh, and H. Boon. 2006. 'How Far Can Complementary and Alternative Medicine Go? The Case of Chiropractic and Homeopathy', *Social Science & Medicine* 63: 2617–27.

Kickbusch, I. 1989. 'Self-Care in Health Promotion', *Social Science & Medicine* 29: 125–30.

Kim, K.K., and P.M. Moody. 1992. 'More Resources, Better Health? A Cross-National Perspective', *Social Science & Medicine* 34, 8: 837–42.

Kinderman, P., E. Setzu, F. Lobban, and P. Salmon. 2006. 'Illness Beliefs in Schizophrenia', *Social Science & Medicine* 63, 7: 1900–11.

Kirsch, M.H. 2000. *Queer Theory and Social Change*. London: Routledge.

Klein, R. 2005. *Premier's Speech to the Canadian Club*. 11 January: AB.

Kliewer, E., and A. Kazanjian. 2000. *The Health Status and Medical Services Utilization of Recent Immigrants to Manitoba and British Columbia: A Pilot Study*. Vancouver: BC Office of Health Technology Assessment.

Koehn, S. 2005. 'Ethnic Minority Seniors Face a Double Whammy in Health Care Access', Vancouver: Providence Health Care.

Kontos, P.C. 2000. 'Resisting Institutionalization: Constructing Old Age and Negotiating Home', in J. Gubrium and J. Holstein, eds, *Aging and Everyday Life*. Oxford: Blackwell Publishing.

Kopec, J.A., I.A. Williams, T. To, and P.C. Austin. 2001. 'Cross-Cultural Comparisons of Health Status in Canada Using the Health Utilities Index', *Ethnicity & Health* 6, 1: 41–50.

Korsch, B., and V. Negrete. 1972. 'Doctor–Patient Communication', *Scientific American* 227, 2: 66–74.

Kralik, D., T. Koch, K. Price, and N. Howard. 2004. 'Chronic Illness Self-Management: Taking Action to Create Order', *Clinical Nursing* 13, 2: 259–67.

Krick, J., and J. Sobal. 1990. 'Relationships between Health Protective Behaviors', *Journal of Community Health* 15: 19–34.

Krieger, N.A. 2003. 'Does Racism Harm Health? Did Child Abuse Exist before 1962? On Explicit Questions, Critical Science, and Current Controversies: An Ecosocial Perspective', *American Journal of Public Health* 93, 2: 194–9.

Krosnick, J., L. Chang, S. Sherman, L. Chassin, and C. Presson. 2006. 'The Effects of Beliefs about the Health Consequences of Cigarette Smoking on Smoking Onset', *Journal of Communication* 56: S18–37.

Labonte, R., M. Polanyi, N. Muhajarine, T. McIntosh, and A.Williams. 2005. 'Beyond the Divides: Towards Critical Population Health Research', *Critical Public Health* 15, 1: 5–17.

Lafrenière, S.A., Y. Carrière, L. Martel, and A. Bèlanger. 2003. 'Dependent Seniors at Home: Formal and Informal Help', *Health Reports* (Statistics Canada Catalogue No. 82-003-XIE) 14, 4: 31–9.

Lalonde, M. 1974. *A New Perspective on the Health of Canadians*. Ottawa: Information Canada.

Lantz, P.M., J. House, J.M. Lepowski, D.R. Williams, R.P. Mero, and J. Chen. 1998. 'Socioeconomic Factors, Health Behaviors, and Mortality', *The Journal of the American Medical Association* 279: 1703–08.

Lavis, J.N. 2002. 'Ideas at the Margin or Marginalized Ideas? Nonmedical Determinants of Health in Canada', *Health Affairs* 21: 107–12.

Lawton, J. 2002. 'Colonising the Future: Temporal Perceptions and Health-Relevant Behaviours across the Adult Lifecourse', *Sociology of Health & Illness* 24, 6: 714–33.

———. 2003. 'Lay Experiences of Health and Illness: Past Research and Future Agendas', *Sociology of Health & Illness* 25: 23–40.

Layder, D. 1994. *Understanding Social Theory*. London: Sage.

Lee, G.R. 1985. 'Theoretical Perspectives on Social Networks', in W.J. Sauer and R.T. Coward, eds, *Social Support Networks and the Care of the Elderly*. New York: Springer Publishers, 21–37.

Le Petit, C., and J.-M. Berthelot. 2005. *Obesity: A Growing Issue. Healthy Today, Healthy Tomorrow? Findings from the National Population Health Survey* (Catalogue No. 82-618-MWE2005003). Ottawa: Statistics Canada.

Leventhal, E.A., and T.R. Prohaska. 1986. 'Age, Symptom Interpretation, and Health Behavior', *Journal of the American Geriatrics Society* 34, 3: 185–91.

Levin, L.S., and E.L. Idler. 1983. 'Self-Care in Health', *Annual Review of Public Health* 4: 181–201.

Lexchin, J. 1993. 'The Effect of Generic Competition on the Price of Prescription Drugs in the Province of Ontario', *Canadian Medical Association Journal* 148: 35–8.

———. 2001. 'Pharmaceuticals: Politics and Policy', in P. Armstrong, H. Armstrong, and D. Coburn, eds, *Unhealthy Times: Political Economy Perspectives on Health and Care in Canada*. Don Mills, ON: Oxford University Press, 31–44.

Li, P.S. 1998. *The Chinese in Canada*, 2nd edn. Don Mills, ON: Oxford University Press.

Light, D., and S. Levine. 1988. 'The Changing Character of the Medical Profession: A Theoretical Overview', *The Milbank Quarterly* 66 (Supplement 2): 10–32.

Lindsay, C. 1999. *A Portrait of Seniors in Canada*, 3rd edn. Ottawa: Statistics Canada.

Lindstrom, M. 2004. 'Social Capital, the Miniaturization of Community and Self-Reported Global and Psychological Health', *Social Science & Medicine* 59: 595–607.

Link, B.G., and J.C. Phelan. 2000. 'Evaluating the Fundamental Cause Explanation for Social Disparities in Health', in C.E. Bird, P. Conrad, and A.M. Fremont, eds, *Handbook of Medical Sociology*, 5th edn. Upper Saddle River, NJ: Prentice Hall, 33–46.

Linnel, M., and S. Easton. 2006. 'Malingering, Perceptions of Illness, and Compensation Seeking in Whiplash Injury: A Comparison of Illness Beliefs between Individuals in Simulated Compensation Scenarios and Litigation Claimants', *Journal of Applied Social Psychology* 36, 11: 2619–34.

Litva, A., and J. Eyles. 1994. 'Health or Healthy: Why People are Not Sick in a Southern Ontario Town', *Social Science & Medicine* 19: 1083–91.

Lochner, K., E. Pamuk, D. Makuc, B.P. Kennedy, and I. Kawachi. 2001. 'State-Level Income Inequality and Individual Mortality Risk: A Prospective, Multi-Level Study', *American Journal of Public Health* 91, 3: 385–91.

Lock, M. 1986. 'Introduction'. *Culture, Medicine and Psychiatry* 10: 1–5.

Lorber, J. 2005. 'Women Get Sicker, but Men Die Quicker', in G.E. Henderson, S.E. Estroff, L.R. Churchill, N.M.P. King, J. Oberlander, and R.P. Strauss, eds, *The Social Medicine Reader: Social and Cultural Contributions to Health, Difference, and Inequality*, 2nd edn. Durham: Duke University Press, 164–90.

Lovaas, K.E., J.P. Elia, and G.A. Yep. 2006. 'Shifting Ground(s): Surveying the Contested Terrain of LGBT Studies and Queer Theory', in *LGBT Studies and Queer Theory: New Conflicts, Collaborations, and Contested Terrain*. New York: Harrington Park Press, 1–18.

Low, J. 2004. 'Managing Safety and Risk: The Experiences of People with Parkinson's Disease who Use Alternative and Complementary Therapies', *Health: An Interdisciplinary Journal for the Study of Health, Illness and Medicine* 8, 4: 445–63.

Lundgren, R.I., and C.H. Browner. 1990. 'Caring for the Institutionalized Mentally Retarded: Work Culture and Work-Based Social Support', in E.K. Abel and M.K. Nelson, eds, *Circles of Care, Work and Identity in Women's Lives*. New York: State University of New York Press, 150–72.

Lupton, D. 1997. 'Foucault and the Medicalisation Critique', in A. Petersen and R. Bunton, eds, *Foucault, Health and Medicine*. London: Routledge, 94–110.

Lynch, J.W., P. Due, C. Muntaner, and G.D. Smith. 2000. 'Social Capital—Is It a Good Investment Strategy for Public Health?', *Journal of*

Epidemiology and Community Health 54, 6: 404–08.

———, and G.A. Kaplan. 2000. 'Socioeconomic Position', in L.F. Berkman and I. Kawachi, eds, *Social Epidemiology*. Oxford: Oxford University Press.

———, ———, and J.J. Salonen. 1997. 'Why Do Poor People Behave Poorly? Variation in Adult Health Behaviors and Psychosocial Characteristics by Stage of the Socioeconomic Lifecourse', *Social Science & Medicine* 44: 809–19.

Lynch, S.A. 1998. 'Who Supports Whom? How Age and Gender Affect the Perceived Quality of Support from Family and Friends', *Gerontologist* 38, 2: 231–8.

McCann, R., and H. Giles. 2002. 'Ageism in the Workplace: A Communication Perspective', in T.D. Nelson, ed, *Ageism: Stereotyping and Prejudice against Older Persons*. Cambridge, MA: MIT Press, 163–200.

McCormack, D. 2003. 'An Examination of the Self-Care Concept Uncovers a New Direction for Healthcare Reform', *Nursing Leadership* 16, 4: 48–65.

McCormick, R., R. Nedan, P. McNicoll, and J. Lynam. 1997. 'Taking Back the Wisdom: Moving Forward to Recovery and Action', *Canadian Journal of Community Mental Health* 16, 2: 5–8.

McDaniel, S.A. 2002. 'Women's Changing Relations to the State and Citizenship: Caring and Intergenerational Relations in Globalizing Western Democracies', *Canadian Review of Sociology and Anthropology/RCSA* 39, 2: 125–49.

———. 2006. 'Putting Humpty-Dumpty Together: Aging Policy for a New Age. Roundtable on Policy for an Aging Society', *Canadian Sociology and Anthropology Association* May/June.

McDonald, A.D., J.C. McDonald, N. Steinmetz, P.E. Enterline, and V. Salter. 1973. 'Physician Services in Montreal before Universal Health Insurance', *Medical Care* 11: 269–86.

McDonald, J.T., and S. Kennedy. 2004. 'Insights into the "Healthy Immigrant Effect": Health Status and Health Service Use of Immigrants to Canada', *Social Science & Medicine* 59, 8: 1613–27.

McDonald, L., U. George, J. Daciuk, M. Yan, and H. Rowan. 2001. *A Study on the Settlement Related Needs of Newly Arrived Immigrant Seniors in Ontario*. Toronto: Centre for Applied Social Research, University of Toronto.

McDonough, P., G.J. Duncan, D. Williams, and J. House. 1997. 'Income Dynamics and Adult Mortality in the United States, 1972 through 1989', *American Journal of Public Health* 87, 9: 1476–83.

———, and P. Berglund. 2003. 'Histories of Poverty and Self-Rated Health Trajectories', *Journal of Health and Social Behavior* 44, 1: 98–214.

McDowell, I. 2006. *Measuring Health: A Guide to Rating Scales and Questionnaires*, 3rd edn. New York: Oxford University Press.

McFarland, B., D. Bigelow, B. Zani, J. Newsom, and M. Kaplan. 2002. 'Complementary and Alternative Medicine Use in Canada and the United States', *American Journal of Public Health* 92, 10: 1616–18.

McGregor, M.J., M. Cohen, K. McGrail, A.-M. Broemeling, R.N. Adler, M. Schulzer, L. Ronald, Y. Cvitkovich, and M. Beck. 2005. 'Staffing Levels in Not-For-Profit and For-Profit Long-Term Care Facilities: Does Type of Ownership Matter?', *Canadian Medical Association Journal* 172, 5: 645–9.

McKee, M. 2001. 'Europe and North America: A Clash of Cultures?', in A. Ostry and K. Cardiff, eds, *Trading Away Health? Globalization and Health Policy*. Report from the 14th Annual Health Policy Conference of the Centre for Health Services and Policy Research. HPRU 2002:10D. November 9, Vancouver, BC, 25–8.

McKeown, T. 1975. *Medicine in Modern Society*. London: Allen and Unwin.

———. 1976. *The Role of Medicine: Dream, Mirage or Nemesis?* London: Nuffield Provincial Hospitals Trust.

———, R.G. Record, and R.D. Turner. 1975. 'An Interpretation of the Decline in Mortality in England and Wales during the Twentieth Century', *Population Studies* 29: 391–422.

McKinlay, J.B., and S.M. McKinlay. 1977. 'The Questionable Contribution of Medical Measures to the Decline of Mortality in the United States', *The Milbank Memorial Fund Quarterly (Health and Society)* 55, 3: 405–28.

———, and ———. 1987. 'Medical Measures and the Decline of Mortality', in H.D. Schwartz, ed, *Dominant Issues in Medical Sociology*, 2nd edn. New York: Random House.

———, D.B. Potter, and H.A. Feldman. 1996. 'Non-Medical Influences on Medical Decision-Making', *Social Science & Medicine* 45, 2: 769–76.

———, and J. Stoeckle. 1998. 'Corporatization and the Social Transformation of Doctoring', *International Journal of Health Services* 18: 191–205.

McKinnon, A.L., J.W. Gartrell, L.A. Derksen, and G.K. Jarvis. 1991. 'Health Knowledge of Native Indian Youth in Central Alberta', *Canadian Journal of Public Health* 82, 6: 429–33.

McLaughlin, L.A., and K.L. Braun. 1998. 'Asian and Pacific Islander Cultural Values: Considerations for Health Care Decision Making', *Health and Social Work* 23, 2: 116–26.

McMullin, J.A. 2004. *Understanding Social Inequality: Intersections of Class, Age, Gender, Ethnicity and Race in Canada*. Don Mills, ON: Oxford University Press.

Magliano, L., A. Fiorillo, C. De Rosa, M.M. Malangone, and The National Mental Health Project Working Group. 2005. 'Family Burden in Long-Term Diseases: A Comparative Study in Schizophrenia vs. Physical Disorders', *Social Science & Medicine* 61, 2: 313–22.

Malacrida, C. 2004. 'Medicalization, Ambivalence and Social Control: Mothers' Descriptions of Educators and ADD/ADHD', *Health: An Interdisciplinary Journal for the Social Study of Health, Illness and Medicine* 8, 1: 61–80.

Manga, P. 1978. 'The Income Distribution Effect of Medical Insurance in Ontario' (Occasional Paper No. 6). Toronto: Ontario Economic Council.

———, R.W. Broyles, and D.E. Angus. 1987. 'The Determinants of Hospital Utilization under a Universal Public

Insurance Program in Canada',
Medical Care 25, 7: 658–70.

Markey, C., P. Markey, C. Schneider, and
S. Brownlee. 2005. 'Marital Status and
Health Beliefs: Different Relations for
Men and Women', *Sex Roles* 53, 5/6:
443–51.

Marmor, T.R., and K. Sullivan. 2000.
'Canada's Burning! Media Myths
about Universal Health Coverage',
Washington Monthly July/August.

Marmot, M., and E. Brunner. 2004.
'Cohort Profile: The Whitehall II
Study', *International Journal of
Epidemiology* 34, 2: 251–56.

Martel, L., A. Bélanger, J.M. Berthelot,
and Y. Carrière. 2005. *Healthy Aging.
Healthy Today, Healthy Tomorrow?
Findings from the National Population
Health Survey* (Catalogue No. 82-618-
MWE2005004). Ottawa: Statistics
Canada.

Martin-Matthews, A. 2007. 'Situating
"Home" at the Nexus of the Public
and Private Spheres: Ageing, Gender
and Home Support Work in Canada',
Current Sociology 55: 229–49.

Masotti, P.J., R. Fick, A. Johnson-Masotti,
and S. MacLeod. 2006. 'Community
Matters in Healthy Aging. Healthy
Naturally Occurring Retirement
Communities: A Low-Cost Approach
to Facilitating Healthy Aging',
American Journal of Public Health 96,
7: 1164–70.

Mead, G.H. 1934. *Mind, Self, and
Society*. Chicago: University of
Chicago Press.

Meadows, L.M., W.E. Thurston, and C.A.
Berenson. 2001. 'Health Promotion
and Preventive Measures: Interpreting
Messages at Midlife', *Qualitative
Health Research* 11, 4: 450–63.

Medjuck, S., J.M. Keefe, and P.J. Fancey.
1998. 'Available but not Accessible, an
Examination of the Use of Workplace
Policies for Caregivers of Elderly Kin',
Journal of Family Issues 19, 3: 274–99.

Meeker, W.C., and S. Haldeman. 2002.
'Chiropractic: A Profession at the
Crossroads of Mainstream and
Alternative Medicine', *Annals of
Internal Medicine* 136: 216–27.

Mendelson, M., and P. Divinsky. 2002.
*Canada 2015: Globalization and the
Future of Canada's Health and Health
Care*. Prepared for the Future of
Global and Regional Integration
Project, Institute of
Intergovernmental Relations.
Kingston, ON: Queen's University.

Merzel, C., and J. D'Afflitti. 2003.
Reconsidering Community-Based
Health Promotion: Promise,
Performance, and Potential', *American
Journal of Public Health* 93, 4: 557–74.

Meyer, J.W. 2000. 'Globalization—Sources
and Effects on National States and
Societies', *International Sociology,
Journal of the International
Sociological Association* 15, 2: 233–48.

Mhatre, S.L., and R.B. Deber. 1992. 'From
Equal Access to Health Care to
Equitable Access to Health: A Review
of Canadian Provincial Health
Commissions and Reports',
*International Journal of Health
Services* 22, 4: 56–68.

Miles, R. 1982. *Racism and Migrant
Labour*. London: Routledge.

Millar, W.J. 2001. 'Patterns of Use—
Alternative Health Care Practitioners',
Health Reports 13, 1: 9–21.

Mills, C.W. 1959. *The Sociological
Imagination*. New York: Oxford
University Press.

Mirowsky, J., and C.E. Ross. 1998. 'Education, Personal Control, Lifestyle and Health: A Human Capital Hypothesis', *Research on Aging* 20, 4: 415–59.

Mishler, E.G. 1981. 'Viewpoint: Critical Perspectives on the Biomedical Model', in E. Mishler, L.R. Amarsingham, S.D. Osherson, S.T. Hauser, N.E. Waxler, and R. Liem, eds, *Social Contexts of Health, Illness, and Patient Care*. Cambridge: Cambridge University Press.

———. 1989. 'Critical Perspectives on the Biomedical Model', in P. Brown, ed, *Perspectives in Medical Sociology*. Newbury Park: Sage, 153–66.

Mishra, G.D., K. Ball, A.J. Dobson, and J.E. Byles. 2004. 'Do Socioeconomic Gradients in Women's Health Widen over Time with Age?', *Social Science & Medicine* 58, 9: 1585–95.

Mitchell, B.A. 2000. 'The Refilled "Nest": Debunking the Myth of Families in Crisis', in E.M. Gutman and G.M. Gutman, eds, *The Overselling of Population Aging: Apocalyptic Demography, Intergenerational Challenges, and Social Policy*. Don Mills, ON: Oxford University Press, 80–99.

———, and E.M. Gee. 1996. 'Young Adults Returning Home: Implications for Social Policy', in B. Galaway and J. Hudson, eds, *Youth in Transition to Adulthood: Research and Policy Implications*. Toronto: Thompson Educational Publishing, 61–71.

———, A.V. Wister, and E.M. Gee. 2002. '"There's no Place like Home": An Analysis of Young Adults' Mature Coresidency in Canada', *International Journal of Aging and Human Development* 54: 57–84.

Mitchell, L., N.P. Roos, and E. Shapiro. 2005. 'Patterns of Home Care Use in Manitoba', *Canadian Journal on Aging* 24 (Supplement 1): S59–68.

Mizrahi, T. 1986. *Getting Rid of Patients: Contradictions in the Socialization of Physicians*. New Brunswick, NJ: Rutgers University Press.

Moore, E.G., and M.W. Rosenberg, 1990. 'Residential Mobility and Migration Among Canada's Elderly', in V. Marshall and B. McPherson, eds, *Aging: Canadian Perspectives*. Peterborough, ON: Broadview Press, 51–69.

Moriarty, J., and J. Butt. 2004. 'Social Support and Ethnicity in Old Age', in A. Walker and C. Hagan Hennessy, eds, *Growing Older: Quality of Life in Old Age*. Maidenhead: Open University Press.

Mullan, P. 2000. *The Imaginary Time Bomb: Why an Ageing Population is not a Social Problem*. London: IB Tauris.

Mulvany, J. 2000. 'Disability, Impairment or Illness? The Relevance of the Social Model of Disability to the Study of Mental Disorder', *Sociology of Health & Illness* 22, 5: 582–601.

Muntaner, C., C. Borrell, A. Kuns, H. Chung, J. Benach, and S. Ibrahim. 2006. 'Social Class Inequalities in Health: Does Welfare State Regime Matter?', in D. Raphael, T. Bryant, and M. Rioux, eds, *Staying Alive: Critical Perspectives on Health, Illness and Health Care*. Toronto: Canadian Scholars' Press, 139–58.

Murphy, R.F. 1987. *The Body Silent*. New York: Henry Holt.

Murray, C. J., and A.D. Lopez. 1997. 'Global Mortality, Disability, and the

Contribution of Risk Factors: Global Burden of Disease Study', *The Lancet* 349: 1436–42.

Myles, J.F. 1978. 'Institutionalization and Sick Role Identification among the Elderly', *American Sociological Review* 43: 508–21.

Myles, J. 1984. *Old Age in the Welfare State: The Political Economy of Public Pensions*. Boston: Little, Brown and Company.

Nabalamba, A., and W.J. Millar. 2007. 'Going to the Doctor', *Health Reports* (Catalogue no. 82-003) 18, 1: 23–35.

Nagarajan, K.V. 2004. 'Rural and Remote Community Health Care in Canada: Beyond the Kirby Panel Report, the Romanow Report and the Federal Budget of 2003', *Canadian Journal of Rural Medicine* 9, 4: 245–51.

Napolitano, M.A., H. Lerch, G. Papandonatos, and B.H. Marcus. 2006. 'Worksite and Communications-Based Promotion of a Local Walking Path', *Journal of Community Health* 31: 326–42.

National Forum on Health. 1997. *Canada Health Action: Building on the Legacy*. Ottawa: Health Canada.

National Institutes of Health. 2007. *What is CAM?* Available at: http://nccam.nih.gov/health/whatiscam/#d6. Accessed 15 December 2007.

Navarro, V. 1976. *Medicine Under Capitalism*. New York: Prodist.

———. 1985. 'U.S. Marxist Scholarship in the Analysis of Health and Medicine', *International Journal of Health Services* 15, 4: 413–35.

———. 1988. 'Professional Dominance or Proletarianization? Neither', *The Milbank Quarterly* 66 (Supplement 2): 57–75.

———. 2002a. 'Neoliberalism, "Globalization", Unemployment, Inequalities and the Welfare State, in *The Political Economy of Social Inequalities: Consequences for Health and Quality of Life*. Amityville, NY: Baywood Publishing Company, 33–107.

———. 2002b. 'The Political Economy of the Welfare State in Developed Capitalist Countries', in *The Political Economy of Social Inequalities: Consequences for Health and Quality of Life*. Amityville, NY: Baywood Publishing Company, 121–69.

———, C. Borrell, J. Benach, C. Muntaner, A. Quiroga, M. Rodrigues-Sanz, N. Vergés, J. Gumá, and M.I. Pasarin. 2004. 'The Importance of the Political and the Social in Explaining Mortality Differentials among the Countries of the OECD, 1950–1998', in *The Political and Social Contexts of Health*. Amityville, NY: Baywood Press, 11–86.

———, and L. Shi. 2001. 'The Political Context of Social Inequalities and Health', *Social Science & Medicine* 52, 3: 481–91.

Nayak, A. 2006. 'After Race: Ethnography, Race and Post-Race Theory', *Ethnic and Racial Studies* 29, 3: 411–30.

Nazroo, J., M. Bajekal, D. Blane, and I. Grewal. 2004. 'Ethnic Inequalities', in A. Walker and H.C. Hennessy, eds, *Growing Older: Quality of Life in Old Age*. Maidenhead: Open University Press, 35–59.

Neal, M.B., N.J. Chapman, B. Ingersall-Dayton, and A.F. Emlen. 1993. *Balancing Work and Care for Children, Adults, and Elders*. Newbury Park, CA: Sage.

Netemeyer, R.G., J.C. Andrews, and S. Burton. 2005. 'Effects of Antismoking Advertising-Based Beliefs on Adult Smokers' Consideration of Quitting', *American Journal of Public Health* 95, 6: 1062–66.

Newbold, K.B. 2005. 'Self-Rated Health within the Canadian Immigrant Population: Risk and the Healthy Immigrant Effect', *Social Science & Medicine* 57: 1981–95.

———, and J. Danforth. 2003. 'Health Status and Canada's Immigrant Population', *Social Science & Medicine* 57: 1981–95.

Ng, E., R. Wilkins, F. Gendron, and J. M. Berthelot. 2005. *Dynamics of Immigrants' Health in Canada: Evidence from the National Population Health Survey* (Catalogue No. 82-618). Ottawa: Statistics Canada.

Noh, S., and V. Kaspar. 2003. 'Diversity and Immigrant Health', in P. Anisef and M. Lanphier, eds, *The World in a City*. Toronto: University of Toronto Press, 316–53.

Northcott, H.C. 2002. 'Health Care Restructuring and Alternative Approaches to Health and Medicine', in B.S. Bolaria and H.D. Dickinson, eds, *Health, Illness, and Health Care in Canada*, 3rd edn. Scarborough, ON: Nelson Thomson, 460–74.

Novack, D.H., R. Plumer, R.L. Smith, H. Ochitill, G.R. Morrow, and J.M. Bennett. 1979. 'Changes in Physicians' Attitudes toward Telling the Cancer Patient', *Journal of the American Medical Association* 241: 897–900.

Nutbeam, D. 1986. 'Health Promotion Glossary', *Health Promotion* 1: 113–27.

Obermeyer, C.M., M. Schulein, A. Hardon, L.L. Sievert, K. Price, A.C. Santiago, et al. 2004. 'Gender and Medication Use: An Exploratory, Multi-Site Study', *Women & Health* 39, 4: 57–73.

Oliver, M. 1983. *Social Work with Disabled People*. London: Macmillan.

O'Malley, M.S., J.A. Earp, M.J. Hawley, M.J. Schell, H.F. Mathews, and J. Mitchell. 2001. 'The Association of Race/Ethnicity, Socioeconomic Status, and Physician Recommendations for Mammography: Who Gets the Message about Breast Cancer Screening?', *American Journal of Public Health* 91, 1: 49–54.

Omran, A.R. 1971. 'The Epidemiologic Transition: A Theory of the Epidemiology of Population Change', *Milbank Memorial Fund Quarterly* 49: 509–38.

Park, J. 2005. 'Use of Alternative Health Care', *Health Reports* 16, 2: 39–42.

Parke, B.B. 2007. 'Understanding the Hospital Environment and Older People: A Social Ecological Analysis'. PhD Dissertation, University of Victoria, 2007.

Parke, R.D. 1996. *Fatherhood*. Cambridge, MA: Harvard University Press.

Parsons, T. 1951. *The Social System*. New York: Free Press.

Pearlin, L.I., J.T. Mullin, S.J. Semple, and M.M. Skaff. 1990. 'Caregiving and the Stress Process: An Overview of Concepts and their Measures', *The Gerontologist* 30: 583–491.

Pederson, A., and D. Raphael. 2006. 'Gender, Race, and Health Inequalities', in D. Raphael, T. Bryant, and M. Rioux, eds, *Staying Alive: Critical Perspectives on Health, Illness and Health Care*. Toronto: Canadian Scholars' Press, 159–91.

Pejlert, A. 2001. 'Being a Parent of an Adult Son or Daughter with Severe Mental Illness Receiving Professional Care: Parent's Narratives', *Health & Social Care in the Community* 9, 4: 194–204.

Penning, M.J. 1998. 'In the Middle: Parental Caregiving in the Context of Other Roles', *Journals of Gerontology: Social Sciences* 53B: S188–197.

———. 2001. 'Health of the Elderly: From Institutional Care to Home and Community Care', in B.S. Bolaria and H.D. Dickinson, eds, *Health, Illness and Health Care in Canada*, 3rd edn. Toronto: Harcourt Brace and Company, 292–308.

———, D.E. Allan, and M.E. Brackley. 2001. 'Health Care Restructuring: Impact on Home Care Service Utilization among Older Adults in British Columbia'. Paper presented at the International Association of Gerontology, Vancouver, BC.

———, M.E. Brackley, and D.E. Allan. 2006. 'Home Care and Health Reform: Changes in Home Care Utilization in One Canadian Province, 1990–2000', *The Gerontologist* 46, 6: 744–58.

———, ———, C. Zheng, and D.E. Allan. (forthcoming). 'Geography, Home Care, and Health Care Reform in British Columbia, 1991–2000', in D. Cloutier-Fisher, L. Foster, and D. Hultsch, eds, *Health and Aging in British Columbia: Vulnerability and Resilience, Canadian Western Geographical Series*. Victoria, BC: Western Geographical Press.

Pérez, C.E. 2002. 'Health Status and Health Behaviour among Immigrants', *Health Reports* 13: 1–12.

Pescosolido, B.A. 1992. 'Beyond Rational Choice: The Social Dynamics of How People Seek Help', *American Journal of Sociology* 97: 1096–1138.

———, S.A. Tuch, and J.K. Martin. 2001. 'The Profession of Medicine and the Public: Examining Americans' Changing Confidence in Physical Authority from the Beginning of the "Health Care Crisis" to the Era of Health Care Reform', *Journal of Health and Social Behaviour* 42, 1: 1–16.

Petersen, A., and R. Bunton. 1997. *Foucault, Health and Medicine*. London: Routledge.

Peterson, D.M. 2002. 'The Potential of Social Capital Measures in the Evaluation of Comprehensive Community-Based Health Initiatives', *American Journal of Evaluation* 23, 1: 55–64.

Petts, J. 2004. 'Health, Responsibility, and Choice: Contrasting Negotiations of Air Pollution and Immunization Information', *Environment and Planning* A37: 791–804.

Pflanz, M. 1974. 'A Critique of Anglo-American Medical Sociology', *International Journal of Health Services: Planning, Administration, Evaluation* 4, 3: 565–74.

———. 1975. 'Relations between Social Scientists, Physicians and Medical Organizations in Health Research', *Social Science & Medicine* 9: 7–13.

Pick, S., Y.H. Poortinga, and M. Givaudan. 2003. 'Integrating Intervention Theory and Strategy in Culture-Sensitive Health Promotion Programs', *Professional Psychology: Research and Practice* 34, 4: 422–29.

Pickard, L. 2001. 'Carer Break or Carer-Blind? Policies for Informal Carers in the UK', *Social Policy & Administration* 35, 4: 441–58.

———, R. Wittenberg, A. Comas-Herrera, B. Davies, and R. Darton. 2000. 'Relying on Informal Care in the New Century? Informal Care for Elderly People in England to 2031', *Ageing and Society* 20, 6: 747–72.

Pickett, W., M.J. Garner, W.F. Boyce, and M.A. King. 2002. 'Gradients in Risk for Youth Injury Associated with Multiple-Risk Behaviours: A Study of 11,329 Canadian Adolescents', *Social Science & Medicine* 55, 6: 1055–68.

Picot, G. 2004. *The Deteriorating Economic Welfare of Immigrants and Possible Causes*. Ottawa: Statistics Canada.

Pillemer, K., and D. Finkelhor. 1988. 'The Prevalence of Elder Abuse: A Random Sample Survey', *The Gerontologist* 28: 51–7.

Plummer, K. 2003. 'Queers, Bodies and Postmodern Sexualities: A Note on Revisiting the "Sexual" in Symbolic Interactionism', *Qualitative Sociology* 25, 4: 515–28.

Popay, J., and M. Bartley. 1993. 'Conditions of Formal Domestic Labour', in S. Platt, H. Thomas, S. Scott, and G. Williams, eds, *Locating Health: Sociological and Historical Explanations*. Brookfield, VT: Avenury, 97–120.

———, G. Williams, C. Thomas, and A. Gatrell. 1998. 'Theorising Inequalities in Health: The Place of Lay Knowledge', *Sociology of Health & Illness* 20, 5: 619–44.

Population Reference Bureau. 2005. *2005 World Population Data Sheet*. Washington, DC. Available at: http://www.prb.org/Publications/Data sheets/2005/2005WorldPopulation DataSheet.aspx.

Potter, S.J., and J.B. McKinley. 2005. 'From a Relationship to Encounter: An Examination of Longitudinal and Lateral Dimensions in the Doctor–Patient Relationship', *Social Sciences & Medicine* 61, 2: 465–79.

Pritchard, J. 2002. *Male Victims of Elder Abuse: Their Experiences and Needs*. York, UK: Joseph Rowntree Foundation.

Pruett, K.D. 2000. *Fatherneed: Why Father Care is as Essential as Mother Care to Your Child*. New York: The Free Press.

Prus, S.G., and E. Gee. 2002. *Gender Differences in the Influence of Economic, Lifestyle and Psychosocial Factors on Later-Life Health*. Hamilton, ON: Program for Research on Social and Economic Dimensions of an Aging Population, McMaster University.

Public Health Agency of Canada. 2002. 'Education as a Determinant of Health'. Available at: http//www.pha-caspc.gc.ca/ph-sp/phdd/overview_implications /10_education.html. Accessed 19 April 2005.

Putnam, R.D., with R. Leonardi and R. Nanetti. 1993. *Making Democracy Work: Civic Traditions in Modern Italy*. Princeton, NJ: Princeton University Press.

———. 2000. *Bowling Alone: The Collapse and Revival of American Community*. New York: Simon & Schuster.

Qualls, S.H. 1993. 'Family Therapy with Older Adults', *Generations* 17: 73–4.

Rachlis, M., and C. Kushner. 1989. *Second Opinion: What's Wrong with Canada's Health Care System and How to Fix It*. Toronto: Collins.

Rajaram, S.S., and A. Rashidi. 1998. 'Minority Women and Breast Cancer Screening: The Role of Cultural Explanatory Models', *Preventive Medicine* 27: 747–64.

Raphael, D. 1999. 'Health Effects of Economic Inequality: Overview and Purpose', *Canadian Review of Social Policy* 44: 25-40.

———. 2004. *Social Determinants of Health: Canadian Perspectives.* Toronto: Canadian Scholars' Press.

———. 2006. 'Social Determinants of Health: An Overview of Concepts and Issues', in D. Raphael, T. Bryant, and M. Rioux, eds, *Staying Alive: Critical Perspectives on Health, Illness and Health Care.* Toronto: Canadian Scholars' Press, 115–38.

Raphael, D., and T. Bryant. 2002. 'The Limitations of Population Health as a Model for a New Public Health', *Health Promotion International* 17, 2: 189–99.

———, J. Macdonald, R. Colman, R. Labonte, K. Hayward, and R. Torgerson. 2005. 'Researching Income and Income Distribution as a Determinant of Health in Canada: Gaps between Theoretical Knowledge, Research Practice, and Policy Implementation', *Health Policy* 72: 217–32.

Redefining Progress. 1994. *The Genuine Progress Indicator Redefining Progress.* San Francisco.

Rein, M. 1969. 'Social Class and the Utilization of Medical Care Services: A Study of British Experience under the National Health Service', *Hospitals* 43, 13: 43–54.

Reverby, S. 1996. 'A Caring Dilemma: Womanhood and Nursing in

Historical Perspective, in P. Brown, ed, *Perspectives in Medical Sociology*, 2nd edn. Prospect Heights, IL: Waveland Press, 667–83.

Rier, D.A. 2000. 'The Missing Voice of the Critically Ill: A Medical Sociologist's First-Person Account', *Sociology of Health & Illness* 22, 1: 68–93.

Riley, J.C. 2001. *Rising Life Expectancy: A Global History.* Cambridge: Cambridge University Press.

Riska, E., and K. Wegar, eds. 1993. *Gender, Work and Medicine. Women and the Medical Division of Labour.* London: Sage.

Romanow, R. J., Commissioner. 2002. *Building on Values. The Future of Health Care in Canada.* Ottawa: Commission on the Future of Health Care in Canada.

Roos, L.L., J. Magoon, S. Gupta, S, Chateau, and P.J. Veugelers. 2004. 'Socioeconomic Determinants of Mortality in Two Canadian Provinces: Multilevel Modeling and Neighborhood Context', *Social Science & Medicine* 59: 1435–47.

Rosenstock, L.M. 1974. 'Historical Origins of the Health Belief Model', *Health Education Monographs* 2: 1–8.

Rosenthal, C.J. 1986. 'Differentiation of Multigenerational Households', *Canadian Journal on Aging* 5, 27–42.

———. 2000. 'Aging Families: Have Current Changes and Challenges been "Oversold?"', in E.M. Gurman and G.M. Gutman, eds, *The Overselling of Population Aging: Apocalyptic Demography, Intergenerational Challenges, and Social Policy.* Don Mills, ON: Oxford University Press, 45–63.

Ross, C.E. and C.-L. Wu. 1996. 'Education, Age and the Cumulative

Advantage in Health', *Journal of Health and Social Behavior* 37, 1: 104–20.

Rubin, H.J., and I.S. Rubin. 2001. *Community Organizing and Development*, 3rd edn. Boston: Allyn and Bacon.

Rubinstein, R.L. 1990. 'Culture and Disorder in the Home Care Experience: The Home as Sickroom', in J.F. Gubrium and A. Sankar, eds, *The Home Care Experience, Ethnography and Policy*. London: Sage, 37–57.

Sadler, G.R., S.K. Dhanjal, N.B. Shah, R.B. Shah, C. Ko, M. Anghel, M., et al. 2001. 'Asian Indian Women: Knowledge, Attitudes and Behaviors toward Breast Cancer Early Detection', *Public Health Nursing* 18, 5: 357–63.

St. John, P.D., B. Havens, C.H.M. van Ineveld, and M. Finlayson. 2002. 'Rural–Urban Differences in Health Status of Elderly Manitobans', *Canadian Journal of Rural Medicine* 7, 2: 89–93.

Saks, M. 2001. 'Alternative Medicine and Health Care Division of Labour: Present Trends and Future Prospects', *Current Sociology* 49, 3: 119–34.

Sanders, C., J. Donovan, and P. Dieppe. 2002. 'The Significance and Consequences of Having Painful and Disabled Joints in Older Age: Co-Existing Accounts of Normal and Disrupted Biographies', *Sociology of Health & Illness* 24, 2: 227–53.

Scheff, T.J. 1966. *Being Mentally Ill: A Sociological Theory*. Chicago: Aldine.

Schopler, E., and B.G. Mesibov. 1994. *Behavioral Issues in Autism*. New York and London: Plenum Press.

Segall, A. 1990. 'A Community Survey of Self-Medication Activities', *Medical Care* 28: 301–10.

———. 1997. 'Sick Role Concepts and Health Behavior', in D.S. Gochman, ed, *Handbook of Health Behavior Research I: Personal and Social Determinants*. New York: Plenum Press, 289–301.

———, and N.L. Chappell. 2000. *Health and Health Care in Canada*. Toronto: Prentice Hall.

———, and J. Goldstein. 1989. 'Exploring the Correlates of Self-Provided Health Care Behaviour', *Social Science & Medicine* 29: 153–61.

Sellers, D.E., S.A. McGraw, and J.B. McKinlay. 1994. 'Does the Promotion and Distribution of Condoms Increase Teen Sexual Activity? Evidence from an HIV Prevention Program for Latino Youth', *American Journal of Public Health* 84, 12: 1952–59.

Settersten, R.A., and G.O. Hagestad. 2001. 'What's the latest? II. Cultural Age Deadlines for Educational and Work Transitions', *The Gerontologist* 36, 5: 602–13.

Shakespeare, T., and N. Watson. 2001. 'The Social Model of Disability: An Outdated Ideology?', in S. Barnartt and B. Altman, eds, *Exploring Theories and Expanding Methodologies: Where Are We and Where Do We Need to Go?* Oxford: JAI Press.

Sharma, U. 1992. *Complementary Medicine Today: Practitioners and Patients*. London: Tavistock/ Routledge.

Sharpe, P.A., N.M. Clark, and N. Janz. 1991. 'Differences in the Impact and Management of Heart Disease between Older Men and Women', *Women & Health* 17: 25–43.

Shields, M., and S. Tremblay. 2002. 'The Health of Canada's Communities', *Health Reports* (Supplement 13): 1–25.

Shortt, S.E.D., and R.A. Shaw. 2003. 'Equity in Canadian Health Care: Does Socioeconomic Status Affect Waiting Times for Elective Surgery?', *Canadian Medical Association Journal* 168, 4: 413–16.

Siddiqi, A., and C. Hertzman. 2007. 'Towards an Epidemiological Understanding of the Effects on Long-Term Institutional Changes on Population Health: A Case Study of Canada versus the USA', *Social Science & Medicine* 64: 589–603.

Simon, J.G., J.B. De Boer, I.M.A. Joung, H. Bosma, and J.P. Mackenbach. 2005. 'Perceived Health: How is Your Health in General? A Qualitative Study on Self-Assessed Health', *European Journal of Public Health* 15, 2: 200–08.

Sinding, C. 2003. 'Disarmed Complaints: Unpacking Satisfaction with End-of-Life Care', *Social Science & Medicine* 57: 1375–85.

Smaje, C. 2000. 'Race, Ethnicity, and Health', in C.E. Bird, P. Conrad, and A.M. Fremont, eds, *Handbook of Medical Sociology*, 5th edn. Upper Saddle River, NJ: Prentice Hall, 114–128.

Smedley, B.D., A.Y. Stith, and A.R. Nelson. 2005. 'Unequal Treatment: What Healthcare Providers Need to Know about Racial and Ethnic Disparities in Healthcare', in G.E. Henderson, S.E. Estroff, L.R. Churchill, N.M.P. King, J. Oberlander,

and R.P. Strauss, eds, *The Social Medicine Reader: Social and Cultural Contributions to Health, Difference, and Inequality*, 2nd edn. Durham: Duke University Press, 123–32.

Smith, R.L. 1969. *At Your Own Risk: The Case against Chiropractic.* Available at: http://www.chirobase.org/05RB/AYOR/00c.html. Accessed 30 August 2007.

Soldo, B.J., and M.S. Hill. 1995. 'Family Structure and Transfer Measures in the Health and Retirement Study', *Journal of Human Resources* 30 (Supplement): S108–37.

Srinivasan, S., L. O'Fallon, and A. Dearry. 2003. 'Reviewing the Evidence. Creating Healthy Communities, Healthy Homes, Healthy People: Initiating a Research Agenda on the Built Environment and Public Health', *American Journal of Public Health* 93, 9: 1446–50.

Stacey, C.L. 2005. 'Finding Dignity in Dirty Work: The Constraints and Rewards of Low-Wage Home Care Labour', *Sociology of Health & Illness* 27, 6: 831–54.

Stannard, C. 1973. 'Old Folks and Dirty Work: The Social Conditions for Patient Abuse in a Nursing Home', *Social Problems* 20, 3: 329–42.

Starr, P. 1982. *The Social Transformation of American Medicine.* New York: Basic Books.

Statistics Canada 1992. *Report on the Demographic Situation in Canada, 1992.* Current Demographic Analysis. Ottawa: Ministry of Industry, Science and Technology.

———. 1994. *Health Status of Canadians.* (Catalogue no. 11-612E). Ottawa: Statistics Canada.

———. 1995. *Births and Deaths*. Ottawa: Statistics Canada.

———. 1996. *National Population Health Survey, 1994/95*. Ottawa: Statistics Canada, Health Statistics Division.

———. 1998. *National Population Health Survey, 1996/97*. Ottawa: Statistics Canada, Health Statistics Division.

———. 1999. *Personal Health Practices: Smoking, Drinking, Physical Activity and Weight* (Catalogue no. 82-003). Ottawa: Statistics Canada.

———. 2000. *National Population Health Survey, 1998/99*. Ottawa: Statistics Canada, Health Statistics Division.

———. 2001a. *Health Indicators, December 2001* (Catalogue no. 82-221-XIE). Ottawa: Statistics Canada.

———. 2001b. *Health Reports* 12, 3 (April) (Catalogue no. 82-003-XPE). Ottawa: Statistics Canada.

———. 2001c. *Self-Esteem, by Age Group and Sex, Household Population aged 12 and over, Canada Excluding Territories, 1994/95* (Catalogue no. 82-221-XIE). Ottawa: Statistics Canada.

———. 2002a. *National Population Health Survey, 2000/01*. Ottawa: Statistics Canada, Health Statistics Division.

———. 2002b. *A Profile of Disability in Canada* (Catalogue no. 89-577-XIE). Ottawa: Minister of Industry.

———. 2002c. *Canada at a Glance* (Catalogue no. 82-617). Ottawa: Statistics Canada.

———. 2002d. *Canadian Community Health Survey—Mental Health and Well-Being* (Catalogue no. 82-617). Ottawa: Statistics Canada.

———. 2002e. *Family Violence in Canada: A Statistical Profile* (Catalogue no. 85-224). Ottawa: Statistics Canada.

———. 2002f. *How Healthy are Canadians? A Summary. 2002 Annual Report* (Catalogue no. 82-03-SIE). Ottawa: Statistics Canada.

———. 2002g. *Leading Causes of Death at Different Ages, Canada, 1999* (Catalogue no. 84F0503XPB). Ottawa: Statistics Canada.

———. 2002h. *Taking Charge: Perceptions of Control over Life*. Ottawa: Statistics Canada. Available at: http://www.statcan.ca/english/freepub/11-008-XIE/2006001/main_mastery.htm#younger.

———. 2003. 'Canadian Community Health Survey: Mental Health and Well-Being', *The Daily* 3 September 2003. Available at: http://www.statcan.ca/Daily/English/030903/d030903a.htm. Accessed 14 January 2005.

———. 2004a. *The Daily* 27 September 2004. Available at: http://www.statcan.ca/Daily/English/040927/d040927a.htm. Accessed 10 September 2005.

———. 2004b. *e-Book* (Catalogue no. 11-404-XIE). Ottawa: Supply and Services Canada. Available at: http://142.206.72.67/02/02b/02b_008d_e.htm. Accessed 24 April 2007.

———. 2004c. CANSIM, Table 102-0552 and Catalogue no. 84F020009X for 2004 data.

———. 2005. *Life Expectancy at Birth*. Available at: http://www.statcan.ca/english/Pgdb/health26.htm. Accessed 13 January 2005.

———. 2006a. *The Daily* 20 December 2006. Available at: http://www.statcan.ca/Daily/English/061220/d061220b.htm. Accessed 4 January 2007.

———. 2006b. *Residential Care Facilities, 2003/2004* (Catalogue no. 83-237-XIE). Ottawa: Minister of Industry.

Stein, L. 1967. 'The Doctor–Nurse Game', *Archives of General Psychiatry* 16: 699–703.

Stewart, M. 2003. 'Questions about Patient-Centered Care: Answers from Quantitative Research', in M. Stewart, J.B. Brown, W.W. Weston, I.R. McWhinney, C.L. McWilliam, and T.R. Freeman, eds, *Patient-Centered Medicine: Transforming the Clinical Method*, 2nd edn. Abingdon, UK: Radcliffe Publishing, 263–8.

Stewart, W.H., and P.E. Enterline. 1961. 'Effects of the NHS on Physician Utilization and Health in England and Wales', *New England Journal of Medicine* 265: 1187–94.

Stokols, D. 1996. 'Translating Social Ecological Theory into Guidelines for Community Health Promotion', *American Journal of Health Promotion* 10: 282–98.

Stone, L.O., C.J. Rosenthal, and I.A. Connidis. 1998. *Parent-Child Exchanges of Supports and Inter-generational Equity* (Catalogue no. 89-557-XPE). Ottawa: Statistics Canada.

Stoneman, Z. 2001. 'Supporting Positive Sibling Relationships During Childhood', *Mental Retardation & Developmental Disabilities Research Reviews* 7: 134–42.

Straus, R.R. 1957. 'The Nature and Status of Medical Sociology', *The American Sociological Review* 22: 200–04.

Strauss, A.L., and B.G. Glaser. 1975. *Chronic Illness and the Quality of Life.* St. Louis, MI: Mosby.

Street, R.L. 1991. 'Information-Giving in Medical Consultations: The Influence of Patients' Communicative Styles and Personal Characteristics', *Social Science & Medicine* 32, 5: 541–8.

Sullivan, M.J., and Y. Scattolon. 1995. 'Health Policy Planning: A Look at Consumer Involvement in Nova Scotia', *Canadian Journal of Public Health* 86, 5: 317–20.

Sutton, D.L., and D. Persaud. 1989. *Minority Elderly New Yorkers: The Social and Economic Status of Rapidly Growing Population.* Albany, NY : New York State Office for Aging, Division of Program Development and Evaluation, Research and Analysis Unit.

Sword, W., S. Watt, and P. Krueger. 2006. 'Postpartum Health, Service Needs, and Access to Care Experiences of Immigrant and Canadian-Born Women', *Journal of Obstetric, Gynecologic and Neonatal Nursing* 35, 6: 717–27.

Szinovacz, M. 1997. 'Adult Children Taking Parents into Their Homes: Effects of Childhood Living Arrangements', *Journal of Marriage and the Family* 59: 700–17.

Takamura, J. 2002. 'Social Policy Issues and Concerns in a Diverse Aging Society: Implications of Increasing Diversity', *Generations* 26, 3: 33–8.

Talberth, J., C. Cobb, and N. Slattery. 2006. 'The Genuine Progress Indicator 2006: A Tool for Sustainable Development'. Available at: http://www.rprogress.org/publications/2007/GPI%202006.pdf.

Tamblyn, R., and R. Perreault. 2000. 'Prescription Drug Use and Seniors', *Canadian Journal on Aging* 19 (Supplement 1): 143–75.

Tennstedt, S., and B.H. Chang. 1998. 'The Relative Contribution of Ethnicity versus Socioeconomic Status in Explaining Differences in Disability and Receipt of Informal Care', *Journal of Gerontology* 53B, 2: S61–70.

Thomas, C. 2001. 'Feminism and Disability: The Theoretical and Political Significance of the Personal and Experiential', in L. Barton, ed, *Disability, Politics and the Struggle for Change*. London: David Fulton.

Thommasen, H.V. 2000. 'Physician Retention and Recruitment Outside Urban British Columbia', *BC Medical Journal* 42, 6: 304–08.

Thompson, C.J. 2003. 'Natural Health Discourses and the Therapeutic Production of Consumer Resistance', *The Sociological Quarterly* 44, 1: 81–107.

Torrance, G.W. 1998. 'Hospitals as Health Factories', in D. Coburn, C. D'Arcy, and G.M. Torrance, eds, *Health and Canadian Society: Sociological Perspectives*. Toronto: University of Toronto Press, 438–55.

Tousjin, W. 2006. 'Beyond Decline: Consumerism, Managerialism and the Need for a New Medical Professionalism', *Health Sociology Review* 15, 5: 469–80.

Townsend, P., and N. Davidson, eds. 1982. *Inequalities in Health: The Black Report*. Harmandsworth, UK: Penguin.

Trovato, F. 2001. 'Aboriginal Mortality in Canada, the United States and New Zealand', *Journal of Biosocial Science* 33: 67–86.

———, and N.M. Lalu. 1996. 'Narrowing Sex Differentials in Life Expectancy in the Industrialized World: Early 1970s to Early 1990s', *Social Biology* 43, 1–2: 20–37.

Tucker, J.S., P.L. Ellickson, and D.J. Klein. 2002. 'Smoking Cessation during the Transition from Adolescence to Young Adulthood', *Nicotine & Tobacco Research* 4, 3: 321–32.

Turner, B.S. 1997. *The Body in Society: Explorations in Social Theory*, 2nd edn. London: Sage.

Twaddle, A. 1994. 'Disease, Illness and Sickness Revisited', in A. Twaddle and L. Nordenfelt, eds, *Disease, Illness and Sickness: Three Central Concepts in the Theory of Health*. Linköping, Sweden: Linköping University Press, 1–18.

Ungerson, C. 2000. 'Thinking about the Production and Consumption of Long-Term Care in Britain: Does Gender Still Matter?', *Journal of Social Policy* 29, 4: 623–43.

United Nations. 2005. *World Population Prospects: The 2004 Revisions*. New York: United Nations, Department of Economic and Social Affairs—Population Division.

Ursula, H. 2004. 'Effects of Informal Care on Paid-Work Participation in Great Britain: A Lifecourse Perspective', *Aging and Society* 24, 6: 851–80.

van de Mheen, H., K. Stronks, C.T.M. Schrijvers, and J.P. Mackenbach. 1999. 'The Influence of Adult Ill Health on Occupational Class Mobility and Mobility out of and into Employment in the Netherlands', *Social Science & Medicine* 49, 4: 509–518.

van Doorslaer, E., C. Masseria, and X. Koolman. 2006. 'Inequalities in Access to Medical Care by Income in Developed Countries', *Canadian Medical Association Journal* 174, 2: 177–83.

van Ryn, M., and J. Burke. 2000. 'The Effect of Patient Race and

Socioeconomic Status on Physicians' Perceptions of Patients', *Social Science & Medicine* 50, 6: 813–28.

Van Ziegert, S. 2002. 'Global Spaces of Chinese Culture: A Transnational Comparison of Diasporic Chinese Communities in the United States and Germany', PhD dissertation, Rice University, Houston, TX.

Vaughan, B. 2001. 'Handle with Care: On the Use of Structuration Theory within Criminology', *British Journal of Criminology* 41: 185–200.

Veenstra, G. 2001. 'Social Capital and Health', *Isuma* 2, 1: 72–81.

———. 2002. 'Social Capital and Health (Plus Wealth, Income Inequality and Regional Health Governance)', *Social Science & Medicine* 54, 6: 849–68.

———. 2003. 'Economy, Community and Mortality in British Columbia, Canada', *Social Science & Medicine* 56, 8: 1807–16.

———. 2006. 'Neo-Marxist Class Position and Socioeconomic Status: Distinct or Complementary Determinants of Health?', *Critical Public Health* 16, 2: 111–29.

Verhoef, M.J., H.S. Boon, and D.R. Mutasingwa. 2006. 'The Scope of Naturopathic Medicine in Canada: An Emerging Profession', *Social Science & Medicine* 63, 2: 409–17.

Veugelers, P.J., A.M. Yip, and G. Kephart. 2001. 'Proximate and Contextual Socioeconomic Determinants of Mortality: Multilevel Approaches in a Setting with Universal Health Care Coverage', *American Journal of Epidemiology* 154, 8: 725–32.

Virchow, R. 1848. 'Report on the Typhus Epidemic in Upper Silesia', in L.J. Rather, ed, *Rudolph Virchow: Collected Essays on Public Health and Epidemiology* 1: 205–20. Cantor, MA: Science History.

Wadsworth, L.A., and A.M. Thompson. 2005. 'Media Literacy: A Critical Role for Dietetic Practice', *Canadian Journal of Dietetic Practice and Research* 66, 1: 30–6.

Wadsworth, M.E.J., and D.J.L. Kuh. 1997. 'Childhood Influences on Adult Health: A Review of Recent Work from the British 1946 National Birth Cohort Study, the MRC National Survey of Health and Development', *Paediatric and Perinatal Epidemiology* 11, 1: 1365–3016.

Wagner, L.S., and T.H. Wagner. 2003. 'The Effect of Age on the Use of Health and Self-Care Information: Confronting the Stereotype', *The Gerontologist* 43, 3: 318–24.

Wainwright, S. P., and A. Forbes. 2000. 'Philosophical Problems with Social Research on Health Inequalities', *Health Care Analysis* 8, 2: 259–77.

Waitzkin, H. 1985. 'Information Giving in Medical Care', *Journal of Health and Social Behavior* 26: 81–101.

———. 2000. 'Changing Patient–Physician Relationships in the Changing Health-Policy Environment', in C.E. Bird, P Conrad, and A.M. Fremont, eds, *Handbook of Medical Sociology*, 5th edn. Upper Saddle River, NJ: Prentice Hall, 271–83.

Waldram, J.B., D.A. Herring, and T.K. Young. 2006. *Aboriginal Health in Canada: Historical, Cultural and Epidemiological Perspectives*. Toronto: University of Toronto Press.

Walker, A. 1996. 'Social Services for Older People in Europe', in R. Bland, ed,

Developing Services for Older People and Their Families. London: Jessica Kingsley Publishers.

———. 2004. 'Reexamining the Political Economy of Aging: Understanding the Structure/Agency Tension', in J. Baars, D. Dannefer, C. Phillipson, and A. Walker, eds, *Aging, Globalization, and Inequality: The New Critical Gerontology*. New York: Baywood Publishing Company, 59–80.

Walker, B.L., N.J. Osgood, J.P. Richardson, and P.H. Ephross. 1998. 'Staff and Elderly Knowledge and Attitudes toward Elderly Sexuality', *Educational Gerontology* 24, 5: 471–89.

Watson, D., H. Krueger, D. Mooney, and C. Black. 2005. *Planning for Renewal: Mapping Primary Health Care in British Columbia*. Vancouver: Centre for Health Services and Policy Research, University of British Columbia.

Weiss, G.L., and L.E. Lonnquist. 1997. *The Sociology of Health, Healing and Illness*. Upper Saddle River, NJ: Prentice Hall.

Weiss, J.M. 2002. 'Hardiness and Social Support as Predictors of Stress in Mothers of Typical Children, Children with Autism, and Children with Mental Retardation', *Autism* 6, 1: 115–30.

Weitz, R. 1996a. *The Sociology of Health, Illness and Health Care: A Critical Approach*. Belmont: Thomson Learning.

———. 1996b. 'Life with AIDS', in P. Brown, ed, *Perspectives in Medical Sociology*, 2nd edn. Prospect Heights, IL: Waveland Press, Inc., 727–40.

Welsh, S., M. Kelner, B. Wellman, and H. Boon. 2004. 'Moving Forward? Complementary and Alternative

Practitioners Seeking Self-Regulation', *Sociology of Health & Illness* 26, 2: 216–41.

Wen, S.W., V. Goel, and J.I. Williams. 1996. 'Utilization of Health Care Services by Immigrants and Other Ethnic/Cultural Groups in Ontario', *Ethnicity and Health* 1, 1: 99–109.

Wennemo, I. 1993. 'Infant Mortality, Public Policy and Inequality—A Comparison of Industrialized Countries, 1950–1985', *Sociology of Health & Illness* 15, 4: 429–46.

White, K. 2002. *An Introduction to the Sociology of Health & Illness*. London: Sage.

Whitehead, M. 1988. 'The Health Divide', in P. Townsend and N. Davidson, eds, *Inequalities in Health: The Black Report and the Health Divide*. Harmondsworth, UK: Penguin Books, 215–356.

Whittle K.L., and K.L. Inhorn. 2002. 'Rethinking Difference: A Feminist Reframing of Gender/Race/Class for the Improvement of Women's Health Research', *International Journal of Health Services* 31, 1: 147–65.

Whyte, M.K. 2004. 'Filial Obligations in Chinese Families: Paradoxes of Modernization', in C. Ikels, ed, *Filial Piety, Practice and Discourse in Contemporary East Asia*. Stanford: Stanford University Press, 106–27.

Wiehe, V.R. 1998. 'Elder Abuse', in *Understanding Family Violence: Treating and Preventing Partner, Child, Sibling, and Elder Abuse*. Thousand Oaks, CA: Sage, 127–65.

Wilkins, K., and E. Park. 1998. 'Home Care in Canada', *Health Reports* (Statistics Canada Catalogue no. 82-003) 10, 1: 29–37.

Wilkins, R., J.-M. Bertholet, and E. Ng. 2002. 'Trends in Mortality by Neighbourhood Income in Urban Canada from 1971 to 1996', *Health Reports—Supplement* (Statistics Canada Catalogue no. 82-003-XPE) 13: 1–28.

Wilkinson, R., and M. Marmot. 2003. 'The Social Determinants of Health: The Solid Facts'. Copenhagen: World Heath Organization Regional Office for Europe. Available at: http://www.who.int/social_determinants/links/publications/en/. Accessed 14 June 2007.

Wilkinson, R.G. 1996. *Unhealthy Societies: The Afflictions of Inequality*. New York: Routledge.

Williams, A.M. 1996. 'The Development of Ontario's Home Care Program: A Critical Geographical Analysis', *Social Science & Medicine* 42, 6: 937–48.

Williams, A.P., R. Deber, P. Baranek, and A. Gildiner. 2001. 'From Medicare to Home Care: Globalization, State Retrenchment, and the Profitization of Canada's Health-Care System', in P. Armstrong, H. Armstrong, and D. Coburn, eds, *Unhealthy Times: Political Economy Perspectives on Health and Care in* Canada. Don Mills, ON: Oxford University Press, 7–30.

———, K. Domnick, and E. Wayda. 1998. 'Women in Medicine: Toward a Conceptual Understanding of the Potential for Change', in D. Coburn, C. D'Arcy, and G.M. Torrance, eds, *Health and Canadian Society: Sociological Perspectives*. Toronto: University of Toronto Press, 347–58.

Williams, C. 2005. 'The Sandwich Generation', *Canadian Social Trends*:

16–24. This article is an adaptation of 'The Sandwich Generation', *Perspectives on Labour and Income* (Statistics Canada Catalogue no. 75-001-XIE, vol. 5, no. 9). Available at: www.statcan.ca:8096/bsolc/english/bsolc?catno=75-001-X20041097033. Accessed 14 June 2007.

———. 2006. 'Still Missing? Comments on the Twentieth Anniversary of "The Missing Feminist Revolution in Sociology"', *Social Problems* 53, 4: 454–8.

Williams, D.R. 1990. 'Socioeconomic Differentials in Health: A Review and Redirection', *Social Psychology Quarterly* 53: 81–99.

Williams, G.H. 1984. 'The Genesis of Chronic Illness: Narrative Re-Construction', *The Sociology of Health & Illness* 6, 2: 176–200.

———. 2003. 'The Determinants of Health: Structure, Context and Agency', *The Sociology of Health & Illness* 25: 131–54.

Williamson, D. 2000. 'Health Behaviors and Health: Evidence that the Relationship is not Conditional on Income Adequacy', *Social Science & Medicine* 51, 12: 1741–54.

Willis, E. 2006. 'Introduction: Taking Stock of Medical Dominance', *Health Sociology Review* 15, 5: 421–31.

Wilson, G. 2000. *Understanding Old Age*. London: Sage.

Wilson, K., and M.W. Rosenberg. 2002. 'The Geographies of Crisis: Exploring Accessibility to Health Care in Canada', *Canadian Geographer* 46, 3: 223–34.

Wister, A.V. 2005a. *Baby Boomer Health Dynamics: How Are We Aging?* Toronto: University of Toronto Press.

———. 2005b. 'Built Environment, Health, and Longevity: Multilevel Salutogenic and Pathogenic Pathways', *Journal of Housing for the Elderly* 19, 2: 49–70.

———, and C. Moore. 1998. 'First Nations Elders in Canada', in A.V. Wister and G.M. Gutman, eds, *Health Systems and Aging in Selected Pacific Rim Countries: Cultural Diversity and Change*. Vancouver: Simon Fraser University Gerontology Research Centre, 103–24.

Wolff, T. 2003. 'The Healthy Communities Movement: A Time for Transformation', *National Civic Review* 92, 2: 95–111.

Wolinsky, F.D. 1988. 'The Professional Dominance Perspective, Revisited', *The Milbank Quarterly* 66 (Supplement 2): 33–47.

World Health Organization (WHO). 1946. Constitution of the World Health Organization, Signed on 22 July 1946 in New York City, *International Organization* 1, 1: 225–39.

———. 1958. *The First Ten Years of the World Health Organizatio*n. Geneva: WHO.

———. 1977. Resolution WHA40.43— Technical Cooperation. Geneva: WHO.

———. 1984. *Health Promotion: A Discussion Document on the Concept and Principles*. Geneva: WHO, Working Group on Concept and Principles of Health Promotion.

———. 1986. *Ottawa Charter for Health Promotion*. Copenhagen: WHO Regional Office for Europe.

———. 1998. *Health Promotion Glossary*. Geneva: WHO.

———. 2007. *International Classification of Diseases and Related Health Problems, 10th Revision*. Available at: http://www.who.int/classifications/apps/icd/icd10online/. Accessed 10 December 2007.

Wotherspoon, T. 2002. 'Nursing Education: Professionalism and Control', in B.S. Bolaria and H.D. Dickinson, eds, *Health, Illness and Health Care in Canada*, 3rd edn. Scarborough, ON: Nelson Thomson Learning, 82–101.

Wright, E.O. 1979. *Class, Crisis and the State*. London: Verso.

Yach, D. 1998. 'Health and Illness: The Definition of the World Health Organization', *Ethik in der Medizin* 10, 1: S7–13. Available at: http://www.medizin-ethik.ch/publik/health_illness.htm. Accessed 14 December 2007.

Yamato, R. 2006. 'Changing Attitudes towards Elderly Dependence in Postwar Japan', *Current Sociology* 54, 2: 273–91.

Yates, M.E., S. Tennstedt, and B.-H. Change. 1999. 'Contributors to and Mediators of Psychological Well-Being for Informal Caregivers', *Journal of Gerontology: Psychological Sciences* 54B, 1: P12–22.

Yen, I.A., and G.A. Kaplan. 1999. 'Neighbourhood Social Environment and Risk of Death: Multilevel Evidence from the Alameda County Study', *American Journal of Epidemiology* 149, 10: 898–907.

Yew, L.K. 2000. *From Third World to First: The Singapore Story: 1965–2000*. New York: HarperCollins.

Yong, H.H., R. Borland, and M. Siahpush. 2005. 'Quitting-Related Beliefs, Intentions, and Motivations of Older Smokers in Four Countries: Findings from International Tobacco Control Policy Evaluation Survey', *Addictive Behaviors* 30, 4: 777–88.

Young, J.T. 2004. 'Illness Behaviour: A Selective Review and Synthesis', *Sociology of Health & Illness* 26, 1: 1–21.

Zaner, R. 1994. 'Experience and Moral Life: A Phenomenological Approach to Bioethics', in E. DuBose, R. Hamel, and L.J. O'Connell, eds, *A Matter of Principles? Ferment in US Bioethics.* Valley Forge, PA: Trinity Press International.

Zelek, B., and S.P. Phillips. 2003. 'Gender and Power: Nurses and Doctors in Canada', *International Journal for Equity in Health* 2:1.

Ziersch, A.M. 2005. 'Health Implications of Access to Social Capital: Findings from an Australian Study', *Social Science & Medicine* 61: 2119–31.

Zola, I.K. 1972. 'Medicine as an Institution of Social Control', *Sociological Review* 20: 407–584.

———. 1973. 'Pathways to the Doctor— From Person to Patient', *Social Science & Medicine* 7: 677–89.

———. 1983. *Socio-Medical Inquiries.* Philadelphia, PA: Temple University Press.

Zong, L., and P.S. Li. 1994. 'Different Cultures or Unequal Life Chances: A Comparative Analysis of Race and Health, Racial Minorities Medicine and Health'. Halifax: Fernwood, 113–26.

Zussman, R. 1992. *Intensive Care: Medical Ethics and the Medical Profession.* Chicago: University of Chicago Press.

———. 1993. 'Life in the Hospital: A Review', *The Milbank Quarterly* 71, 1: 167–85.

Index

Themes in Canadian Sociology Series

Scott Davies and Neil Guppy
The Schooled Society: An Introduction to the Sociology of Education (2006)
ISBN 9780195421088

Maureen Baker
Choices and Constraints in Family Life (2007)
ISBN 9780195421057

Vic Satzewich and Nikolaos Liodakis
'Race' and Ethnicity in Canada: A Critical Introduction (2007)
ISBN 9780195421316

William O'Grady
Crime in Canadian Context: Debates and Controversies (2007)
ISBN 9780195422955

Suzanne Staggenborg
Social Movements (2008)
ISBN 9780195423099

Janet Siltanen and Andrea Doucet
Gender Relations in Canada: Intersectionality and Beyond (2008)
ISBN 9780195423204

Neena L. Chappell and Margaret J. Penning
Understanding Health, Health Care, and Health Policy in Canada: Sociological Perspectives (2009)
ISBN 9780195424768